PSYCHOLOGICAL ASPECTS
OF CHILDHOOD CANCER

PSYCHOLOGICAL ASPECTS OF CHILDHOOD CANCER

Edited by

JONATHAN KELLERMAN, Ph.D.

Associate Clinical Professor of Pediatrics (Psychology)
University of Southern California
School of Medicine
Director, Psychosocial Program, Division of Hematology-Oncology
Childrens Hospital
Los Angeles, California

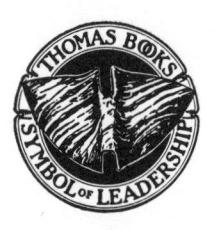

CHARLES C THOMAS • PUBLISHER
Springfield • Illinois • U.S.A.

Published and Distributed Throughout the World by
CHARLES C THOMAS • PUBLISHER
Bannerstone House
301-327 East Lawrence Avenue, Springfield, Illinois, U.S.A.

©1980, by CHARLES C THOMAS • PUBLISHER
ISBN 0-398-03989-5
Library of Congress Catalog Card Number: 79-23154

Library of Congress Cataloging in Publication Data

Main entry under title:

Psychological aspects of childhood cancer.

   Bibliography: p.
   Includes index.
   1. Tumors in children — Psychological aspects.
I. Kellerman, Jonathan. [DNLM: 1. Neoplasms — In
infancy and childhood. 2. Neoplasms — Psychology.
QZ200.3 P974]
RC281.C4P73   1980   618.9′29′940019   79-23154
ISBN 0-398-03989-5

Printed in the United States of America
C-1

CONTRIBUTORS

GORDON D. ARMSTRONG, Ph.D.: Research Associate, School of Nursing, University of Minnesota, Minneapolis, Minnesota.

JAMES ARONSON: Diagnosed with Ewing's Sarcoma in May, 1975, and treated, successfully, from 1975 to 1977, James Aronson is currently in Peru collecting plants for the Missouri Botanical Garden.

JERRY D. DASH, Ph.D.: Senior Psychologist, Psychosocial Program, Division of Hematology-Oncology, Children's Hospital of Los Angeles; Assistant Clinical Professor of Pediatrics (Psychology), University of Southern California, Los Angeles, California.

HELEN DESMOND, Ph.D.: Research Clinical Associate, Los Angeles Psychoanalytic Society and Institute; Consultant, Kaiser-Permanente Hospice Care Program, Norwalk, California; Consultant, Pediatric Cancer Research Program, Childrens Hospital of San Diego, California; Psychologist in private practice, Los Angeles, California.

STEPHEN P. HERSH, M.D.: Assistant Director for Children and Youth, National Institute of Mental Health, Rockville, Maryland.

ALBERT R. HOLLENBECK, Ph.D.: Postdoctoral Fellow, Laboratory of Developmental Psychology, National Institute of Mental Health, Bethesda, Maryland.

ERNEST R. KATZ, M.A.: Research Associate, Psychosocial Program, Division of Hematology-Oncology, Childrens Hospital of Los Angeles; Doctoral candidate, clinical psychology, University of Southern Calofornia, Los Angeles, California.

JONATHAN KELLERMAN, Ph.D. (Editor): Associate Clinical Professor of Pediatrics and Psychology, University of Southern California School of Medicine; Director, Psychosocial Program, Division of Hematology-Oncology, Childrens Hospital of Los Angeles, California.

GERALD P. KOOCHER, Ph.D.: Assistant Professor of Psychology, Harvard Medical School; Chief Psychologist, Sidney Farber Cancer Institute, Boston, Massachusetts.

ARTHUR S. LEVINE, M.D.: Chief, Pediatric Oncology Branch, National Cancer Institute, Bethesda, Maryland.

IDA MARTINSON, R.N., Ph.D.: Professor of Nursing and Director of Research, School of Nursing; and Lecturer, Department of Physiology,

School of Medicine, University of Minnesota, Minneapolis, Minnesota.

KATHLEEN McCUE, M.A.: Patient Activity Specialist, Psychosocial Program, Division of Hematology-Oncology, Childrens Hospital of Los Angeles, California.

HOWARD A. MOSS, Ph.D.: Research Psychologist, Laboratory of Developmental Psychology, National Institute of Mental Health, Bethesda, Maryland.

ELLEN D. NANNIS, M.S.W.: Research Assistant, Laboratory of Developmental Psychology, National Institute of Mental Health, Bethesda, Maryland.

PHILLIP A. PIZZO, M.D.: Senior Investigator, Pediatric Oncology Branch, National Cancer Institute, Bethesda, Maryland.

DAVID RIGLER, Ph.D.: Professor of Psychiatry, Pediatrics and Psychology, University of Southern California School of Medicine; Chief Psychologist, Division of Psychiatry, Childrens Hospital of Los Angeles, California.

BETSY SACHS, M.S.W.: Clinical Social Worker, Behavioral Science Division, Department of Social Service, Childrens Hospital of Pittsburgh, Pennsylvania.

STUART E. SIEGEL, M.D.: Associate Professor of Pediatrics, University of Southern California School of Medicine; Head, Division of Hematology-Oncology, Childrens Hospital of Los Angeles, California.

BARBARA M. SOURKES, Ph.D.: Clinical Psychologist, Sidney Farber Cancer Institute, Department of Pediatric Oncology, Children's Hospital Medical Center of Boston, Department of Psychiatry and Harvard Medical School, Boston, Massachusetts.

JOHN J. SPINETTA, Ph.D.: Professor of Psychology, San Diego State University; Director, Pediatric Cancer Psychosocial Research Program, Childrens Hospital and Health Center of San Diego, California.

BARBARA E. STROPE, B.S.: Social Science Analyst, Laboratory of Developmental Psychology, National Institute of Mental Health, Bethesda, Maryland.

ELIZABETH J. SUSMAN, R.N., Ph.D.: Assistant Professor of Nursing, The Pennsylvania State University, University Park, Pennsylvania; Consultant, Laboratory of Developmental Psychology, National Institute of Mental Health, Bethesda, Maryland.

LONNIE K. ZELTZER, M.D.: Assistant Professor of Pediatrics and Head, Division of Adolescent Medicine, University of Texas Health Science Center, San Antonio, Texas.

PREFACE

THE PURPOSE OF THIS BOOK is to offer a comprehensive and practical guide to the psychological management of children with cancer. Two themes will be found running repeatedly throughout the book. First is the notion that, due to treatment advances in pediatric oncology, many forms of childhood cancer can be thought of as chronic disease. For this reason, an emphasis has been placed upon psychosocial rehabilitation — helping the child and family return to the prediagnostic adjustment state. The second issue to be considered is that as the medical assault against cancer becomes more and more intensive and technologically advanced, there is an increased need to consider the psychological side effects of treatment.

Needless to say these themes are not independent of each other, for it is precisely because so many children with cancer are living extended lives that the value of examining the quality of those lives has increased. Iatrogenic factors such as procedure-related pain and discomfort, side effects of chemotherapy, central nervous system decrement due to cranial radiation, and the psychological correlates of extended hospitalization and isolation are among the many issues that are relevant in this regard.

While it is clear that no book can or should offer "cookbook" remedies to complex problems, there is a clear emphasis in this book upon practical approaches. For this reason, most of the contributors to the present volume write from backgrounds of extensive clinical experience in various aspects of pediatric oncology. Along these lines, clinical case presentations have been generously used.

The reader may be puzzled at the relative dearth of material related to death and dying. This is not because of a failure to recognize that many children with cancer do die of their disease but is due, rather, to the wealth of research on thanatology that has been presented, often excellently, in other books. One chapter in the present volume has been devoted to the child with cancer who dies but even in this instance the theme of maintaining family integrity through psychosocial rehabilitation has not been abandoned, for the emphasis is upon helping the child die at home.

It is my hope that this book will aid the health professional in understanding some of the ways that cancer impacts psychologically upon the child and family, and point toward optimal modes of psychosocial care. In addition, if this volume is successful, it will raise more questions than it answers and stimulate further research in this vital and fascinating area.

JONATHAN KELLERMAN, Ph.D.

ACKNOWLEDGMENTS

I WOULD LIKE TO THANK the contributors to this volume, who took time out from busy academic and clinical schedules in order to provide original material, as well as to express my appreciation to authors and editors who gave me permission to reprint previously published material.

In addition, I wish to thank Dr. Stuart E. Siegel, Head, Division of Hematology-Oncology for his support of psychosocial care, in general, and for his encouragement of an atmosphere of applied research, one of the results of which is the compiling of this volume. Special acknowledgement of the secretarial assistance of Ms. Lourdes Centeno and Ms. Lea Butterfield is in order, as are thanks to the Psychosocial Staff, Division of Hematology-Oncology, Childrens Hospital of Los Angeles, whose competence and dedication freed me sufficiently from administrative duties to be able to devote time to the tasks of writing and editing.

My wife, Dr. Faye Kellerman was constantly supportive, encouraging, and patient throughout the task of compiling this book, as she has been during our wonderful years together. Once again, I thank her.

Finally, I would like to express my respect for the hundreds of children with malignant disease that I have encountered in the course of clinical and research activities, and their families, and to offer hope that this volume will be one small step in the effort to achieve and maintain increased quality of life for them.

J.K.

CONTENTS

PSYCHOLOGICAL ASPECTS
OF CHILDHOOD CANCER

SECTION I

IMPACT OF ILLNESS AND TREATMENT

Chapter One

THE CURRENT OUTLOOK FOR CHILDHOOD CANCER — THE MEDICAL BACKGROUND

STUART E. SIEGEL

THE NEED FOR A DEFINITIVE text dealing with the psychosocial aspects of childhood cancer is itself a statement on the current status of therapy for these diseases which were in the past universally fatal. Only a brief thirty years ago, the median survival for acute lymphoblastic leukemia, the most common malignancy in children, was three to six months (Tivey, 1951; Fernbach, 1973). Currently, 60 percent of such children survive five years from diagnosis (Hammond, 1978; Simone, 1974), and increasing numbers are alive and free of disease ten, fifteen, and even twenty years from diagnosis. It is in this rapidly changing context that the child with cancer and his or her family must be viewed, one which holds the hope and real possibility of prolonged survival and in some cases cure but does not yet guarantee this outcome for all children.

Despite these improving survival figures, aside from accidents, cancer remains the most common cause of death in children following the neonatal period (Silverberg, 1979). The importance of cancer as a cause of death in childhood overshadows the fact that it is, fortunately, a much rarer occurrence in children than adults with an incidence of 11/100,000 children aged 0-15 years/year (Sutow, 1973). While a variety of solid tumors, e.g. lung, breast, ovarian, gastrointestinal, cervical, and uterine cancer are the most common malignancies in the adult population, acute leukemia, specifically acute lymphoblastic leukemia (A.L.L.), is the most frequently diagnosed neoplasm in children (Sutow, 1973; Hammond, 1978; Jones, 1976). (Table 1-I). Progress in this disease over the past thirty years has provided a model for treatment of other malignancies of the hemopoietic system in both children and adults.

Figure 1-1 illustrates the remarkable progressive improvement in the outcome of therapy for A.L.L. over this period of time. This trend has been due to several sequential developments which were the product of intensive clinical research studies in this disease. By far the most important contribution was the development of specific chemotherapeutic agents with sufficient selectivity for the leukemic cell population over normal cells to permit clinical application (Table 1-II). Beginning in 1948 with the use of Aminopterin® by Farber (Farber,

5

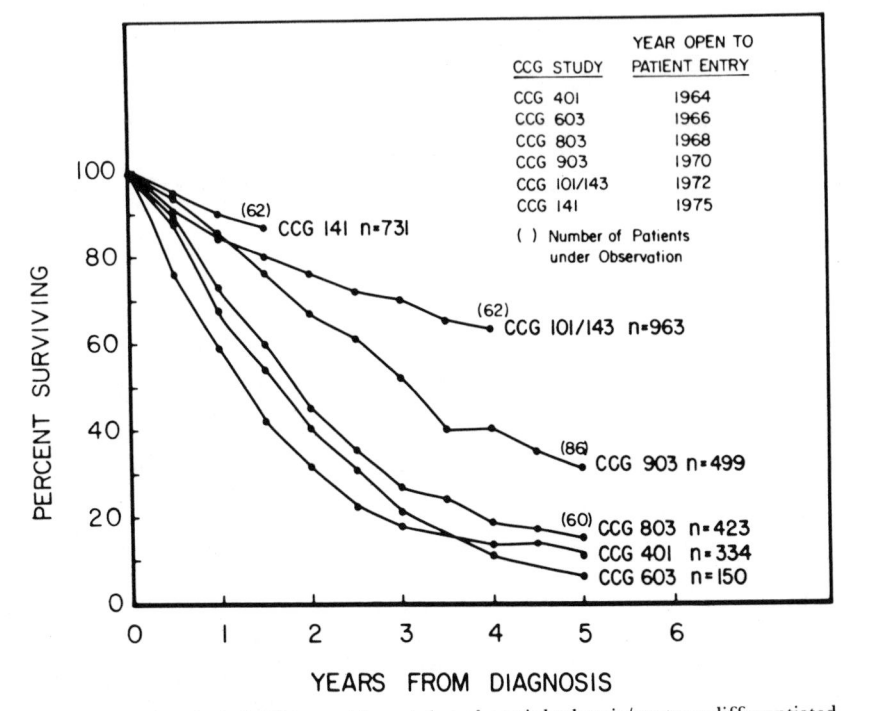

Figure 1-1. Survival of children with acute lymphocytic leukemia/acute undifferentiated
leukemia, Children's Cancer Study Group. From G. D. Hammond, The
Team Approach to the Management of Pediatric Cancer. *Cancer 41:*29-35,
1978. Reprinted by permission.

TABLE 1-I

DISTRIBUTION OF SPECIFIC CANCER DIAGNOSES IN CHILDREN*

Acute lymphoblastic leukemia	30%
Acute myelogenous and myelomonocytic leukemia	8%
Other leukemias	1%
Hodgkin's Disease	3%
Non-Hodgkin's Lymphoma	4%
Wilms' Tumor	6%
Neuroblastoma	9%
Bone Tumors	8%
Soft Tissue Sarcomas	6%
Retinoblastoma	2%
Brain Tumors	14%
Miscellaneous Tumors (i.e. Hepatic, Teratoma)	9%

*Summary adapted from Sutow, W. W., et al., 1973; Hammond, G. D., et al., 1978;
Jones, P. G. and Campbell, P. E., 1976).

TABLE 1-II
CHEMOTHERAPEUTIC AGENTS COMMONLY USED IN CHILDHOOD
CANCER

Type of Malignancy	Agents Employed
Acute Lymphoblastic Leukemia	*Vincristine, 6-Mercaptopurine, Prednisone, Methotrexate, L-asparaginase, Adriamycin, Cyclophosphamide*
Acute Myelogenous Leukemia	*Vincristine, Adriamycin, Prednisone, Daunomycin, Cytosine Arabinoside, 6-Thioguanine, 5-Azacytidine*
Wilms' Tumor	*Vincristine, Cyclophosphamide, Actinomycin-D, Adriamycin*
Neuroblastoma	*Cyclophosphamide, Cis-platinum, Vincristine, VM-26*
Hodgkin's Disease	*Vincristine, Procarbazine, Nitrogen Mustard, Prednisone, Adriamycin, Bleomycin, Cyclophosphamide, CCNU-BCNU*
Non-Hodgkin's Lymphoma	*Vincristine, Cyclophosphamide, Prednisone, Adriamycin, Methotrexate, BCNU, 6-Mercaptopurine, Cytosine Arabinoside, 6-Thioguanine*
Osteogenic Sarcoma	*Methotrexate, Cyclophosphamide, Adriamycin*
Ewing's Sarcoma	*Cyclophosphamide, Actinomycin-D, Vincristine, Adriamycin*
Soft Tissue Sarcomas	*Vincristine, Actinomycin-D, Cyclophosphamide, Adriamycin*
Hepatoblastoma	*Adriamycin, Vincristine, Cyclophosphamide, Actinomycin-D*
Brain Tumors	*? Vincristine, ? CCNU-BCNU ? Procarbazine*

1948), new agents have been tested in increasing numbers and over fifteen have been incorporated into "conventional" treatment programs now in use (Henderson, 1969; Simone, 1974). The second major advance was the realization by Frei, Freireich, Karon, Henderson, and others that combinations of these agents could provide additive and even synergistic antileukemic effects, while producing manageable and generally transient side effects (Frei, 1967; Henderson, 1969; Freireich, 1968). The relatively rapid onset of disease relapse when therapy was discontinued immediately after a remission had been obtained then led to the concept of maintenance chemotherapy for extended periods of time up to five years in the face of continued disease remission (Frei, 1965; Henderson, 1969).

These developments resulted in initial remission rates of 80-90 percent of patients and median remission durations of two to three years. A small fraction, less than 10 percent of children, appeared to remain in long-term continuous remission (>five years) with this therapy (Hammond, 1978; Simone, 1974). When the reasons for ultimate treatment failure were analyzed, it was apparent that initial recurrence in sites "protected" from systemic chemotherapy, the so-called "sanctuaries," was primarily responsible for ultimate systemic relapse and death. The major sanctuary identified was the central nervous system (CNS). Indeed, 50 percent of children with A.L.L. developed central nervous system relapse at some time during the course of the disease (Simone, 1974). The introduction of CNS prophylaxis using combinations of cranial or craniospinal radiation and intrathecal chemotherapy reduced the risk of CNS relapse to less than 10 percent and brought us to the current response status (Simone, 1974; Simone, 1975; Hammond, 1978).

Some of the major avenues of future clinical research in A.L.L. are already apparent at this time. The observation that approximately 15 percent of males remaining in continuous remission three to five years relapse in another sanctuary, the testes, when taken off chemotherapy is leading to closer monitoring of potential testicular involvement and may result in selective prophylaxis (Simone, 1974; Simone, 1975). Analysis of several larger series of children with A.L.L. have now shown that certain patient characteristics present at diagnosis, such as patient age and initial white blood cell count, have prognostic value for remission duration and survival (Coccia, 1976). This information permits design of clinical trials for "good prognosis" patients that seek to reduce the amount of therapy and side effects encountered, while evaluating new therapeutic alternatives for "poor prognosis" patients. Finally, a constant search is being carried out for new chemotherapeutic agents for those patients who will fail current therapeutic programs. Each year approximately 10,000 new compounds are screened for antileukemic activity and toxicity, and 10-20 are eventually found to warrant clinical trial.

The treatment of many solid tumors in childhood has also undergone major changes in the past thirty years, and the results have included a significant cure rate for some of these neoplasms (Figure 1-2). The most notable example of this progress has been the treatment of Wilms' tumor (Figure 1-3). Surgical removal of the tumor resulted in a 10-20 percent cure rate, with the remainder of patients dying of local and systemic metastases. The introduction of radiotherapy to the tumor bed in the 1930s reduced the risk of local recurrence but did not affect the rate of systemic spread. The introduction of single agent chemotherapy, especially the use of Actinomycin-D® in the 1950s, produced a major improvement in survival by reducing the appearance of systemic metastases. Finally, the use of the combination of vincristine and Actinomycin-D in conjunction with surgery and

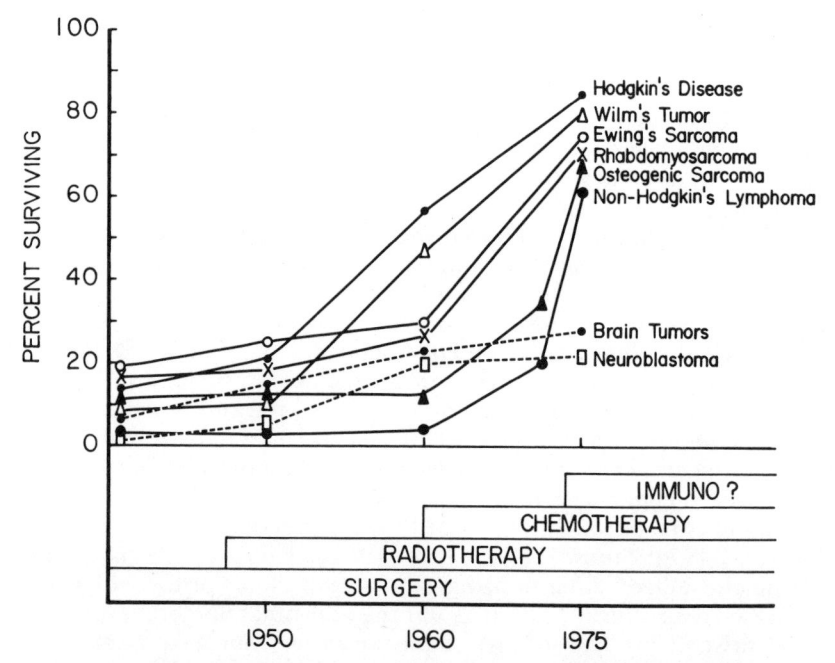

Figure 1-2. Overall improvement in two-year survival in childhood solid tumors indicating striking improvement over the last decade. From G. D. Hammond, The Team Approach to the Management of Pediatric Cancer. *Cancer* *41:*29-35, 1978. Reprinted by permission.

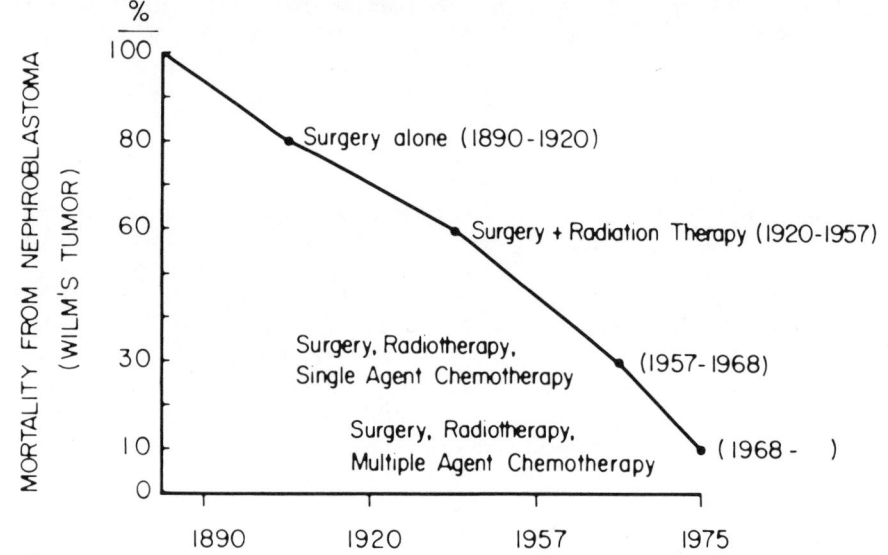

Figure 1-3. Progressive improvement in survival from nephroblastoma (Wilms' tumor) with the development of multidisciplinary therapy over the last century.

radiotherapy has produced long-term survival rates of greater than 80 percent for localized disease, and a five-year survival of 50 percent of patients presenting with distant metastases at diagnosis (D'Angio, 1967; Rosenstock, 1974). Similar advances using a multimodality approach have been noted in patients with rhabdomyosarcoma and other soft tissue sarcomas (Raney, 1974) and lymphomas (Wollner, 1976; Carbone, 1973; Murphy, 1974). Combined modality therapy in these malignancies has often reduced the need for radical surgical and/or radiotherapeutic treatment, and has allowed the maximum preservation of normal body functions (Ortega, 1979).

The treatment of bone tumors remains somewhat controversial. The use of local radiotherapy and chemotherapy, particularly cyclophosphamide, has resulted in major improvements in survival in Ewing's sarcoma and has largely eliminated the need for amputation (Rosen, 1974; Pomeroy, 1975; Nesbit, 1976). The use of high-dose Methotrexate® with citrovorum factor rescue and adriamycin following amputation for osteogenic sarcoma may reduce the rate of occurrence of pulmonary metastases in the first two years after diagnosis (Jaffe, 1978; Kinney, 1974; Sutow, 1978; Cortes, 1978). However, recent studies from the Mayo Clinic utilizing amputation alone produced similar disease-free survival periods as did the adjuvant chemotherapy trials (Gilchrist, 1978). Nevertheless, all major series undertaken since 1970 agree that *overall* survival with this tumor has improved from 20 percent alive at two years in the pre-1970 studies, to 60-75 percent two-year survival in the current studies (Jaffe, 1978; Sutow, 1978). In addition, newer methods of limb preservation for lesions located in accessible areas of long bones are reducing the need for amputation in selective cases (Rosen, 1975; Marcove, 1978; Jaffe, 1978).

As the therapy for childhood cancer has become effective, complications of the diseases and the treatment acquire greater importance in determining the outcome of each disease episode. These "side effects" may be of immediate or late onset in nature (Table 1-III). The immediate effects are generally transient and reversible, though life-threatening complications may result. As an example, infection (usually occurring as a result of impaired host defenses related to the disease and its therapy) is the major proximate cause of death in children with acute leukemia, as well as resulting in significant morbidity and mortality in children with solid tumors (Table 1-III) (Levine, 1974; Hughes, 1974). Other side effects such as hair loss are dramatic in their appearance and psychological effect, but are of little physiological consequence to the child.

Progress in childhood cancer therapy has, therefore, naturally included major improvements in the diagnosis, treatment, and prevention of these untoward effects. The development of newer, more powerful antibiotics and granulocyte transfusion therapy has permitted a more aggressive approach to serious infection in these patients (Levine, 1974). The use of sophisticated barrier isolation facilities in

TABLE 1-III

SIDE EFFECTS OF CHILDHOOD CANCER AND ITS THERAPY

Treatment Modality	Immediate Effects	Late Effects
Surgery	Loss of normal function (i.e. organ, limb)	Infection Fibrous scarring and adhesions Fistula formation
Radiation	Acute skin and mucosal inflammation Tissue edema and inflammation Acute radiation pneumonitis Nausea and vomiting Radiation enteritis Bone marrow suppression (with 2° infection and hemorrhage) Alopecia	"Secondary" malignancy Soft tissue and visceral fibrosis Gonadal dysfunction Endocrine gland dysfunction Dental maldevelopment and degeneration Cataracts Inhibition of bony growth ? Brain dysfunction
Chemotherapy	Bone marrow depression (with 2° infection and hemorrhage) Nausea and vomiting Alopecia Mucositis Hepatitis Steroid effects Cardiomyopathy (anthracyclines) Neuropathy (Vinca alkaloids) Cystitis (Cyclophosphamide) Allergic reactions (L-asparaginase) Pancreatitis (L-asparaginase) Pneumonitis (Methotrexate, BCNU)	"Secondary" malignancy Gonadal dysfunction Cirrhosis ? Brain dysfunction ? Chromosomal abnormalities Adrenal dysfunction Chronic cystitis

conjunction with oral and topical antisepsis and antibiotics (the so-called "protected environment") is reducing the risk of infection in patients requiring very intensive therapy for previously resistant neoplasms (Levine, 1974; Levine, 1975). Similarly, the availability of platelet concentrates has dramatically reduced hemorrhagic complications in the past fifteen years (Freireich, 1966; Yankee, 1969).

Thus, the child with cancer must now often be viewed against a background of a relatively rapid improvement in both short- and long-term survival, produced by the use of intensive multimodality treatment programs having both transient and late side effects. The need for a psychosocial approach to these children and their families is now no less important than the requirement for the sophisticated therapeutic intervention just described. The potential for prolonged survival following such an acute and sustained physical and psychological assault on the patient and family provides a challenge and a responsibility for health professionals to develop and test both preventative and therapeutic psychosocial intervention techniques as part of true comprehensive care.

REFERENCES

Bloom, H. J. G.: Combined modality therapy for intracranial tumors. *Cancer, 35:*111, 1975.

Carbone, P. P.: Management of patients with non-Hodgkin's lymphoma. *Ann Intern Med, 131:*455, 1973.

Coccia, P., Sather, H., Nesbit, M., et al.: Inter-relationship of initial WBC, age and sex in predicting prognosis in childhood acute lymphoblastic leukemia. *Am Soc Hematology Meeting* (Abstract) 1976.

Cortes, E. P., Holland, J. F., and Gildewell, O.: Amputation and adriamycin in primary osteosarcoma. A five year report. *Cancer Treat Rep 62:*271, 1978.

D'Angio, G. J., Evans, A. E., Breslow, N., et al.: The treatment of Wilms' tumor — Results of the National Wilms' Tumor Study. *Cancer, 38:*633, 1976.

Evans, A. E., D'Angio, G. J., and Randolph, J.: A proposed staging for children with neurobastoma. *Cancer, 27:*374, 1971.

Farber, S., Diamond, L. K., Mercer, R. D., et al.: Temporary remissions in acute leukemia in children produced by folic acid antagonist, 4-aminopteroyl-glutamic acid (Aminopterin). *N Eng J Med 238:* 787, 1948.

Fernbach, D. J.: Natural history of acute leukemia. In Sutow, W. W., Vietti, T. J. and Fernbach, D. J. *Clinical Pediatric Oncology,* Saint Louis, The C. V. Mosby, 1973, pp. 153-193.

Frei, E. III, Karon, M., Levin, R. H., Freireich, E. J., et al.: The effectiveness of combinations of antileukemic agents in inducing and maintaining remission in children with acute leukemia. *Blood, 26:*642, 1965.

Freireich, E. J.: Effectiveness of platelet transfusion in leukemia and aplastic anemia. *Transfusion, 6:*50, 1966.

Freireich, E. J., Henderson, E., Karon, M., and Frei, E. III: The treatment of acute leukemia considered with respect to cell population kinetics. In *The Proliferation and Spread of Neoplastic Cells.* Baltimore, Williams and Wilkins, 1968, p. 441.

Hammond, G. D., Bleyer, A., Hartmann, J. R., Hays, D. M., and Jenkin, R. D. T.: The team approach to the management of pediatric cancer. *Cancer, 41:*29, 1978.

Henderson, E.: Treatment of acute leukemia. *Semin Hematol 6:*271, 1969.

Hughes, W. T., Feldman, S., and Cox, F.: Infectious diseases in children with cancer. *Pediatr Clin N Am, 21:*583, 1974.

Jaffe, N., Frei, E. III, and Watts, H.: High-dose Methotrexate in osteogenic sarcoma: A five year experience. *Cancer Treat Rep 62:*259, 1978.

Jaffe, N., Watts, H., Fellows, K. E., et al.: Local en bloc resection for limb preservation. *Cancer Treat Rep 62:*217, 1978.

Jones, P. G. and Campbell, P. E.: Malignant disease in childhood. In *Tumors of Infancy and Childhood,* Oxford, Blackwell Scientific, 1976, pp. 1-34.

Kinney, T. R. and Chung, S. M. K.: Advances in the treatment of tumors arising in bone. *Semin Oncol 1:*47, 1974.

Levine, A. S., Schimpff, S. C., Graw, P. G. Jr., and Young, R. C.: Hematologic malignancies and other bone marrow failure states: Progress in the management of complicating infections. *Semin Hematol 11:*141, 1974.

Levine, A. S., Robinson, R. A., and Hauser, J. M.: Analysis of studies on protected environments and prophylactic antibiotics in adult acute leukemia. *Eur J Cancer, 11 Suppl. 57:*1975.

Marcove, R. C.: En bloc resections for osteogenic sarcoma. *Cancer Treat Rep 62:*225, 1978.

Murphy, S. B. and Davis, L. W.: Hodgkin's disease and the non-Hodgkin's lymphomas in childhood. *Semin Oncol. 1:*17, 1974.

Nesbit, M. E.: Ewing's sarcoma. *CA 26:*174, 1976.

Nesbit, M. E., Kersey, J., Finklestein, J., et al.: Immunotherapy and chemotherapy in children with neuroblastoma. *J Natl Cancer Inst 57:*717, 1976.

Ortega, J. A.: A therapeutic approach to childhood pelvic rhabdomyosarcoma without pelvic exenteration. *J Pediatr 94:*205, 1979.

Pomeroy, T. C. and Johnson, R. E.: Combined modality therapy of Ewing's sarcoma. *Cancer 35:*14, 1973.

Raney, R. B. Jr., Schnaufer, L. and Donaldson, M. H.: Soft-tissue sarcoma in childhood. *Semin Oncol 1:*57, 1974.

Rosen, G., Wollner, N., Tan. C., et al.: Disease-free survival in children with Ewing's sarcoma treated with radiation therapy and adjuvant four-drug sequential chemotherapy. *Cancer 33:*384, 1974.

Rosenstock, J. G. and Bishop, H. C.: Wilms' tumor and its treatment. *Semin Oncol 1:*27, 1974.

Silverberg, E.: Cancer Statistics, 1979. *CA 29:*6, 1979.

Simone, J.: Acute lymphoblastic leukemia in childhood. *Semin Hematol 11:*25, 1974.

Simone, J. V., Aur, R. J. A., Hustu, O., et al: Combined modality therapy of acute leukemia. *Cancer, 35:*25, 1975.

Sutow, W. W.: General aspects of childhood cancer. In Sutow, W. W., Vietta, T. J., and Fernbach, D. J. *Clin Pediatr Oncol,* Saint Louis, The C. V. Mosby Co., 1973, pp. 1-6.

Sutow, W. W., Gehan, E. A., Dyment, P. G., et al.: Multidrug adjuvant chemotherapy for osteosarcoma. *Cancer Treat Rep 62:*265, 1978.

Wilson, C. B., Gutin, P., Boldrey, E. B., et al.: Single-agent chemotherapy of brain tumors. *Arch Neurol 33:*739, 1976.

Wollner, N., Burchenal, J. H., Lieberman, P. H., et al.: Non-Hodgkin's lymphoma in children. *Cancer 37:*123, 1976.

Yankee, R. A., Grument, F. C. and Rogentine, G. N.: Platelet transfusion therapy. The selection of compatible platelet donors for refractory patients by lymphocyte HLA typing. *N Engl J Med 281:*1208, 1969.

Chapter Two

ILLNESS IMPACT AND SOCIAL REINTEGRATION

ERNEST R. KATZ

DUE TO INCREASING long-term survival and potential for cure in children with cancer, the qualitative nature of life experience has become an area of growing concern (Lansky et al., 1975; Goggin et al., 1976). This has resulted in a shift in psychosocial emphasis, from that of coping with imminent death to helping the child and family *live* with a chronic illness (Koch et al., 1974), and has led to the recognition of the importance of psychosocial rehabilitation and reintegration (Wilbur, 1975; Kagan-Goodheart, 1977; Katz et al., 1977; Rusk, 1977).

The literature on chronic illness in children has generally noted a higher degree of socio-emotional and school difficulties in ill children than their healthy peers (Pless and Roughmann, 1971; Bakwin and Bakwin, 1972; Myers, 1975; Pless and Pinkerton, 1975). Though current evidence does not support the notion that chronically ill children are especially vulnerable to classical psychopathology (Tavormina et al., 1976), the potential for increased psychological stress related to illness seems well documented (Pless and Pinkerton, 1975; Magrab, 1978). Numerous authors have attempted to define the nature of stress related to pediatric chronic illness, as well as the types of problems they may create or exacerbate, and develop preventative therapeutic approaches (Maddision and Raphael, 1971; Steinhauer, 1974; Grave and Pless, 1974; Becker, 1975; Pless and Pinkerton, 1975; Travis, 1976; Magrab, 1978).

Serious illness in childhood such as cancer, requiring prolonged intensive medical treatment, can prove very disruptive to the child's behavior pattern, contributing to alterations in self-concept, social isolation, and other psychosocial problems (Becker, 1972; Hoffman and Becker, 1973; Stubblefield, 1974; Pless and Pinkerton, 1975; Battle, 1975; Kellerman et al., 1979; Koocher and Sallan, 1978; Zeltzer et al., 1979). The diagnosis and treatment of cancer in a child may lead to a reduction or cessation of normal, non-illness related activity. This may result in preoccupation with illness and reduce the chances of effective rehabilitation (Travis, 1976).

The purpose of this chapter is to acquaint the reader with factors identified in the literature and clinical experience as influencing children's responses to their diagnosis and treatment of cancer. With the goal of facilitating maximal adjustment to illness, special emphasis will

14

be placed on the importance of social reintegration and the primary need for continued school experience.

PREMORBID DETERMINANTS OF ADJUSTMENT

An important first step in understanding the child's response to illness is an evaluation of the personal and social history of the child and his family (Pless and Pinkerton, 1975). Steinhauer et al. (1974) have noted how a child's development and adjustment prior to the onset of illness will influence his responses after diagnosis. The child who has had difficulty separating from his parents may have significant problems coping with hospitalization. The previously phobic child is likely to develop intense fears of medical procedures, while the hyperactive child may have difficulty tolerating forced immobilization. Other examples include the child who has had difficulty in relating to authority figures and may thus be more likely to develop problems in his relationships with doctors and nurses, and the previously shy and withdrawn child, whose illness involves physical disability or deformity, who may become increasingly self-conscious, resulting in further impairments in social functioning (Steinhauer et al., 1974). In summary, it is suggested that increased stress brought about by illness may exacerbate preexisting psychological disturbance (Pless and Pinkerton, 1975; Katz et al., 1977). The following represent areas of inquiry that are likely to prove useful in identifying predictors of adaptation to illness.

Self-Concept (Self-Esteem)

The individual's self-esteem is a personal judgment of self-worth that is expressed in the attitudes he holds toward himself (Coopersmith, 1967). Self-concept, or the overall perception one has of himself, is viewed as a basic and primary component of personality functioning (Mussen, Conger and Kagan, 1974). Lazarus (1966) has pointed out that positive self-esteem may be assumed to reduce vulnerability to threat and facilitate healthy or adaptive forms of coping. Mussen et al. (1974) noted that a favorable self-concept is essential to personal happiness and effective functioning, both in the child and adult.

Conversely, poor self-concept has been associated with feelings of inadequacy, unworthiness, and subsequent behavioral problems. Children with poor self-esteem tend to have difficulty developing and maintaining fulfilling social relationships and to feel isolated and alone (Coopersmith, 1967). High levels of anxiety tend to correlate positively with a negative conception of the self (Phillips et al., 1960). Ruebush (1960) found that anxious children have a tendency to derogate themselves and have a reduced image of their bodily integrity and adequacy. Impairment in school adjustment and subsequent academic progress has also been positively related to a poor self-concept, though it is often unclear which comes first, poor school performance or poor self-concept (Phillips, 1960). Coopersmith (1967), in studying a large number of preadolescent boys attending public schools in Connecticut, found that those high in self-esteem approached tasks and persons with a greater expectation for success and positive experiences than did their peers with poor self-concept.

Several authors have evaluated the impact of serious chronic illness on self-concept in children. Stubblefield (1974) pointed out that the increased frustration and disappointments faced by a chronically ill child in his daily life may lead to self-doubts relating to problem-solving skills. The chronically ill child's forced dependence upon parents and medical staff, along with restrictions of activity and a possible lack of accurate information regarding the etiology and prognosis of his condition, can lead to a severe sense of worthlessness (Maddison and Raphael, 1971). Among adolescents with chronic illness, Weinberg (1970) noted the degree to which the disability interferes with mastery and control, and places the youth in a dependent state. He suggests that this can be particularly damaging to the body-integrity of males. Meissner et al. (1967) found that physical problems of high impact and visibility interfered particularly with the development of normal self-concept among adolescent girls.

In evaluating the concept of adjustment in children with chronic disorders, Pless and Pinkerton (1975) hypothesized that the stress of illness leads to an altered self-concept resulting from both physical change factors and socio-emotional responses of family and others. This change is seen as influencing adaptation to the illness and is mediated by the child's resources and abilities.

Bakwin and Bakwin (1972) noted how a chronic illness may make a child feel different than his peers, thereby reducing his self-esteem. In a controlled study of chronically ill children, Tavormina et al. (1976) noted no significant decrease in self-concept within a sample skewed toward relatively mild disability. Preliminary results of a study currently in progress with seriously chronically ill adolescents tends to indicate a positive relationship between perceived severity of illness and reduced self-esteem (Zeltzer et al., 1979).

The effects on self-concept in a child diagnosed with cancer are similar to those generally reported for children with other chronic illnesses. In addition, however, the generally *acute onset* and *life-threatening* nature of the disease can make postdiagnostic adjustment extremely traumatic for the oncology patient (Oakley and Patterson, 1968). Based on clinical experience, the author suggests that possession of a positive self-concept prior to the onset of illness allows a greater potential for maintaining a higher self-concept during illness with fewer problems in adjustment.

Case One

Ronald, diagnosed with Stage IV lymphoma one year earlier, was nine years old when his attending oncologist referred him for psychological intervention to help with withdrawn behavior and extreme nausea. This behavior became acute every second week, just prior to his receiving chemotherapy.

In interviewing Ronald, the psychologist became aware of Ronald's low self-esteem and lack of confidence. This was manifested by his inability to describe any activity he felt competent with, and his description of himself as a child no one wanted to play with or befriend. His premorbid school history was one of unenthusiastic performance and social isolation. His mother described him as a "finicky" child, a characteristic that became more pronounced since his illness, with increased irritability and refusal to attend school due to unsubstantiated medical complaints.

Ronald's preexisting poor self-concept appeared to be further reinforced by his illness and treatment. This resulted in his focusing upon the disabling aspects of his illness leading to withdrawal from school, peers, and nonillness related activities. Ronald's potential for successfully adapting to his illness was severely impaired, and supportive psychotherapy was instituted to help reduce his anxiety and increase involvement in normal childhood experiences.

After several months of psychological intervention, Ronald was noticeably more involved in school and social activities, displaying less treatment-related anxiety at home and in the clinic. In addition, he was noted to recover more quickly from the toxic effects of his chemotherapy.

Case Two

Jo Anne was ten years of age when diagnosed with acute lymphocytic leukemia. She was in the fifth grade of a private school for high achieving children. She was very involved with her parents in recreational activities that often included other children and their families. Jo Anne had many friends that expressed their concern for her by inundating her with get-well cards while she was in the hospital. Jo Anne was anxious to return to school and take up horseback riding, an activity that she had planned well in advance of her illness.

Jo Anne received much emotional support from her parents, school, and peers. She succeeded in maintaining a high level of social involvement even while undergoing intensive outpatient care at the hospital.

Premorbid Family Interaction Patterns

The manner in which the child and parents interact affects adaptation to illness. This is by no means unrelated to self-esteem and, in fact seems to interact strongly with it. Coopersmith (1967) found that children with high self-esteem seemed to have parents who were also high in self-esteem. These parents were also more emotionally stable, more self-reliant, and more effective in their attitudes regarding child care than parents with low self-esteem. Interactions between parents of high self-esteem children tended to be marked by greater compatibility and ease, with clear definitions of each parent's areas of authority and responsibility. These parents tended to have high expectations for their children, while providing consistency in modeling, encouragement, and support. Mothers who valued the opinions and expressions of their children tended to have children with higher self-esteem.

In contrast, mothers of children low in self-esteem tended to be inattentive and neglectful, producing an environment that was often emotionally impoverished. Such mothers tended to depreciate their children and treat them as a burden. Emotional responses to their children ranged from hostility to indifference.

In evaluating the parent-child relationship after the diagnosis of cancer, it is useful to assess the nature of the premorbid relationship in order to alert the clinician to potential difficulties (Becker, 1972; Pless and Pinkerton, 1975). Extreme parental fear and anxiety about their child that predates the illness can have the effect of sensitizing parents and child to the disabling aspects of the illness (Futterman and Hoffman, 1970; Lansky et al., 1975).

Case Three

Bill was twelve years of age when diagnosed with acute lymphocytic leukemia. He was the youngest of two sons and always appeared frail in his parent's estimation. His parents noted that Bill never displayed the physical prowess or behavioral independence that his older brother did. As a result, they had attempted to watch Bill carefully at all times, fearing that he would be unable to care for himself without regular parental supervision.

When Bill was first diagnosed, his parents felt that their estimation of his weakness had been validated. They allowed him to do whatever he wished, and his mother quit her job to care for him full-time. Bill's parents accepted his decision to remain out of school until he was ready to return. They had few expectations for healthy behavior, nor did they feel it appropriate to impose any limits.

After nine months, Bill became extremely overdemanding, irritable, and socially isolated. His parents began to resent what they viewed as manipulative behavior, and requested psychological assistance.

Steinhauer et al. (1974) described the particular threat to family equilibrium brought about when chronic disease occurs in a child whose family relationships are already strained. Koocher and Sallan (1978) commented upon the extreme familial stress that accompanies the diagnosis of cancer in a child, emphasizing how preexisting emotional problems can be exacerbated by the diagnosis. The existence of *premorbid marital stress* is another factor noted by Steinhauer et al. (1974) as particularly upsetting to family equilibrium. In a recent study on marital discord and divorce in parents of a child with cancer, Lansky et al. (1978) concluded that heightened marital stress among parents of children with cancer was a common experience, but that the incidence of divorce was not found to be greater than that in the general population.

Case Four

Jonathan was four years of age when his one-and-a-half year old sister was diagnosed with a Wilms' tumor, Stage III. Jonathan was referred for psychological counseling because of his repeated physical abuse of his sister, including hitting, biting, and pulling of her hair. An assessment of their premorbid interaction pattern revealed that Jonathan had much difficulty adjusting to the birth of his new sister and had always been extremely jealous of any special attention given to her. After the diagnosis, Jonathan's jealousy became more intense as both parents left him for several days at a time with a babysitter while staying with his sister in the hospital.

In addition, it was discovered that the parents had experienced major marital difficulties prior to their daughter's illness. These problems had increased at the time of psychological referral to the point where separation was being considered. Jonathan understood that his parents disagreed often and blamed his sister for causing the increasing family strain as well as what he perceived as his own abandonment.

Jonathan's parents became involved in marital therapy with a hospital social worker. Jonathan was scheduled to be seen regularly by the author for supportive psychotherapy, but distance and transportation problems precluded successful follow-through with this plan.

A referral was made for Jonathan to be seen at a local child guidance clinic.

School and Social History

The child's premorbid school and social history influence subsequent adaptation and may be predictive of later problems (Steinhauer et al., 1974). Katz et al. (1977) found a significant incidence of learning and school problems in children with cancer that had their origins in the child's premorbid experience. This was particularly evident in children who hesitated to return to school when judged medically able. The child and his parents who have found school to be a rewarding, enjoyable experience before the onset of illness will have a stronger inclination to return to school after diagnosis than the child with a history of school attendance and/or socio-academic difficulties.

Mattson (1972) has noted how virtually all children with a chronic disability will occasionally take advantage of their disease in order to avoid unpleasant situations. Children with preexisting negative attitudes about school may find that their illness gives them an acceptable excuse to avoid this experience.

Parents with little premorbid school involvement may not perceive the importance of continued academic participation nor possess the ability to help the child reintegrate. In addition, parents who were ambivalent about their child's school attendance prior to illness onset may now experience even less resolve to have their child participate regularly.

Case Five

George was fourteen years of age when diagnosed with acute lymphocytic leukemia. He had not returned to school for two months after beginning treatment, although his physician had recommended school reintegration three weeks after diagnosis. In evaluating his premorbid school history, it was noted that George had attended four schools in the two years preceding his illness. Records indicated that George was having difficulty following through with assignments and his parents engineered the school transfers in an attempt to help him find a teacher who "could motivate him." Psychometric testing revealed George to be of above-average intelligence and ability.

After diagnosis, George refused to attend school. His parents supported this

decision on the grounds that he was too ill and didn't need to be "bothered." Seven
months later, George was bored and began to be a nuisance to his parents. They
then realized that George was not facing imminent death and that he needed to be
involved in normal activities with appropriate limits on his behavior.

The child's premorbid involvement in social activities and hobbies,
i.e., scouts, church, arts and crafts, sports, can be a rich source of
information about interests, talents, resources, and coping style. The
patient who has established many gratifying social relationships prior
to his diagnosis has much to look forward to in his return to normal life
experiences and may be more likely to aggressively pursue a rehabilitative course than his withdrawn peer.

Case Six

Monica was seven years old when diagnosed with a non-Hodgkin's lymphoma,
Stage III. She was hospitalized for initial inductive chemotherapy in a reverse
isolation Laminar Airflow Unit for approximately five weeks.

Prior to the onset of her illness, Monica was very involved in caring for her horse
and entering him in riding competitions. When she became ill and was hospitalized, her parents brought pictures of her horse and related objects to the
hospital. They helped her maintain a positive attitude regarding her treatment,
seeing it as potentially controlling her illness and allowing her to return to her
horse and shows.

Hospital staff found that Monica's interests in horses helped them establish
rapport with her. They regularly engaged her in active discussion about her horse
and gave her the opportunity to redirect her attention from the anxiety of
hospitalization and treatment.

Upon discharge, Monica was delighted to be able to return to her horse and
began riding as soon as her physician felt she was able to do so. Her active
equestrian interest continued to provide a recreational focus for her as she
followed-through with extended outpatient care.

The nature of the child's premorbid interests can have a positive
interaction with illness, as in the case above, where the interest can be
maintained and even strengthened. However, where the illness directly impairs postdiagnostic participation in premorbid interests, this
can prove very disturbing and lead to depressive reactions.

Case Seven

Janet was fourteen years of age when diagnosed with osteogenic sarcoma. She
underwent an above-the-knee amputation of her right leg soon after, followed by
intensive chemotherapy that required periodic hospitalization.

Prior to her illness, Janet had been an accomplished dancer and was trying out
for her high school's cheerleading squad. After her surgery, Janet was determined
to master the use of her prosthetic device and return to cheerleading. This goal
was at first a source of great hope, but led to despair when she realized that her
rehabilitation would be slow. Her frustration led to withdrawal and depression.
Janet was assisted, through ongoing psychological support, to ventilate her feelings and develop alternative, more moderate and obtainable goals.

Prior Medical Experience

Becker (1972), in discussing childhood responses to hospitalization, noted how previous history of hospitalization is an important predictive variable. The child who has had previously stressful medical experiences may be particularly sensitive to the intensive medical care required to treat his malignancy.

Prior medical experience of parents and other family members can affect their response to the ill child (Pless and Pinkerton, 1975). Parents who may have experienced the diagnosis and treatment of cancer in themselves, a relative, or a friend, may have different expectations for their child's adjustment than parents without such prior experience.

Case Eight

James was diagnosed with acute lymphocytic leukemia when eleven years of age. The confirmation of this diagnosis proved especially difficult to accept for James' father, as he had a brother who had died of leukemia when fifteen years of age.

James' father became oversolicitous of him, no longer expecting any type of school performance or other behavior he now felt was too strenuous. The father felt that James had no chance for survival, based on his prior experience with his brother but not reflecting actual medical prognosis. This attitude was detected by James even though there was never any direct discussion concerning both of their fears. James became withdrawn and isolated and was referred for psychological support.

Regular therapeutic sessions were held with James to help him regain motivation for goal-directed behavior. Initial progress was made in school reintegration. However, the attitude of his parents remained ambivalent, and they continuously reinforced any dependent behavior that James would demonstrate. Parents were not amenable to family or individual therapy to help them encourage James' attempts to become reinvolved in active experiences. Under the circumstances, it was not possible to help James achieve his potential for school reintegration, though he did develop several supportive social relationships and continued his academic program with a home teacher.

THE NATURE OF THE ILLNESS AND ITS TREATMENT

The child's potential for social and academic reintegration is directly related to the realities of his illness. The term "cancer" refers to a group of diseases having basic similarities in terms of development and effect on the host organism, but they are distinctive from each other in very specific ways. Cancers differ from each other by cell type, site of origin, rapidness of growth, impact on the host, age of the host at onset, responsiveness to treatment, and prognosis (Mozden, 1965, Koocher and Sallan, 1978). These factors plus others (such as available medical resources) will determine the exact nature of treatment selected. Treatment is usually disease-specific, although general treatment approaches and drugs may be similar for different cancers (Sutow et al., 1977).

Disease Process and Prognosis

It is difficult to make a general statement about the typical pediatric response to cancer because of the specificity of each medical situation, treatment, and individual child. When assessing psychosocial response to illness, it is of the utmost importance that the *specific* disease process and its treatment be understood (Pless and Pinkerton, 1975; Travis, 1976; Magrab and Calcagno, 1978, Koocher and Sallan, 1978). For example, a child diagnosed with acute lymphocytic leukemia may have a very good chance of obtaining a fairly rapid and extended remission of his illness soon after treatment is initiated (Pinkel, 1976). However, the requirement of regularly scheduled bone marrow aspirations and lumbar punctures can be very anxiety provoking to the leukemic patient, who may experience more pain and discomfort from his treatment than the illness itself (Katz et al., in press).

A child diagnosed with osteogenic sarcoma may require an amputation as well as intensive chemotherapy and radiotherapy. A relatively longer period of adjustment may be expected for a child undergoing an amputation, and the probability of long-term survival is currently low (Jaffe, 1975).

For the child who presents at time of diagnosis with a Stage IV widely disseminated malignancy, social reintegration may be unrealistic until the medical situation stabilizes. In contrast, the patient with a Stage I localized malignancy can generally be expected to resume premorbid activities fairly quickly.

Whether the patient's condition and prognosis are excellent or poor, it is imperative that continuing needs of childhood development be recognized. The possibilities for maximizing potential for positive, adaptive experiences must not be overlooked for any youngster, even the child facing imminent death (Kagan-Goodheart, 1977; Burton, 1974).

Case Nine

Greg was twelve years of age when diagnosed with a hepatoblastoma, Stage III, initially treated with intensive chemotherapy and radiation therapy. He and his family had arrived in the United States less than one year prior to his illness, and Greg had not had the opportunity to become well acculturated to his new school and community. As Greg felt poorly most of the time, his parents were reluctant to try to direct his behavior toward any type of school or social reintegration, particularly because he felt negatively about school. They did allow for a home teacher to work with Greg on a limited academic curriculum.

After approximately one year, a surgical resection of the tumor was performed, after which Greg's ability to survive was in question due to medical complications. Greg's parents understood the severity of their son's illness but were unable to be with him regularly due to their employment requirements. Greg regularly complained of high levels of pain and appeared depressed and withdrawn.

The psychologist who had previously interacted with Greg on a limited basis around the issue of school reintegration was requested to assist with his current difficulties. Daily sessions with Greg in his hospital room, involving nondirective recreational activities and general emotional support, succeeded in the establishment of good rapport. Greg began to spend less time focusing on the anxiety and discomfort of his illness and was taught self-hypnosis to further increase relaxation and comfort. This coincided with an improvement in his medical condition allowing previously high levels of pain medications to be reduced.

The psychologist and medical staff communicated with Greg's parents about the importance of family support and encouragement. In addition, they were helped to understand that Greg could be maintained at home, if the family could adjust to his medical needs and provide alternative supervision during working hours. School reintegration began to be discussed, and parents were encouraged to raise their expectations of Greg's quality of life, even if he was still at significant medical risk.

Greg began to sense a change in the attitudes of parents and staff regarding his potential. He responded by becoming increasingly active in the hospital recreation room and began making plans for his return home.

Once home, Greg and his family were encouraged to follow through with school reintegration after his physician determined this was appropriate on an initially limited basis. Greg became worried about school but was assisted through ongoing psychological support to reduce his fears and see school as an opportunity to be a normal person. After his return to school, he and his parents reported a positive alteration in his mood and activity level. He was reported to be doing well academically and was noticeably more calm and relaxed during successive medical appointments.

Tumor Site

The site of a tumor may cause specific emotional difficulties related to its visibility, physical impairment, or previous sociodevelopmental experiences involving that physical area (Adsett, 1963). Tumors involving the genitalia, for example, may elicit conflictual feelings regarding later procreative ability (Adsett, 1963; Kellerman and Katz, 1977). Parents may be more affected by the emotional implications of the tumor site than the patient himself and may project their own symbolic meanings and anxieties onto the child.

Case Ten

Robert was diagnosed with a localized, Stage I testicular sarcoma at four years of age. His mother was visibly and understandably upset when informed of Robert's need to have one testicle removed to reduce the threat of tumor spread.

After the surgery, despite an excellent prognosis and no physical impairment, his mother treated him as a disabled child. She explained that she had the belief that he could never be "normal" with only one testicle, as he might be sexually sterile and unable to bear children.

Through supportive counseling and her involvement in a program to help reduce Robert's anxiety to needles and medications, the mother was helped to understand how procreative ability was only *one* aspect of a normal life. She became aware of how her expectations and attitudes were preventing Robert from being able to behave in a manner appropriate for a child of his age.

Counseling of the mother was followed by a reduction of her reinforcement of Robert's sick-role behavior (moaning, psychogenic vomiting), and an increase in her encouragement of regular school participation and consistent behavioral standards at home. Along with play therapy and systematic desensitization, ma-

ternal support helped Robert overcome his intense anxiety related to treatment
and his behavior at home and school returned to its pre-illness pattern.

Treatment Regimen

The treatment regimen selected for a childhood malignancy is specific to the nature and extent of illness, as well as the individual characteristics of the child (Sutow, et al., 1973). Treatment will vary in the combination and quantities of drugs utilized, whether or not surgical intervention is required and to what extent, as well as if and how radiation therapy is used. The treatment program and the child's medical progress will determine how frequently the child needs to be seen for outpatient visits and/or hospitalizations.

In general, the more complex the treatment program, the more factors that may potentially interfere with rehabilitation and reintegration (Pless and Pinkerton, 1975). With the apparent increase in sophisticated and complex multimodal treatment programs, the future challenge to psychosocial adaptation can be expected to increase as well.

Side Effects

One of the most significant paradoxes confronted in the treatment of cancer is the issue of side effects produced by the treatment itself. Most of the anticancer drugs are toxic not only to the proliferating malignancy, but to normal cells as well (Hughes, 1976). This is also true of radiation therapy (Jaffe, 1976). Side effects of surgical intervention are often the most obvious (Wilbur, 1975).

To a child's mind, having to undergo painful medical procedures as well as tolerate noxious medications may seem worse than the disease itself. It can be particularly confusing to a child who is told that the treatment he is receiving is to help make him feel better, when the short range results are usually just the opposite. For this and other reasons, the importance of providing supportive information and answering questions as they arise cannot be overemphasized.

Treatment side effects include (Weiss et al., 1974; Golden, 1975; Hughes, 1976; Jaffe, 1976; Koocher and Sallan, 1978):

CHEMOTHERAPY:

Mouth and lip ulcers
Nausea and vomiting
Hair loss
Weight gain
Fluid retention
Pain and weakness in extremities
Fevers
Tissue burns resulting from injection leakage
Increased susceptibility to disease
Neurotoxicity, with potential cognitive and affective impairment

Hepatic, pulmonary, cardiac, and urinary toxicity
Reduced fertility
Secondary malignancies
RADIATION THERAPY:
   Nausea and vomiting
   Hair loss
   Skin burns and discoloration
   Facial markings from cranial irradiation
   Headaches
   Impaired physical growth and development
   Reduced fertility
SURGICAL INTERVENTION:
   Disfigurement
   Reduced organic function
   Requirement for prosthetic device

Many of the obvious side effects of chemotherapy and radiation therapy are generally of a temporary nature, such as hair loss, weight gain, and nausea. However, as more children survive for longer periods of time, late side effects such as neurotoxicity and damage to other organs are becoming more prevalent (Jaffe, 1976). This points to the need for continued surveillance and investigations to improve the safety and efficacy of treatment.

Aside from the direct effect on the child's physiological functioning and comfort, side effects are capable of eliciting negative social responses (Koocher and Sallan, 1978). This can lead to increased emotional difficulties mediated by the intensity and frequency of treatment, as well as the individual child's personality and perceptions (Clapp, 1976).

Conditioned anticipatory anxiety is a common behavioral response to repeated medical procedures (Kellerman et al., 1979). The child may become anxious in advance of a medical appointment and may vomit or become withdrawn. In addition, such conditioned anxiety may cause the child to have a more severe and prolonged reaction to chemotherapy than is physiologically explainable, thereby increasing discomfort and reducing the child's potential for continued school and social experiences.

Case Eleven

Karen was nine years old when diagnosed with acute myelogenous leukemia. She had adjusted well to her initial treatment regimen, continuing in school and with her social activities. Her illness was in remission for eight months, after which time she had a relapse and was told that intensive reinductive treatment would be required.

Karen became more anxious with each successive visit for chemotherapy. She started to vomit as soon as she received her medication, and soon developed anticipatory vomiting which began when she and her mother arrived in the hospital parking lot. Finally, as she grew increasingly withdrawn and isolated in response to increased anxiety, she began to vomit the night before with emesis continuing well after the cessation of treatment.

In order to help reduce Karen's treatment-related anxiety, regular sessions with a psychologist were initiated. Hypnosis was utilized to help increase feelings of comfort and well-being, and Karen was assisted in learning self-hypnosis that she could use on her own. In addition, systematic desensitization was employed to help reduce the ability of selected environmental cues to evoke high levels of incapacitating anxiety.

Along with the specific interventions noted above, the psychologist helped Karen's mother reduce her reinforcement of Karen's anxious behavior. Rather than running to hold her each time Karen was nauseated, the mother was instructed to assess the situation and take all precautions for Karen's well-being but not to become physically demonstrative. Instead, she was told to hold Karen and demonstrate affection when Karen was feeling well or involved in satisfying activities that were not illness related.

The frequency and intensity of Karen's anxiety responses to treatment reduced noticeably within two weeks. Unfortunately, her medical status deteriorated rapidly and long-term follow-up was not possible.

GEOGRAPHICAL FACTORS

Where local treatment facilities are inadequate or nonexistent, the child may be required to travel extensive distances to receive treatment. This may make even the most routine medical appointment into a full-day outing. By increasing the time required for medical attention, such factors contribute to further disruptions in school and social reintegration (Evans, 1975).

When hospitalizations are required at distant treatment centers, the child may not have the benefit of regular family and friends visiting. This can result in increased isolation and depression.

INTELLECTUAL AND DEVELOPMENTAL FACTORS

The child's ability to comprehend and adjust to his illness will depend on his emotional and intellectual development and resources (Pless and Pinkerton, 1975; Stubblefield, 1974; Becker, 1972; Maddison and Raphael, 1971; Katz et al., 1977; Lubin, 1975; Magrab and Calcagno, 1978).

Developmental Disruption

The psychosocial development of the child is generally accepted as progressing through various stages, usually in a prescribed order of occurrence (Mussen et al., 1974). Lowit (1973) stressed that "chronic disease varies in its impact with the developmental stage at which it first affects the patient." In looking at the incidence of school reintegration difficulties in children with cancer, for example, Kellerman and Katz (unpublished) noted a higher incidence of problems in children just beginning school for the first time. The authors hypothesized that the normal developmental process of separation and individuation was complicated by the diagnosis of a potentially fatal illness (Lansky et al., 1975; Futterman, and Hoffman, 1972).

Garrard and Richmond (1963) have suggested that Erickson's concept of progressive psychosocial development can be useful in highlighting the nature of the crisis presented by serious illness in childhood. Using this model, these authors illustrate how serious illness may result in inadequate resolution of the normal tasks of development. Illness during the period from twelve months to three years may limit the child's opportunities for self-expression, intensify maternal control, and enhance passivity and feelings of helplessness, thus interfering with the *achievement of autonomy*. Illness during ages four to five may produce extreme guilt and lead to an excessive inhibition of initiative, interfering with the *development of conscience*. From six to eleven, the illness may result in a sense of inferiority and inadequacy rather than a progression to the normal sense of *achievement and accomplishment*. Illness in adolescence may interfere with the ability to establish clear concepts of role and identity, with resultant role diffusion (Kellerman and Katz, 1977).

Developmental Response to Physical Change and Treatment

Children's response to physical changes induced by cancer and its treatment vary along cognitive-developmental lines (Katz et. al., 1977). The preschool child rarely experiences baldness or weight gain as a severe disability because of his lack of preoccupation with appearance and due to an ego-centered social perspective (Mussen et al., 1974). The school age child, with an increasing self-awareness and social outlook, is often disturbed by physical changes as it affects how others view him. The adolescent, for whom personal appearance and peer group acceptance are of primary importance, often experiences baldness and other physical changes with the highest level of anxiety (Moore et al., 1969; Kellerman and Katz, 1977).

Responses to difficult medical procedures also appear to vary developmentally. In a study of children with leukemia undergoing repeated outpatient bone marrow aspirations, the behavioral expression of distress was found to vary by age (Katz et al., in press). Young children tended to display a larger variety of behaviors than older children, including more uncontrolled motor movements. Older children exhibited less anticipatory anxiety, and recovered faster at the conclusion of the procedures. Self-report of discomfort during the procedure also varied by age, with younger children reporting more discomfort (Katz et al., in preparation)

Regression

How the child perceives his world at any given point in time has important implications for what he understands about his illness and the types of illness-related information he can readily integrate (Lubin, 1975). Several authors note how the stress of illness can cause a child to temporarily, defensively regress in his behavior and cognitive performance (Lubin 1975; Becker, 1972; Stubblefield, 1974; Maddison and Raphael, 1971). This type of response should not be considered pathological unless it persists and continually disrupts functioning.

The moderate frequency with which regressive behavior under stress occurs has important ramifications for health professionals who transmit information to the child. Repetition of basic information may be necessary to enable the child to comprehend at his own pace.

Sex Differences in Children With Cancer

The sex of the child with cancer may be an important variable in determining overall adjustment to illness. Goggin et al. (1976) found that among children with malignancies, younger boys tended to experience more anxiety than younger girls, but this trend reversed when looking at older children. The authors explained their results as being consistent with general cultural trend of boys being more psychologically at risk at younger ages, with the trend reversing as age increases.

In children with leukemia, girls exhibited significantly more distress behaviors during outpatient bone marrow procedures than boys, across all ages studied (8 months to 18 years: Katz et al., in press). Girls also reported more subjective discomfort (Katz et al., in preparation). These findings are consistent with general sex differences in society which tend to encourage girls to be more expressive of their emotional state than boys (Gotts, 1968; Maccoby & Jacklin, 1974).

Magical Thinking

Piaget, in his studies of cognitive development in children, determined that thinking in young children often tends to have magical characteristics (Elkind, 1974). Thoughts and wishes may be perceived as so powerful that they can cause direct harm to other people, or conversely, may protect them from harm (Elkind, 1974; Maddison and Raphael, 1971). From the age of four or five (the period of conscience development in the Eriksonian schema), the child has a reasonably well-developed sense of what is appropriate behavior, though he may not, in fact, always conform to that standard. Maddison and Raphael (1971) note how a child may perceive his illness as a punishment for unacceptable thoughts, impulses, or behaviors. These distorted ideas may unwittingly be reinforced by punitive parental comments, i.e. "I told you not to go outside without your coat on!", as well as unintentional comments of hospital staff.

Mattson (1972) notes how the preschool child, in particular, has little ability to comprehend the causality and nature of an illness. Pain and other symptoms tend to be interpreted as punishment for being bad. Vernon et al. (1965) point out that children may interpret the separation involved in hospitalization as withdrawal of parental love and affection. For children, chance occurrence of illness is a difficult concept to comprehend, as it often is for adults, and the child is likely to search for reasons for the illness in his immediate past (Freeman, 1968).

Young pediatric patients often attribute illness and injury to recent family interactions. They may see illness as due to their disobedience or because parents failed to protect them and may attribute blame for the illness to themselves or other family members. Mattson (1972) points out how these distorted interpretations of bodily changes may be perpetuated by the child's reluctance to ask questions and vent his anxiety regarding how and why he became ill.

Case Twelve

Manuel was eight-and-a-half years of age when diagnosed with a Ewing's sarcoma, with a primary tumor in his leg. He was seen by a psychologist for vomiting and gagging that began during administration of chemotherapy but continued after each course of therapy ended.

As a routine part of evaluating Manuel's problem, the psychologist asked Manuel why he had to visit the doctor and receive medications. Manuel replied that he had a tumor. When asked what that meant, he replied that it was "like an animal that crawled into my leg and is growing." Manuel proceeded to draw a picture of his tumor which was shaped like an animal and had fish scales and pointed antennae. It became clear that he had allowed his imagination to interpret his mother's explanation to him that he had a "bug" that caused the illness.

Treatment of his vomiting began with the provision of more realistic information to help him comprehend his illness more appropriately. Hypnosis and training in self-hypnosis were utilized to help reduce anxiety and increase feelings of comfort, along with suggestions aimed at reducing his gagging behavior. Concurrently, he was assisted to become more fully reintegrated into school, and his mother was involved to actively support and reinforce his appropriate, healthy behavior.

PARENTAL RESPONSE

Parental attitudes about their child's illness and his ability to adjust have been found to significantly influence postmorbid adjustment (Pless and Pinkerton, 1975; Gravis, 1976). After receiving the diagnosis of cancer in their child, parents commonly manifest signs and symptoms of psychic shock (Koch et al., 1974). This may be accompanied or followed by a deep sense of mourning and grief (Richmond and Waisman, 1955; Myers, 1975). The child is usually able to comprehend that something is seriously wrong with him even in the absence of direct verbal communication (Spinetta, 1973).

This initial period of disorganization is generally followed by a period of reintegration during which defenses are often able to cushion the parent from a direct confrontation with reality (Maddison and Raphael, 1971). This is the time when many parents begin to plan for adjusting to the realities of their child's illness. Suggestions for positive school and social reintegration, at this time, may assist in the family's development of a generally optimistic orientation, rather than a continued focus on mourning and hopelessness (Karon, 1975).

Initial Denial

Defensive denial of the full implications of the child's diagnosis can serve a useful purpose in allowing parents not to overly dwell upon fatality, and thereby, manage in the face of anxiety that might otherwise be overwhelming (Maddison and Raphael, 1971; Travis, 1975). However, the persistence of a high level of unrealistic denial may do a disservice to the child and his management if the parents harbor fantasies about the correct nature of the diagnosis and its severity (Maddison and Raphael, 1971).

A high level of denial may preclude the parents and child from communicating openly and honestly about their fears. This may hamper the family's adjustment and, in the event of later terminal illness and death, lead to unresolved feelings and greater emotional stress upon the survivors (Kubler-Ross, 1973).

Guilt

Parental guilt is a very common reaction, often stemming from the concern about causing the illness or failing to recognize symptoms early enough (Richmond and Waisman, 1955; Karon, 1975; Spinetta et al., 1976). Guilt may also arise from an unconscious "death wish" harbored toward the child, or the belief that he may not have been cared for properly (Karon, 1975), as well as from societal norms establishing parental responsibility for child rearing (Kellerman and Katz, 1978).

Over-Protection

In dealing with sick children, adults may intensify gratification of dependency needs in an attempt to help the child feel more secure and comfortable and as a response to their own anxiety (Maddison and Raphael, 1971; Steinhauer, et al., 1974). While to some extent additional parental support is needed, prolonged and excessive gratification of these needs may prove so satisfying that the child may resist giving it up. This can interfere with normal striving toward mature independence, thereby reducing the development of self-confidence and initiative (Steinhauer, 1974), fostering excessive dependency (Myers, 1975).

Parental overprotectiveness may lead to unnecessary restrictions upon the child's activities and experiences (Myers, 1975). It may also result in a reduction of normal, premorbid standards of discipline and behavior, thereby making the child different from his siblings and peers (Myers, 1975). Reduced parental expectations for their child's ability to continue his premorbid activities, particularly school, may communicate a sense of hopelessness and despair to the child (Moore, 1969; Spinetta et al., 1976).

Fewer behavioral adjustment problems have been found among children with leukemia whose parents continued with normal discipline after the onset of their illness, particularly relating to the child's task-avoidance (Heffron et al., 1973). A patient can quickly sense when his illness allows him to get extra advantages within his family and community, especially when parental demands are inconsistent and favor the sick child (Maddison and Raphael, 1971; Heffron et al., 1973; Myers, 1975). This can result in the child's "using" his illness to get what he wants, and may prevent his giving up of certain illness symptoms which have now become a major source of reinforcement (Weinder, 1970; Maddison and Raphael, 1971).

Over-Identification and Parental Anxiety

In a study of parents of seriously ill children, Korsch et al. (1954) found that parents who reported the highest anxiety in their children tended themselves to voice more anxiety, embarrassment, and guilt about their child's illness than parents who saw their children as less anxious. The possibility exists that some parents may over-identify with their child's situation, imposing their perceptions of the child's illness experience onto him. This may result in parents emphasizing symptoms and disabilities with which the child himself may not be as acutely concerned.

Parental anxiety has been found to influence children's responses to hospitalization (Robinson, 1968) and to outpatient clinic appointments (Hefernan and Azarnoff, 1971). Parental anxiety can effect the content and manner of verbal and nonverbal communication related to hospital and medical experience. This can influence and sensitize the child's perception of his experience and increase his anxiety and maladaptive behavioral responses (Escalona, 1953).

Case Thirteen

Linda was fourteen-and-a-half years of age when diagnosed with osteogenic sarcoma, resulting in the amputation of her left leg above the knee. She was in the ninth grade and her first year at a new high school. Linda was an attractive adolescent who had been very socially active, and had tried-out for cheerleading immediately prior to her diagnosis. After her amputation, Linda's mother insisted that her return to school be delayed until she had completely mastered the use of her prosthesis. In addition, her mother decided against preparing her for the possibility of hair loss, a probable side effect of chemotherapy. This decision was based on her fear that Linda would be too overwhelmed to cope.

Linda encountered several difficulties in her adaptation to the prosthetic device, and continued to postpone her return to school. Her mother was particularly fearful of the possibility that Linda might be ridiculed for looking strangely. Linda's mother was very concerned about her own appearance and appeared to over-identify with her daughter's plight. As such she found it very difficult to be supportive of Linda's social reintegration.

Separation Anxiety

Given the diagnosis of a malignancy and the implied potential for death, separation anxiety in both parents and child is understandable (Richmond and Waisman, 1955). Such anxiety can become particularly acute when there is evidence of deterioration in the child's condition.

How separation anxiety is handled in any particular instance is related to age, the quality of the separation-individuation phase of the child's development, as well as the perceived nature of the danger (Futterman and Hoffman, 1970).

Separation anxiety has been implicated in the development and maintenance of night terrors in a child with leukemia (Kellerman, 1979). Separation anxiety, particularly between the mother and sick child, has been observed in the development and maintenance of *school phobia* in children with cancer, as noted by Futterman and Hoffman (1971) and Lansky, et al. (1975). As these authors point out, both the child and his parents may be fearful of even temporary separation, due to the illness's potential fatality and concerns about permanent separation. Due to the lack of awareness regarding the origin of their anxiety, the mildest symptom of discomfort expressed by the child may result in the parents allowing him to stay home. In this way, parents may unwittingly reinforce dependent behavior, reducing the child's motivation to continue with normal, premorbid activities.

Case Fourteen

Sue, an eleven-year-old girl with acute lymphocytic leukemia, was diagnosed three months after she and her family arrived in the United States from the Far East. Sue had just started the fourth grade when she became ill and did not return to school that year. Her parents were very protective of their daughter and felt school to be an unnecessary burden at that time.

At the start of the next school year, it was discovered that Sue had not been enrolled in school, nor were there any plans for her to do so. A referral was made to the school psychologist, who contacted Sue and her parents. They were quite emphatic that she was not ready for school but agreed that she needed academic instruction. A home teacher was subsequently arranged to work with Sue. Two months later, Sue's physician noticed that she had regressed socially and emotionally. He felt very strongly that Sue's staying home when she was medically capable of attending school was unhealthy and contributed to her perception of herself as helpless and sick, an attitude reinforced by her parents.

Sue was seen by a psychologist to assist in her school reintegration. She was able to ventilate her fears concerning potential ridicule at school and agreed to allow the psychologist to help prepare the school for her return. Sue's parents were seen to enlist their cooperation and support. They explained how they felt it was important for Sue to be in school but did not feel they could make the arrangements themselves. They were very grateful for assistance with this.

Sue returned to school and attended regularly. She became more outgoing and age-appropriate in her behavior, and her parents began to see her as a capable individual and related to her in that manner.

PEER AND COMMUNITY RESPONSES

Peer socialization has been recognized as crucial in the psychological development of children (Campbell, 1964). The peer group provides a primary opportunity to learn social-interaction skills, such as dealing with hostility, dominance, leadership, and conflict resolution (Mussen et al., 1974). The peer group also serves a primary purpose in the development of social attitudes (Hartup, 1970). As such, peer responses can affect the child's emotional response to illness. A review of three epidemiologic studies of chronic disease in children found ill children to be socially isolated more often than their normal peers (Pless and Roughman, 1971).

Maddison and Raphael (1971) have noted the frequent presence of negative attitudes about seriously ill children within the general community. This may result in the child and his family becoming isolated from social, sporting, and leisure activities with peers. Such a reaction may increase the child's guilt about his illness and feelings of rejection. This can be especially difficult for adolescents, experiencing a stage of life when peer group acceptance is of primary concern (Moore, 1969; Kellerman and Katz, 1977).

Attitudes About Cancer

A major factor affecting the ability of the child with cancer to interact successfully and be accepted within his social environment has to do with general attitudes about cancer. Many misconceptions about cancer abound, such as the hopelessness of treatment and imminence of death. Another fallacy is that cancer is contagious and, therefore, an adult or child with cancer must be isolated (Travis, 1976). Mistaken attitudes about cancer are often formed by incomplete and distorted accounts of the disease and its treatment presented in the press, or the emphasis within the media upon dramatic cases rather than on long-term adaptation (Rimer, 1976; Mendelsohn, 1976).

An additional source of mistaken attitudes may be personal experience with cancer or cancer patients that predate modern treatment approaches and improved prognoses. Such incorrect and stereotypic perception may result in the unnecessary and unfair exclusion of children with cancer from normal peer interaction (Lubin, 1975).

Case Fifteen

Jane was diagnosed with acute lymphocytic leukemia when she was eight years of age, and had been in continual remission for eight months. She was becoming withdrawn and depressed as of late, refusing to leave her house for play or school. In interviewing Jane, the psychologist became aware of her fears concerning her peers. She had been taunted about her probable death and several children had told her how their mothers would not allow them to play with her, because they might "catch" her disease. She had also experienced comments from unfamiliar adults about her "strange" appearance.

Case Sixteen

Steve, fourteen years of age, was very concerned about the community's response to his diagnosis of acute lymphocytic leukemia. He felt as if people were looking at him all the time as if he were a "goner." He began to restrict his activity outside of the home, and an increase in physical complaints was also noted. He was particularly disturbed about pen marks on his face for cranial irradiation, and was anxious for that phase of therapy to end.

When Steve began to lose his hair, his immediate concern was for how students at his new school might react. He considered staying out of school until regrowth. Through psychological counseling, Steve was helped to realize that such an action would result in his falling behind academically and unnecessarily reduce his opportunity for social contact with positive experiences. He and his parents met with his teachers to explain his situation and enlist their cooperation to help Steve return to school and participate fully.

SCHOOL AND THE CHILD WITH CANCER

In order to promote optimal rehabilitation, several authors have advised that the pediatric cancer patient be encouraged to return to premorbid activities and environments as soon as is medically feasible (Karon, 1975; Wilbur, 1975; Spinetta et al., 1976; Kagan-Goodheart, 1977; Katz et al., 1977). One particularly important premorbid experience is school, the disruption of which has been related to major problems in postdiagnostic psychosocial adjustment (Moore et al., 1969; Futterman and Hoffman, 1970; Cyphert, 1973; Smith and Grobstein, 1974; Greene, 1975; Lansky et al., 1975; Spinetta et al., 1976; Katz et al., 1977).

Initial entrance into school represents a major milestone in the average child's life (Mussen et al., 1974). His socio-emotional environment is now expanded from the immediate family and related experiences to include teachers and peers. Occupying more than half of the child's waking hours for ten years or more of his life, school becomes a major focal system in the young person's environment as a primary social and educational experience (Stanford and Roark, 1974).

Schooling may be viewed as a primary agent for promoting psychological growth through the integration of cognitive and affective experiences (Zimiles, 1967). As such, it represents the continuation of normal life activities and acts as a bridge between a child's past and his future (Travis, 1976). Because school is a major social experience, it may be useful to utilize the return to school as a model for social reintegration in general.

For the child diagnosed with cancer, continuation of a social and academic program provides an important opportunity to be "normal" (Cyphert, 1973; Karon, 1975; Spinetta, et al., 1976; Travis, 1976; Katz et al., 1977). The child with cancer who is denied school participation is, in effect, being denied a major opportunity to engage in age-appropriate, goal-oriented behavior. Such interference with normal activity can lead to increased frustration (Bakwin and Bakwin, 1972), and reinforcement of hopelessness and despair, thereby obstructing the child's ability to cope with his illness and the rehabilitation process in general (Spinetta et al., 1976). Even for the child facing imminent death, school experience can be useful in providing a sense of emotional well-being (Oswin, 1974).

School Problems of Children With Cancer

The child with cancer whose disease is in remission or under control faces many hardships in his attempt to return to school and maintain normal school performance, even when no medical restrictions exist (Katz et al., 1977). He must spend a good deal of time at treatment centers and compensate for the long absences this can impose. Visible side effects of treatment, as well as the illness itself, are capable of eliciting negative social responses from peers and school personnel, thereby affecting the patient's self-concept and subsequent school and social participation (Kaplan, 1974; Greene, 1975; Katz et al., 1977; Koocher and Sallan, 1978). Inappropriate parental attitudes and behavior may further adversely effect the child's school and social adjustment (Futterman and Hoffman, 1970; Bakwin and Bakwin, 1972; Lansky et al., 1975).

In order to determine the incidence of school problems presented by children with cancer, Kellerman et al. (1979) reviewed a sample of pediatric cancer patients referred for psychological problems at Childrens Hospital of Los Angeles. Out of 101 newly and previously diagnosed children referred over one sixteen-month period, 17.8 percent had difficulty with continuation of their school program that required professional assistance. Another 14 percent of this group had learning disabilities for which assistance was sought. Results from this sample revealed, then, the presence of school-related problems in at least 30 percent of the children who develop psychological problems in response to their illness. School reintegration represented the most frequent challenge to social adjustment.

Specific types of school problems of children with cancer have been discussed by Katz et al. (1977), who noted *four general categories:*

1. The child exhibits school anxiety due to illness and/or treatment-induced physical side effects, i.e. hair loss, weight gain or loss, nausea and vomiting, surgical disfigurement.
2. The child, parents, and school require assistance in school reintegration after prolonged absence.
3. The child presents with illness-related learning disabilities requiring psychological evaluation and possible special school arrangements.
4. The newly diagnosed patient requiring preventative intervention and guidance regarding school reintegration.

The following factors need to be considered when evaluating such problems and devising treatment strategies:

Teacher Variables in School Reintegration

The teacher plays a crucial role in facilitating the ill child's emotional and socio-academic adjustment in school by influencing the tone of the classroom and helping peers understand physical changes, absences, and potential limitations (Greene, 1976; Paul et al., 1977). Several important factors can influence a teacher's ability to be effective in facilitating school reintegration, as follows:

ILLNESS ATTITUDES AND EMOTIONAL RESPONSE: The teacher's ability to tolerate a seriously ill child in a regular class will vary, as few teachers are provided adequate instruction in working with children who have serious medical problems (Greene, 1975). Myers (1975) and Kaplan et al. (1974) have pointed out how a teacher confronted by a seriously ill child may feel the need to avoid the child out of fear of depression about the child's condition. Avoidance of the child with cancer may be eased in that it can be in apparent compliance with school policy. Such policy may exclude the child from regular classes because of technicality, such as repeated absences, perhaps requiring a home teacher even when the child might benefit more from regular class experience. General policies of regular class exclusion are not usually in the child's best interest (Gearheart and Weishahn, 1976).

Teachers and school personnel may be unsure of what childhood cancer means in operational, realistic terms, as it relates to the child's ability to continue regular school participation (Kaplan et al., 1974; Greene, 1975). On numerous occasions, the author has discussed the diagnoses and treatment of childhood cancer with school teachers, administrators and school nurses, after securing the necessary permission from the child and his parents. The purpose of such direct contact is to provide information, answer questions, and help them understand the importance of regular school experience for the child. In addition, potential school problems can be dealt with preventively, thereby helping the teacher be better able to reintegrate the child. Teachers are very often at a loss as to how to make the child feel most comfortable, and may need support regarding classroom issues related to noticeable treatment side effects or the enforcement of discipline for a seriously ill child.

Contacts with school personnel are generally accomplished by phone, with follow-up as indicated. The personal contact afforded by a school visit has proven quite useful in facilitating an ongoing relationship between the hospital and the school.

Case Seventeen

Jerry, age four, was diagnosed with a non-Hodgkin's lymphoma Stage III, and was hospitalized in reverse isolation for two months. The importance of involving him in a normal, preschool experience was discussed with the parents and the child prior to and after discharge. Jerry's parents were somewhat reluctant to consider school return until they felt secure about the stability of his medical condition. When the child no longer showed any evidence of active disease, they were again encouraged to seek a school placement, as yet unarranged.

After several weeks, the mother reported that none of the several preschool directors she spoke to were willing to accept her child due to his cancer. The hospital-based school psychologist called one director to discuss this issue in further depth. The director *assumed* that the child's condition was contagious and did not want to endanger her other charges. When the actual nature of the child's illness, treatment, and current medical status were adequately explained, the director agreed whole-heartedly that Jerry needed the opportunity for normal peer interaction and that her facility and program would be made available.

When Jerry's mother met with the director for the purpose of enrolling Jerry in the program, the director cited Jerry in violation of certain school requirements. Chief among these was the need for each pupil to have received all childhood inoculations prior to beginning school. Jerry had not received all his shots due to his illness, and though his physician was willing to go on record that school posed an acceptable health risk, the director was not comfortable with these circumstances. Jerry's mother was eventually able to locate another preschool that would accommodate Jerry.

TEACHING THE CHILD WITH CANCER: Many teachers are unsure of how to teach a child with cancer. They may feel that the child's illness, treatment, and potential death make him subject to a high level of stress and may unnecessarily reduce their demands for regular school performance. The teacher's expectation of the child's reduced capacity for school work can lead to a self-fulfilling prophecy that may impede the child's motivation to try (Rothbart et al., 1971). By creating a dual set of standards, one for the child with cancer and another for the rest of his peers, the teacher may inadvertently enhance the child's sense of inadequacy (Katz et al., 1977). On the other hand, the teacher who may not be aware of the child's actual abilities in view of his illness and treatment, and does not allow for flexibility or variability in the academic program, may unfairly penalize the child for not keeping up with the rest of his class (Kaplan et al., 1974).

CLASSROOM INTERACTIONS: Teachers are often unclear as to whether and/or how to inform the class about the child's illness (Kaplan et al., 1974). The child may experience ridicule and isolation in the classroom due to his illness or physical side-effects, creating a management dilemma for the teacher. At the other extreme, a teacher may feel the class has become oversolicitous of the sick child to the point where it impedes his ability to progress normally.

By providing classmates with accurate information that focuses on helping them accept their ill peer and understand his needs and experiences, the teacher and the child can help prevent these problems from arising.

Case Eighteen

Louise was diagnosed with acute lymphocytic leukemia when she was thirteen years of age and in the eighth grade. She had been very active, academically, socially, and athletically, prior to her diagnosis. Louise was worried that her classmates would no longer accept her now that she had leukemia and that she might not be able to continue her high level of school involvement. Her teachers and principal were very understanding and assisted her in informing the class about her illness, its treatment, and how she would still be able to be active in school activities. Louise taught the class about leukemia during a science unit dealing with the human body. She was able to continue her school experience with a high level of support from her classmates. The teacher reported that Louise's illness provided him with an excellent opportunity to help his pupils learn about the need for accepting people who are different.

Case Nineteen

Jay suffered a relapse of his acute myelogenous leukemia when he was fourteen and in the ninth grade at a new school. When he lost his hair in the course of chemotherapy, he was subjected to acts of ridicule by a small group of students who followed him around the school yard. With the support of Jay's hospital psychologist, his school counselor was appraised of the situation and asked to intervene. The counselor called the students to a meeting in his office and explained that Jay was receiving medical care for a serious illness and helped them understand how their behavior was making Jay particularly uncomfortable. In addition, Jay was taught to respond directly to any taunts by explaining that he was receiving medical treatment and extinguishing their behavior by not responding further nor expressing any discomfort.

Jay encountered no further problems of this nature for the remainder of his school experience.

The classroom presentation of a child's illness should not be overly detailed, nor should the uncertainty of prognosis be dwelled upon. The emphasis should be on the child's day-to-day experience and how peers will need to tolerate some change in their classmate's appearance or routine. The author knows of several teachers who have found it useful to discuss a particular child's illness within the context of a more general classroom discussion related to physical differences and the need for tolerance.

Problems of ridicule often occur on the playground with children from other classes. The author has found it useful to have the classroom teacher communicate with other teachers as to how they can help modify their students' behavior. Generally, personal communication with the children involved in such activity by their teachers will help reduce such incidents.

Attendance Problems

Frequent absences are a significant school problem for the child with a serious illness (Steinhauer et al., 1974; Travis, 1976; Katz et al., 1977). Absences may occur most often during intensive phases of medical treatment, becoming less frequent as the child's condition stabilizes and/or improves. Absences may range in duration from half or whole days for outpatient medical appointments to extended periods during hospitalization or medical crises. Such disruptions can be a great nuisance for even the most understanding teacher who must continually reintegrate the child when he returns, both academically and socially, often requiring the implementation of an individualized curriculum (Cleveland and Berkowitz, 1975).

Rutter et al. (1970) noted how repeated short absences in chronically ill children can lead to discouragement and lowering of morale and confidence. By causing the child to be constantly behind his classmates and in need of remedial work, absences can alter the child's attitudes regarding school as well as his motivation to continue. Repeated absences may exacerbate preexisting school problems, further reducing the potential for positive school experience.

Alternative School Programs

In the past, children with physical and/or emotional problems were often placed in special classes where it was assumed their unique educational needs could best be met. The current trend regarding special education is to emphasize the mainstreaming approach (assisting handicapped children in their return to the regular classroom). This is accomplished through the provision of appropriate educational materials and consultative assistance to the regular class teacher (Gearheart and Weishahn, 1976). This approach is based on the finding that children who are educationally and socially segregated may have more difficulty fitting into society after being labeled as "deviant."

Healthy children are unable to develop appropriate attitudes about children who are different unless they have an opportunity to interact with them (Paul, Turnbell, and Cruickshank, 1977). Cyphert (1973) stressed the potential benefit that classmates of a child with cancer can gain. Such gains include vicarious learning about living with medical problems and understanding how people may differ externally while maintaining the same internal and emotional needs.

Children with malignancies may require the services of a special school program due to unique circumstances related to their illness (Kirten and Liverman, 1977). Children medically unable to attend school for an extended period due to medical complications often require a home teacher. Telephone classes are also available in many school districts and may enable the home-bound pupil to complete more academic work than is possible with a limited home teacher (generally available only one or two hours a week). These programs should be restricted to children absolutely unable to attend regular school, and one should be aware of the possibility that some children and their parents choose home teaching because of emotional factors (Lansky et al., 1975; Katz et al., 1977).

For children unable to tolerate a full school program, partial day programs can often be arranged that enable the child to receive many of the academic and social benefits of regular school attendance. At the same time, their physical limitations are accommodated, and they need not be over-extended. For a patient who has been out of school for an extended period, or who may be wary of attending regular school, beginning with a partial program that is gradually extended can ease the transition.

Because of illness-related learning disabilities, tutoring or assistance from a learning disabilities program may be helpful. On rare occasions a child may require placement in a self-contained class for physically or educationally handicapped children if he suffers a significant disability that cannot be managed within a regular class setting. Fortunately, even such children can usually be mainstreamed back into a regular classroom for at least part of the day where they may experience less isolation and stigma (Gearheart and Weishohn, 1976).

Intersystem Communication

To best meet the educational needs of the child with cancer, it is imperative that cooperation and communication exist between the major systems that effect the child, i.e. his home, school, and medical facility (Kirten and Liverman, 1977). Several authors note that the most general problems faced by school personnel have to do with their reception of adequate and accurate information regarding the child's illness and its management (Kaplan, 1974; Greene, 1975; Travis, 1976).

Depending on the nature of the parent's premorbid relationship to the teacher and the school, they may or may not inform the school of the child's diagnosis (Kaplan, 1974; Greene, 1975). This may be a particular problem for non-English speaking parents who have never fully communicated with the school due to language barriers. This is supported by an unpublished finding of Kellerman et al. (1979) that children with cancer from Spanish-speaking homes have more difficulty with school reintegration than do children from English-speaking families.

Many parents have expressed concern about giving the school true and accurate information, fearing that their child may be ostracized or mistreated (Greene, 1975). Without this information, however, the teacher may be unable to appropriately understand the child's needs and accommodate them effectively (Kaplan et al., 1974). What parents tell the school, however, may be based on their attitudes of what they think the school should know and may not, in fact, accurately reflect reality (Kaplan et al., 1974). For this reason, follow-up contact with the school by a qualified professional aware of school issues can be very helpful to the child and the school (Katz et al., 1977).

When teachers are not provided with adequate information about a child's condition, they may not know where to turn for assistance. It is reported that teachers frequently feel they receive very little support from others, i.e. school, medical, or support personnel, in handling serious medical problems in their students (Myers, 1975). The teacher may be reluctant to discuss the illness directly with the parents for fear of making them uncomfortable (Greene, 1975).

Pless and Pinkerton (1975) delineate the need for a professional, such as the school nurse, to help coordinate the flow of important and appropriate information between the hospital and school. Travis (1976) suggested the school social worker might be most helpful. Katz et al. (1977) discussed the utility of a hospital-based school psychologist who is familiar with both hospital and school systems, as well as with the home environment.

Problems in coordinating communication are more complex in

junior high and high school where the child has several teachers, none of whom may know him well. The need for coordination may be handled by the guidance counselor or school nurse, but careful follow-up is often needed to maintain continued cooperation between the various teachers.

Case Twenty

Robert was four years of age when he was diagnosed with a testicular sarcoma, Stage I. After undergoing surgery and chemotherapy, his condition was very good, and his prognosis for total cure was excellent.

Robert attended a preschool for two years during the course of his treatment. Every month, during his eight-day outpatient course of chemotherapy, Robert would return to school and vomit very frequently, becoming withdrawn and debilitated. His teachers never requested assistance with his behavior, assuming that he was dying of his cancer and that his behavior was no longer under his control. A behavioral analysis of Robert's school behavior during chemotherapy revealed that his symptoms were followed by a high level of teacher and peer reinforcement: he was able to do whatever he liked during those periods and was often held and rocked in the arms of one of the teachers.

When provided with accurate information as to Robert's condition, the teachers were able to modify their perception of him as dying. They understood that their focus of attention on his "sick" behavior may have led to its being reinforced. When they began to withdraw reinforcement of his "ill" behavior and reinforced alternative, regular classroom behavior, the frequency of his vomiting reduced dramatically. In addition, he became more out-going during chemotherapy treatments and was no longer as withdrawn and isolated.

SUMMARY AND CONCLUSION

Variables associated with a child's response to the diagnosis and treatment of cancer have been reviewed, along with selected case histories. It is recognized that comprehensive coverage of each issue raised has not been possible within this forum, nor is it assumed that only the factors mentioned are those which warrant further attention. The reader is encouraged to view the material presented in this chapter as a beginning comprehensive approach to the area and to more thoroughly investigate areas of particular interest.

Much progress in identifying stressful factors and the development of useful preventative and treatment approaches for children with cancer have been made. Yet, more research of a controlled, prospective nature is needed to help clarify predictive relationships. For example, social reintegration, i.e. continued school experience, is one critical variable that has been cited in the clinical literature as both an independent and dependent variable with regard to psychosocial adjustment. Though it would not be possible to randomize children for an experimental confirmation of the role school experience plays in adjustment, the comparison of outcomes in children matched for diagnosis, age, sex, and socioeconomic status that participate in school to varying degrees might help us to draw other than speculative conclusions.

The importance of regular assessment and intervention cannot be overemphasized in terms of clinical utility. Many stressful aspects of the illness and treatment are amenable to amelioration and prevention, and helping professionals should not withhold intervention until a crisis has occurred. Ongoing psychosocial follow-up and periodic reassessment is also vital because of the dynamic nature of pediatric cancer with the child's needs often changing with the passage of time.

Providing for the emotional needs of children with cancer is a demanding task but one that offers the opportunity for satisfaction and impact, through the visible reduction of psychological distress. Medical realities of the child's condition must not prevent constant attempts to maximize potential for satisfying, growth-engendering experiences. Through supportive care and involvement, health professionals can provide a model for significant people in the child's life to facilitate ongoing development. But even more importantly, such a model can do much to help the child maintain hope and encourage his struggle to live and grow in the face of potentially extreme stress.

REFERENCES

Adsett, C. A.: Emotional reactions to disfigurement from cancer therapy. *Can Med Assoc J* 89:385, 1963.

Bakwin, H. and Bakwin, R. M.: *Behavior Disorders in Children.* Philadelphia, W. B. Saunders, 1972.

Battle, C. U.: Chronic physical disease: Behavioral aspects. *Pediatr Clin North Am* 22:525, 1975.

Becker, R. D.: Therapeutic approaches to psychopathic reactions to hospitalization. *Int J Child Psychother* 1:65, 1972.

Burton, L.: *Care of the Child Facing Death.* London, Routledge & Kegan Paul, 1974.

Campbell, J. D.: Peer relations in childhood. Review of Child Development Research. New York, Russel Sage Foundation, 1:289, 1964.

Clapp, M. J.: Psychosocial reactions of children with cancer. *Nurs Clin North Am* 11:1, 73, 1976.

Cleveland, J. O. and Berkwitz, A. J.: Educational implications. In R. M. Peterson & J. O. Cleveland (Eds.): *Medical Problems in the Classroom: An Educators Guide.* Springfield, Thomas, p. 275, 1975.

Connor, F. P.: Education for the handicapped child. In J. A. Downey & N. L. Low (Eds.): *The Child with Disabling Illness.* Philadelphia, W. B. Saunders, 519, 1974.

Coopersmith, S.: *The Antecedents of Self Esteem.* San Francisco, Freeman, 1967.

Cyphert, F. R.: Back to school for the child with cancer. *J Sch Health,* 43:215, 1973.

Elkind, D.: *Children and Adolescents: Interpretive Essays of Jean Piaget.* New York, Oxford University Press, 1974.

Escalona, S.: Emotional development in the first year of life. In M. J. E. Senn (Ed.) *Problems of Injury and Childhood.* Josiah Mary Jr. Found. Conf., Transcript VI, 11, 1953.

Evans, A. E.: Practical care for the family of a child with cancer. *Cancer, 35:* March supplement, 871, 1975.

Ferguson, L. R.: *Personality Development.* Belmont, Brooks/Cole, 1970.

Freeman, R. D.: Emotional reactions of handicapped children. In S. Chess & A. Thomas (Eds.): *Annual Progress in Child Psychiatry and Child Development.* New York, Bruner Mazel, 379, 1968.

Futterman, E. H., and Hoffman, I.: Transient school phobia in a leukemic child. *J Am Acad Child Psychiatry, 9:*477, 1970.

Garrard, S. D. and Richmond, J. B.: The psychological aspects of the management of chronic disease and handicapping conditions in childhood. In H. I. Lief, V. F. Lief & N. R. Lief (Eds.) *Psychological Basis of Medical Practice.* New York, Hoeber, 370, 1963.

Gearheart, B. R., and Weishahn, M. W.: *The Handicapped Child in the Classroom.* Saint Louis, C. V. Mosby, 1976.

Goggin, E. L., Lansky, S. B. and Hassanein, K.: Psychological reactions of children with malignancies. *J Am Acad Child Psychiatry, 15:*314, 1976.

Golden, S.: Cancer chemotherapy and management of patient problems. *Nursing Forum, 14:*278, 1975.

Gotts, E. E.: A note on cross cultural by age-group comparisons of anxiety scores. *Child Development, 39:*945, 1968.

Grave, G. D., and Pless, I. V. (Eds.): *Chronic childhood illness: Assessment of outcome.* DHEW Publ. No. (NIH) 76-877, 1974.

Greene, P.: The child with leukemia in the classroom. *Am J Nurs, 75:*86, 1975.

Hartup, W. W.: Peer interactions and school organization. In P. H. Mussen (Ed.) *Carmichael's Manual of Child Psychology.* New York, John Wiley & Sons, 361, 1970.

Hefernan, N. and Azarnoff, P.: Factors in reducing children's anxiety about clinical visits. *HSMHA Health Reports 86:*1131, 1971.

Heffron, W. A., Bommelaere, K. and Masters, R.: Group discussions with the parents of leukemic children. *Pediatr, 52:*831, 1973.

Hoffman, A. D., and Becker, R. D.: Psychotherapeutic approaches to the physically ill adolescent. *Int J Child Psychother 2:*492, 1973.

Hughes, W. T.: Early side effects in treatment of childhood cancer. *Pediatr Clin North Am, 23:*1, 1976.

Jaffee, N.: Malignant bone tumors. *Pediatr Ann 4:*10, 1975.

Jaffee, N.: Late side effects of treatment: skeletal, genetic, central nervous system and oncogenic. *Pediatr Clin North Am, 23:*1, 1976.

Kagen-Goodheart, L.: Reentry: Living with childhood cancer. *Am J Orthopsychiatry 47:*651, 1977.

Kaplan, D. M., Smith, A. and Grobstein, R.: School management of the seriously ill child. *J. of School Health, 44:*250, 1974.

Karon, M.: Acute leukemia in childhood. In H. F. Conn (Ed.) *Current Therapy, 1975.* Philadelphia, W. B. Saunders, 274, 1975.

Katz, E. R., Kellerman, J., Rigler, D., Williams, K., and Siegel, S. E.: School intervention with pediatric cancer patients. *J Pediatr Psychology 2:*72, 1977.

Katz, E. R., Kellerman, J., and Siegel, S. E.: Distress behavior in children with leukemia undergoing medical procedures: developmental considerations. *J Consult Clin Psychol,* in press.

Katz, E. R., Kellerman, J., and Siegel, S. E.: The relationship between objective and subjective measures of distress in children with leukemia undergoing medical prodecures. In preparation.

Kellerman, J.: Behavioral treatment of night terrors in a child with acute leukemia. *J Nerv Ment Dis.* 167, 182-185, 1979.

Kellerman, J. and Katz, E. R.: The adolescent with cancer: theoretical clinical and research issues. *J Pediatr Psychology 2:*127, 1977.

Kellerman, J., and Katz, E. R.: Attitudes toward the division of child rearing responsibility. *Sex Roles 4:*505, 1978.

Kellerman, J., Katz, E. R. and Siegel, S. E.: Psychological problems of children with cancer. Submitted for publication. 1979.

44   *Psychological Aspects of Childhood Cancer*

Kirten, D. and Liverman, M.: Special educational needs of the child with cancer. *J Sch Health 47:*170, 1977.

Koch, C. R., Hermann, J. and Donaldson, M. H.: Supportive care of the child with cancer and his family. *Semin Oncol 1:*81, 1974.

Koocher, G. R. and Sallan, S. E.: Pediatric oncology. In P. T. Magrab (Ed.) *Psychological Management of Pediatric Problems.* Vol. I. Baltimore, University Park Press, 283, 1978.

Korsch, B. M., Frood, L. E. and Barnett, H. L.: Pediatric discussions with parent groups. *J Pediatr. 14:*171, 1954.

Kubler-Ross, E.: *On Death and Dying.* N.Y., Macmillian Co. 1969.

Lansky, S. B., Lowman, J. T., Vats, T. and Gyulay, J.: School phobias in children with malignant neoplasms. *Am J Dis Child 129:*42, 1975.

Lansky, S. B., Cairns, N. U., Hassanein, R., Wehr, J. and Lowman, J. T.: Childhood cancer: parental discord and divorce. *Pediatrics 62:*184, 1978.

Lazarono, R. S.: *Psychological Stress and the Coping Process.* New York, McGraw-Hill, 1966.

Lindsay, J. and MacCarthy, D.: Caring for the brothers and sisters of a dying child. In L. Burton (Ed.) *Care of the Child Facing Death.* London, Routledge and Kegan Paul, 189, 1974.

Lowit, Z.: Social and psychological consequences of chronic illness in children. *Developmental Medicine and Child Neurology 15:*75, 1973.

Lubin, G. I.: Emotional implications. In R. M. Peterson and J. O. Cleveland (Eds.) *Medical Problems in the Classroom: An Educator's Guide.* Springfield, Thomas, 267, 1975.

Maccoby, E. E., and Jacklin, C. N.: *The Psychology of Sex Differences.* Palo Alto, Ca., Stanford U Pr, 1974.

Maddison, D. and Raphael, B.: Social and psychological consequences of chronic disease in childhood. *Med J Aust 2:*1265, 1971.

Magrab, P. R. (Ed.): *Psychological Management of Pediatric Problems.* Baltimore, University Park Press, 1978.

Magrab, P. R. and Calcagno, P. L.: Psychological impact of chronic pediatric conditions. In P. R. Magrab (Ed.) *Psychological Management of Pediatric Problems.* Vol. I. Baltimore, University Park Press, 3, 1978.

Mattson, A.: Long-term physical illness in childhood: a challenge to psychosocial adaptations. *Pediatrics 50:*801, 1972.

Meissner, A. L., Thoreson, R. W. and Butler, A. J.: Relation of self concept to impact and obviousness of disability among male and female adolescents. *Perceptual Motor Skills. 24:*1099, 1967.

Mendelsohn, H.: Mass communications and cancer control. In J. W. Cullen, B. H. Fox & R. N. Isom (Eds.) *Cancer: the Behavioral Dimensions.* N.Y., Raven Press. 197, 1976.

Moore, D. L., Holton, C. P. and Marten, Q. W.: Psychologic problems in the management of adolescents with malignancy. *Clin Pediatr 8:*464, 1969.

Mozden, P. J.: Neoplasms. In J. S. Myers (Ed.) *An Orientation to Chronic Disease and Disability.* N.Y., Macmillan, 323, 1965.

Mussen, P. H., Conger, J. J. and Kagan, J.: *Child Development and Personality.* Fourth Ed. N.Y., Harper & Row, 1974.

Myers, B. R.: The child with a chronic illness. In R. H. Halsam & P. J. Valletutti (Eds.) *Medical Problems in the Classroom: The Teachers Role in Diagnosis and Management.* Maryland, University Pard Press. 97, 1975.

Oakley, G. P., and Patterson, R. B.: The psychological management of leukemic children and their families. *N C Med J 27:*186, 1968.

Oswin, M.: The role of education in helping the child with a potentially fatal disease. In L. Burton (Ed.) *Care of the Child Facing Death.* London, Routledge and Kegan Paul, 101, 1974.

Paul, J. L., Turnbull, A. P., and Cruickshank, W. M.: *Mainstreaming: A Practical Guide.* Syracuse University Press, 1977.

Phillips, B. N., Hindsman, E. and Jennings, E.: Influence of intelligence on anxiety and perception of self and others. *Child Development. 31:*41, 1960.

Pinkel, D.: Curability of childhood cancer. *JAMA, 235:*1049, 1976.

Pless, I. B. and Pinkerton, P.: *Chronic Childhood Disorder: Promoting Patterns of Adjustment.* Chicago, Henry Kimpton, 1975.

Pless, I. B., and Roghmann, K. J.: Chronic illness and its consequences: observations based on three epidemiologic surveys. *J Pediatrics 79:*351, 1971.

Richmond, J. B. and Waisman, H. A.: Psychologic aspects of management of children with malignant diseases. *Am J Dis Child, 89:*42, 1955.

Rimer, I.: The impact of mass media on cancer control programs. In J. W. Cullen, B. H. Fox & R. N. Isom (Eds.) *Cancer: The Behavioral Dimensions.* N.Y., Raven Press, 179, 1976.

Robinson, D.: Mothers fear their children's well-being in hospital, and the study of illness behavior. *Br J Soc Med 22:*228, 1968.

Rothbart, M., Dalfen, S. S. and Barnett, R.: Effects of a teacher's expectancy on student-teacher interaction. *J Educ Psychol 62:*49, 1971.

Ruebush, B. K.: Children's behavior as a function of anxiety and defensiveness. Unpublished doctoral dissertation, Yale Univ., 1960.

Rusk, H.: *Rehabilitation Medicine.* St. Louis, C. V. Mosby, 1977.

Rutter, M. and Graham, P.: Psychiatric aspects of intellectual and educational retardation. In J. Tizard & K. Whitmore, *Education, Health and Behavior.* London, Longman, 1970.

Spinetta, J. J., Rigler, D., and Karon, M.: Anxiety in the dying child. *Pediatr, 52:*841, 1973.

Spinetta, J. J., Spinetta, P. D., Kung, F. and Schwartz, D. B.: Emotional aspects of childhood cancer and leukemia: a handbook for parents. Leukemia Society of America, San Diego Chapter, 1976.

Stanford, G. and Roark, A. E.: *Human Interaction in Education.* Boston, Allyn and Bacon, 1974.

Steinhauer, P. D., Mushin, D. N. and Rae-Grant, A.: Psychological aspects of chronic illness. *Pediatr Clin North Am 21:*825, 1974.

Stubblefield, R. L.: Psychiatric complications of chronic illness in children. In J. A. Downey & N. L. Low (Eds.) *The Child With Disabling Illness.* Philadelphia. W. B. Saunders, 509, 1974.

Sutow, W. W., Vietti, T. J., & Fernbach, D. J.: *Clinical Pediatric Oncology, 2nd Ed.* Saint Louis, C. V. Mosby, 1977.

Tavormina, J. B., Kastner, L. S., Slater, P. M. and Watt, S. L.: Chronically ill children: a psychologically and emotionally deviant population? *J Abnorm Child Psychol. 4:*99, 1976.

Travis, G.: *Chronic Illness in Children.* Stanford University Press, 1976.

Van Eys, J.: Supportive care for the child with cancer. *Pediatr Clin North Am, 23:*215, 1976.

Vernon, D. T. A., Foley, J. M., Sipowicz, R. R., and Shulman, J. L.: *Psychological Responses of Children to Hospitalization and Illness.* Springfield, Thomas, 1965.

Weinberg, S.: Seminars in nursing, care of the adolescent. *Nursing Outlook. 16:*18, 1968.

Weinberg, S.: Suicidal intent in adolescence: a hypothesis about the role of physical illness. *J Pediatrics 77:* 579, 1970.

Weiner, I.: *Psychological Disturbance in Adolescence.* Interscience Series. N.Y., John Wiley, 1970.

Weiss, H. D., Walker, M. D., and Wiernik, P. H.: Neurotoxicity of commonly used antineoplastic agents. *N Engl J Med 291:*75, 1974.

Wilbur, J. R.: Rehabilitation of children with cancer. *Cancer. 36:*809, 1975.

Wolfish, M. G. and McLean, J.: Chronic illness in adolescents. *Pediatr Clin North Am, 21:*1043, 1974.

Zeltzer, L., Kellerman, J., Ellenberg, L., Dash, J., and Rigler, D.: Objective identification of illness impact and self concept in adolescents with cancer and other chronic disease: implications for health delivery. Paper presented at the Southern Society for Pediatric Research, January 1979.

Zimiles, H.: Preventive aspects of school experience. In E. L. Cowen, E. A. Gardiner & M. Zax (Eds.) *Emergent Approaches to Mental Health Problems.* New York, Appleton-Century-Crofts, 239, 1967.

Chapter Three

SIBLINGS OF THE PEDIATRIC CANCER PATIENT

BARBARA M. SOURKES

I feel so selfish. I always used to yell at Cindy that I wanted my own room. And now I have it — two twin beds — and I'm so lonely . . .

EMBEDDED IN THESE WORDS is a complex of feelings about the sibling experience of living with a child with cancer, and the aftermath of loss. Despite the growing plethora of literature on the child with a life-threatening illness, and the effect on the family, there has been little specific focus on well siblings. In the literature brothers and sisters stand outside the spotlight, although they live through the illness experience with the same intensity as the patient and parents. Part of the reason for their neglect has been that the clinical literature does not originate from a systems view of the family. Most articles focus on the patient, or, at most, on the ill child-parent dyad. Tangential mention is made of the effect on the siblings. However, within a family-systems view, stress in any one part of the family is seen as affecting all other members. When dealing with a child with a life-threatening illness, "the patient is the family." Full attention to the siblings is then a natural consequence.

This chapter examines the experience of siblings of the pediatric cancer patient, both in living with the illness and in bereavement. The focus is on the issues which the siblings face, and the adaptive means they mobilize to negotiate this unique life stress. Illustrations from psychotherapeutic work with siblings indicate the direction for future inquiry and intervention.

REVIEW OF THE LITERATURE

The clinical literature on siblings of the pediatric cancer patient may be classified into three categories. One set of articles presents observations on families, with a section devoted to sibling behavior patterns and symptoms. Retrospective studies on sibling problems, based upon parental report, psychiatric records, and sibling interviews, comprise the second category. The third group of articles comprises accounts of individual psychotherapy with a sibling of a patient.

Observations of Siblings Within the Family

The focus of these articles is on the reactions and symptoms manifested by the well siblings, with some recommendations for management. Most of the data are based upon parental report.

A chapter devoted to siblings of the dying child by Lindsay and MacCarthy (1974) presents issues within a developmental framework. The authors stated that the sibling who is an infant at the time another child is ill is at the highest risk. At a critically formative time, the mother, because of her preoccupation with the patient, may be unable to adapt to and be aware of the infant's cues. The toddler, too young for comprehensive verbal explanation, may see the parental preoccupation as a rejection. The child then may feel badly about himself or herself and regress in development. The child who is older and verbal may feel a complex of resentment, anger and guilt in addition to the rejection, and must learn to cope with the elevated level of anxiety in the family. This child may act out as a defense against depression, or withdraw into daydreams and anxious thoughts. In turn, school performance can be adversely affected. Psychosomatic symptoms often set in: the child sees the illness as a means of getting attention; yet is simultaneously frightened of being ill like the patient. The sibling may show a preferred stress reaction, such as an exaggeration of asthma. Feelings of preoccupation and low self-worth may lead to increased accident proneness. School phobia, the endpoint of a continuum of disturbance, represents the child's cumulative anxiety about separation from mother, about illness, and the fear of the power of the unacceptable anger toward the patient and the parent. The older child may take over care of the patient in a form of identification with parents. Lindsay and MacCarthy point out that this caregiving may be a reaction formation, a costly defense against acknowledging intense resentment.

If the sibling is older than the patient, then rivalries from the time of the sick child's birth may be reactivated. Wiener (1970) also states that competition and rivalry are a developmental aspect of the relationship between a school-aged and a younger child, and may be exacerbated by the stress of illness. If the sibling is younger than the patient, increased envy may arise around the patient's privileges and accomplishments.

Lindsay and MacCarthy point out the ebb and flow nature of the parents' preoccupation with the sick child. Its intensity is highest at the time of diagnosis and during exacerbation or relapse of the illness. The parents' loss of confidence in their parenting skills once they have an ill child may generalize to feeling inadequate with the siblings as well.

At the time of the patient's death, the siblings may quickly seek a substitute. They may find a new friend, imagine a fantasied relationship, or ask the parents for a new baby in the family.

Lindsay and MacCarthy suggest ways to help the well siblings. These children should get information directly from the doctors or their parents, in order to minimize their misconceptions about the illness. Their visits should be encouraged, and they can be included in ward play activities. Parents need help in clarifying priorities in the needs of the patient and the siblings.

Wiener (1970) lists the factors which influence the reaction of siblings to the fatal illness of a child. Included are sibling age and maturity, ability to integrate the meaning of the illness, relationship to the patient, place and adjustment in the family, honesty of communication, and how the sibling is involved in the family adaptation to crisis. Wiener stresses that guilt will lead to depressive symptoms, nightmares, and reactive aggression. By the staff's expressed interest in the siblings, the parents will be encouraged to focus on the needs of these children. The siblings' attendance at the funeral provides an important concrete experience to counterbalance their fantasies about death.

Share (1972) discusses the meaning of the illness to the well siblings. She stresses that siblings lose customary attention, both by the parents' physical absence, as well as by the emotional realignments which occur within the family. Valued family routines and activities are changed. The siblings are angry at the parents and competitive toward the ill child. Most of the anger toward the patient will surface while the child is in remission. The siblings may then be overcome by guilt and fear during the patient's hospitalization. Hendin (1973) also discusses the guilt and resentment and makes a unique point: children may be ashamed of having their family be "different" due to having a dying member.

Koch, Hermann, and Donaldson (1974) describe sibling issues in terms of stages of the patient's illness. At the time of diagnosis, the parents must explicitly state that nothing anyone did, said, or thought was responsible for the disease. During the patient's remission, siblings' visits to the clinic help dispel any mystique. During the terminal phase, the siblings may visit on a voluntary basis when the patient is free from pain or asleep. The parents should be present at these times.

Spinetta, Spinetta, Kung, and Schwartz (1976), in their handbook for parents, stress that siblings should be reassured that the disease was not of their doing, nor is it contagious. Parents can anticipate the children's anger for their "allowing" this to happen, and must be ready to answer questions throughout the disease process.

Kagen-Goodheart (1977) focuses on the problems of living with childhood cancer. When the patient comes home from the hospital, the siblings are confronted with an extremely difficult transition: they expect all to be as before; and yet, it is not. The siblings must be prepared for the fact that the patient will require extra attention even at home. However, the siblings can be reassured that they would get the same attention were they sick and that their cooperation is appreciated. Siblings need the opportunity to discuss their jealousy and anger privately with the parents. It is important to reiterate to the siblings that bad behavior cannot cause illness. Kagen-Goodheart makes a critical point not mentioned in most articles: the patient may express anger toward the siblings for being well. Thus, the resentment is bidirectional.

Townes and Wold (1977) studied the impact of the degree of parental communication about the patient's diagnosis and prognosis on the healthy siblings. Twenty-two siblings of eight leukemic patients were included. Three siblings were under four years of age; eleven were between five and eight years; and eight were nine years or older. Six of the eight patients were preschoolers. The siblings were tested, and parents were interviewed at ten, twenty, and thirty-two months post diagnosis. On a Communication Questionnaire, the parents rated each sibling's awareness that the child with leukemia was ill, had leukemia, and might die. The parents further indicated how much the sibling had been told, had actively questioned, and how much they thought the sibling knew about the patient's disease. They filled out a quantitative Symptom Checklist of the sibling's academic and social functioning. On the Silhouette Test, the siblings estimated the adequacy of their own health and that of the patient, and their expectations for their own longevity and that of the patient.

The overall finding was that the sibling's evaluation of the patient's disease as life-threatening was related to increased parental communication about the implication of the disease and the experience of living with the illness in the family. At ten months, the oldest group of siblings had received the most communication, and understood best the seriousness and short lifespan implication of the illness. The youngest group had received the least information, thought the patient was not very sick, and would live for a long time. By a year later, all the siblings saw the patient as very sick, and as having an abbreviated lifespan. By thirty-two months, five of the eight patients had died, and all the siblings understood the diagnosis and prognosis.

Early in the illness, poor adjustment was associated with little communication from the mother about the nature of the disease, regardless of sex. Following the death of the patient, poor adjustment was associated with age and sex: boys and older children had more problems.

Retrospective Studies

Binger, Ablin, Feuerstein, Kushner, Zoger and Mikkelsen (1969) and Binger (1973) conducted a retrospective study of the impact on families of losing a child from leukemia. Of twenty-three families contacted, twenty agreed to participate in parent interviews. In about half the families, one or more previously well-adjusted siblings had shown evidence of difficulty during the patient's illness. The symptoms included enuresis, headaches, abdominal pain, school problems, depression, and separation anxiety. These symptoms increased in severity after the child's death. Feelings of rejection, guilt, and fear were common. The siblings' reactions to illness and death were multidetermined. Stage of development, family response of adaptation or conflict around the illness and the natural history of the illness were all important factors. After the patient died, the siblings' concerns centered on their responsibility for the death, the fear of being next to die and resentment toward the parents for their preoccupation and inability to protect the child. The children showed a variety of manifest reactions to the patient's death. Some were verbal, while others expressed themselves through play. Certain siblings who appeared unconcerned at the time of the death then overreacted to a subsequent loss. In conclusion, Binger (1973) points out that the reactions included "immediate physical and psychological symptom associated with grief, but in a number of children, [these] continue toward enduring symptoms with distortion in character structure" (p. 196). These children may become adults at risk for emotional disturbance, with a particular disposition to depression.

Gogan, Koocher, Foster, and O'Malley (1977) assessed the impact on the healthy siblings of living with childhood cancer. They interviewed thirteen siblings between the ages of eight and twenty-eight, with a median age of seventeen. All were born previous to the patient's diagnosis, which had to have occurred at least five years previously. Their median age at the time of the patient's diagnosis was four years. The average span between the time of the interview and the diagnosis was thirteen years. It is critical to note that all the patients were alive and part of a long-term survivor group.

The investigators found that the siblings' understanding of the patient's potential fatality increased as a function of present age and age at diagnosis. Most siblings minimized the impact of the illness at the time it had occurred ("Seven-year-olds don't have feelings about those things"). None claimed to remember feeling abandoned. Some rivalry was described, although little guilt was expressed. Most siblings said that the patient had changed as a result of the illness (for example, more nervous, more dependent); but they denied any change in themselves. That the patients were all long-term survivors may have permitted the siblings a more comfortable, less stressful retrospection than in studies where the patients had died.

Cain, Fast, and Erickson (1964) reviewed children's disturbed reactions to the death of a sibling. They gathered clinical data from fifty-eight psychiatric inpatient and outpatient files (developmental history, psychological testing, interviews, therapy process notes). At the time of treatment, the children were between two and fourteen years of age. The majority, if not all, of their symptoms had been attributed to the death of a sibling.

At least half the children expressed much guilt, even five years after the sibling's death. They felt responsible for the death, and asserted that they should have died instead or also. Their deterioration in school performance was further proof of their low self-worth. Some parents had blamed the children for not mourning appropriately.

Many children held distorted concepts of illness and death. Those who had been told that death comes with old age felt betrayed. Some children regressed in order to escape the equation that "getting older means that you will die." Others rationalized that they could not die at least until the age of their sibling's death. The children feared minor physical symptoms and perceived doctors as impotent in the face of illness and death.

Most of the children manifested a death phobia. Some maintained a transparent defensiveness of "I can't die." Many identified with the dead child to the extent that they predicted their own death at the same age, of the same cause and circumstance. The children's views of their parents as omnipotent protectors were devastated.

Almost half the children showed immediate, prolonged, or hysterical anniversary identification with the dead child's prominent symptoms. Twenty percent had been "misidentified" by the parents: their name had been changed to that of the dead child, or resemblances between them were constantly stressed. The parents often made negative comparisons between the child and the hyperidealized dead sibling, especially with regard to school performance.

Cognitive functioning was adversely affected in many children. Some showed a general "not knowing." Others manifested specific disability around time, causality, knowledge of their own age, and confusion of the concepts of young and old.

With the change in family structure, role realignments had to be made. For many of these children, the major impact was the unavailability of the parents during hospitalizations and then during the mourning period.

The children's reactions to the death of a sibling covered the range of areas of affect, cognition, belief systems, superego functioning, and object relationships. Problems were on intrapsychic, family, peer, neighborhood, school, and community levels. The determinants of the children's reactions included: nature of the death; age and character of the child who died; living child's involvement in the death; relationship to the dead child; immediate impact of the death on the parents; effect on the family structure; availability of support; concurrent family stress; and developmental level of the well child. The authors state: "The effects upon the child obviously are not static, undergoing constant developmental transformation and evaluation" (p. 750).

Accounts of Individual Psychotherapy with a Sibling

Feinberg (1970) described the preventive psychotherapy done with two sisters of a six-year-old leukemic boy during his illness and after his death. Feinberg's therapeutic approach provides a conceptual framework for intervention.

The first goal is the establishment of a therapeutic alliance of forthrightness with the child. The therapist must be ready to tell the truth, and the child is not allowed to maintain a stance of ignorance regarding the reason for being in therapy. Feinberg stresses the importance of eliciting the child's understanding of the patient's illness at an early point in therapy.

Feinberg then initiates "immunizing discussions" about loss, often in displaced fashion from the patient. Allowance for catharsis without severe regression is the next therapeutic goal. The therapist must serve as a substitute for the temporarily absent parents. A reality orientation concerning the facts of the illness is maintained at all times.

The mourning process itself is initiated in therapy, using issues of separation and loss in the transference. Feinberg feels that this form of rehearsal will help the child maintain sadness or anger during actual mourning, and prevent untoward disturbance at a later time.

Rosenblatt (1969) presents the case of a child whose sister died of asthma. The boy had turned to rigid religious beliefs to cope with his feelings. Based upon his own work, the findings of Cain, Fast and Erickson (1964), and the general body of psychiatric literature, Rosenblatt's impression is that "no grounds for optimism about large scale prevention of psychopathology" (p. 335) exist when children have lived through the death of a sibling.

Willis (1974) recommends short-term play therapy for siblings to explore their feelings and fantasies about the patient's illness. By using a controlled focus, the hospitalization and subsequent events can be worked through in dramatized play, and distorted ideas can be re-mediated.

EVALUATION OF THE LITERATURE

The literature on siblings of pediatric cancer patients is at an early stage of conceptualization and methodology. An evaluation of the existing studies can provide direction for future inquiry.

Most of the literature has focused on "the sibling of the dying child" rather than on "the sibling of the child with a life-threatening illness." The distinction reflects medical reality of many types of malignancy: what was once an acutely fatal illness now has the character of a serious chronic disease. Whereas attention has centered on the siblings' reaction to loss, it is now necessary to study their experience of living with the ill child over a prolonged period. Although the threat of separation and death is still omnipresent, it is no longer the overriding focus.

The literature has stressed psychopathology and disturbance in siblings, rather than adaptation. A psychiatric approach highlights the extremes of sibling problems, but gives little sense of the continuum of coping. Ongoing parental reports may be biased in perceiving siblings as "problems" in contrast to the idealized patient. Furthermore, the parents' tolerance threshold will be lower under stress, and thus "symptomatic" behavior on the part of siblings will be acutely salient. Retrospective studies have a built-in time distortion. When parents come in for a psychiatric follow-up interview after the patient's death, there is an implicit or explicit definition of the session as problem-oriented. Thus, they may present family difficulties to the exclusion of the functional coping which has occurred.

Much attention has been devoted to the impact of "telling versus not telling" the diagnosis and prognosis of the illness to the siblings. As the nature of the disease has changed, so too has the manner of communicating information. Less at issue now is "to tell or not to tell." More central is the question: What is the impact on the siblings of living with the knowledge and experience of the patient's life-threatening illness?

The existing literature deals mostly with siblings of leukemia patients. In some articles, the patient's precise diagnosis is not given at all. It is critically important that the various childhood malignancies be surveyed for any differential impact on the siblings.

The methodological limitations in the literature on siblings are similar to those in many fields of clinical inquiry. Larger samples with wider age span and tighter controls are needed. Interviews and observations of the siblings at the time of the patient's illness are critical. Objective measures such as psychological testing, school reports and behavioral checklists should be used in assessment. Any structured technique which specifically evaluates the siblings' reactions to the illness experience must not be threatening in its directness.

The siblings of pediatric cancer patients are a vital concern for intervention and research. Their ongoing experience of living with and adapting to a child with a life-threatening illness can be examined within the framework of the family system.

LIVING WITH CHILDHOOD CANCER

What are the normal and expected concerns of siblings of the pediatric cancer patient? The literature is replete with examples of sibling reactions which have been described as "disturbed" or as "symptoms." However it seems likely that many of these reactions, although disruptive on emergence, may in fact represent an adaptation process to a unique life stress. Many questions and concerns are ubiquitous among a sibling group, although the mode of expression may depend upon the developmental stage, both cognitive and emotional, of the child. The issues raised by the siblings do not begin and end at specific points in the illness of the patient. Rather, in an ebb and flow fashion, certain issues will recede or resurge in importance at different times. As has been pointed out in the literature, reactions are often intensified during periods of diagnosis, exacerbation and relapse of the illness. In the same way that normal stages and reactions are acknowledged in the patient's adaptation, so the siblings' experience must be seen from a "normalized" perspective.

In the following section, themes which have emerged from the author's psychotherapeutic work with pediatric cancer patients and their siblings will be described. The children's own statements and drawings illustrate their concerns most aptly. The intervention strategies can be a means for facilitating communication with siblings, either by a therapist, or by parents and other caregivers. The thematic categories are neither mutually exclusive, nor are they necessarily an exhaustive list. However, they can provide a foundation for further exploration.

Causation of the Illness

Siblings often hold two views about how the patient's illness was caused. One view stems from the medical information which they have heard from their parents and the doctors. The other is their own "private" version, often unarticulated, but to which they cling with tenacity. Their private cause is often fraught with emotional and cognitive confusion. From a cognitive point of view, causality is a difficult concept for young children to grasp. They often construe simultaneity, or unrelated sequence of events, as comprising a cause-effect relationship. Combined with intense emotional factors of fear or guilt, the siblings' thinking often contains magical links as their way to make sense of something overwhelming and incomprehensible. Children, as adults, will supply a cause to fill in the gaps when knowledge is lacking or not fully grasped. Their view of the cause often becomes an undergirding theme in their experience of the patient's illness.

Following are siblings' responses to the question: "What do you think caused your brother's/sister's illness? What made him/her sick?"

> She fell off the slide and broke her arm.
> (Cliff, six; brother of Susan, thirteen, osteogenic sarcoma)

> He got sick because I had a sore throat and he caught it.
> (five-year-old sister of twelve-year-old leukemic patient)

> He had a temperature. He's sick. He's not better yet. He's almost better.
> (Ken, four; brother of Brad, two, leukemia)

> She hurt her leg on the chain of her bike. She didn't even notice it until I pointed it out to her. I don't even ride my bike anymore. One night I went out and broke the chain so I couldn't ride it. I told my mother it broke by itself, but I broke it.
> (Bobby, ten; brother of Cindy, fourteen, osteogenic sarcoma)

> I think maybe it was God's way of telling our family to pull together. There had been a lot of dissension among us, and maybe this was a way to bring us together.
> (Irene, seventeen; sister of Debbie, fifteen, osteogenic sarcoma)

In each of these examples, the siblings have supplied a reason which is either coexistent with or instead of a medical view. The self-references in their explanations are of crucial importance.

The critical intervention is to obtain the sibling's version of the cause of the disease. The sooner this view is obtained, the more quickly misconceptions can be clarified. Most children will be pleased — and relieved — to share their reasoning. It will be important to reiterate the medical view many times during the illness, and to be vigilant for the reemergence of any guilt associated with the child's initial reasoning.

With young children who have cognitive difficulty with causality, basic help with that concept in general may help them to understand the illness situation in specific. In everyday situations, a child can be shown that simultaneity or sequence does not necessarily imply cause. They may then better understand the relative randomness of the patient's illness within a complex of other occurrences.

If the sibling is restricting himself or herself from an activity out of fear (e.g. Bobby's bicycle riding), clarifying explanations or a desensitization approach may facilitate its resumption.

Visibility of the Illness and the Treatment Process

I did a lot of growing up in the moment that Karen first took off her scarf when she came home from the hospital.

(Elaine, sixteen; sister of Karen, thirteen, leukemia)

An issue not mentioned in the literature, but which emerged repeatedly in discussions with the siblings, is the effect of the visibility or the invisibility of the disease. This factor plays a particularly important role in the initial period after diagnosis. An illness which leads to a dramatic physical change such as an amputation provides a visible focus for explanation. Yet, the siblings may grapple with whether the patient is still the same person, despite the altered appearance. Young siblings may be puzzled by the invisibility of a disease like leukemia and supply their own real and imagined symptoms. Loss of hair and weight become visual cues in most illnesses; however, the effect is less enduring than that of an amputation.

The visibility or invisibility of the treatment process is a related issue. Siblings may perceive the hospital and clinic as threatening places. Or, they may envy "outings" to the clinic, resenting the patient's chance for time with the parents, and for missing school. They may not understand that although "treatment" is a word with positive valence, the procedures, in actuality, can be dreadful and painful. In the absence of experience, an integrated understanding is difficult for the siblings to achieve.

The following examples illustrate the interweaving of the visibility/invisibility of the disease with the treatment process. In the first vignette, a child tries to "make visible" what is invisible and mysterious.

Ken drew a picture of Brad, saying: "This is Brad with broken legs and a broken mouth. He has a broken dead face and a booboo mouth. What happens if Brad is dead? Like he got run over when a car comes?" Once Ken had seen Brad in the hospital, he reported: "I saw Brad. He was crying. He was bald. I saw him when he had hair."

(Ken, four; brother of Brad, two, leukemia)

The following statements illustrate the impact of amputation, of visible illness.

I didn't think about Cindy's illness too much until I heard that she would need an amputation. *Then* . . .

(Joanne, seventeen; sister of Cindy, fourteen, osteogenic sarcoma)

I just wanted her to have that tumor out of her body. After the amputation I felt relieved. But now, every time she goes into the hospital for her chemotherapy, it brings the cancer right back in your face . . . "

(Irene, seventeen; sister of Debbie, fifteen, osteogenic sarcoma)

Bobby wrote the following story: "This is my sister (drew a one-legged stick figure) and this is me (drew a two-legged figure). There is a difference. But I still think that this is the same Cindy, and I know that she is not the same to you, and I think that she is beautiful." He then drew a picture of Cindy, stressing her very short hair, and her stump (see Figure 3-1). He expressed much concern about how her stump would look.

(Bobby, ten; brother of Cindy, fourteen, osteogenic sarcoma)

THIS IS CINDY

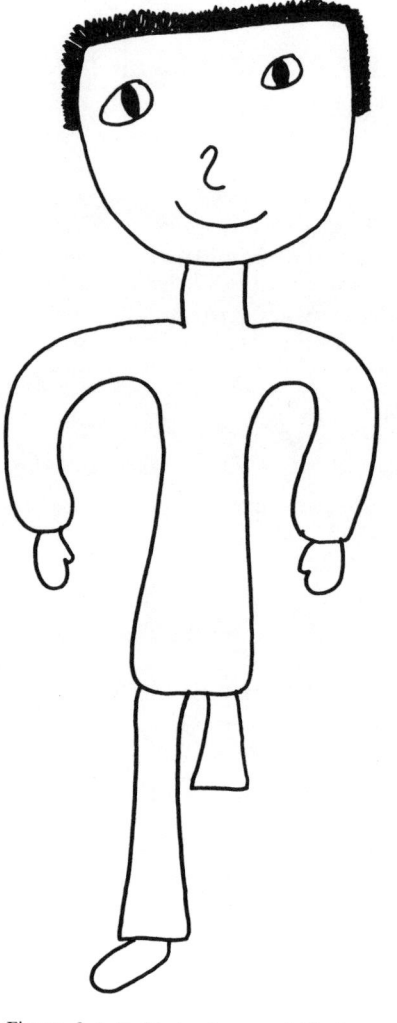

Figure 3-1. Bobby's picture of Cindy.

The siblings' task is to coordinate the concepts of constancy and change, sameness and difference. They must learn that it is the same person who looks so different, or that despite constancy in appearance, inner change is making the child ill.

Drawings are helpful in working with young siblings. How the child portrays the patient — whether changes in appearance are included or omitted — provides a basis for discussion. It is also interesting to compare this drawing with a sibling's self-portrait. In an "invisible" disease such as leukemia, simplified illustrations (of the types of blood cells, for example) can be invaluable for explanation.

Siblings' visits to the hospital and clinic are critical in demystifying the treatment process. In seeing other patients and siblings, they also develop a context for their own experience.

Identification with the Illness

The fear of taking ill with cancer runs high among a sibling group. There is ample reason for this frightening identification. The siblings see many similarities between themselves and the patient. As children in the same family, past experiences that affected one child often affected another. Thus, it is only a matter of extension that an illness which could befall one child could just as easily befall another. This logic is especially true when the siblings cannot stipulate, either cognitively or emotionally, a cause for the illness. The apparent randomness of events leads the sibling to think: "Why not me too?"

> When Bobby was asked if he has any fears or nightmares, he replied: "That my leg will get cut off also. I think about it a lot. I wake up and go into the kitchen. All the time I worry about it." (see Figure 3-2).
> (Bobby, ten; brother of Cindy, fourteen, osteogenic sarcoma)

> Ken described his drawing: "A big rock falls on two boys. They get hurt and bleed and get dead."
> (Ken, four; brother of Brad, two, leukemia)

The siblings need reassurance that there is little likelihood of their getting the same disease, nor is the illness contagious. In order to prevent an overidentification with the patient, siblings must be enabled to pursue their own day-to-day activities and relationships. This independent aspect of their life counterbalances the compelling sense of similarity and identification implied in a sibling relationship.

Guilt and Shame

The siblings' sense of guilt is multifaceted. As seen earlier, many of their views on what caused the patient's illness include either an implicit or explicit self-reference. Beyond the issue of causation, siblings at times feel guilty that they escaped the disease. Acknowledging their relief at being healthy only triggers the guilt more intensely. These children often feel badly when the patient is unable to participate in a particular activity or event because of the illness.

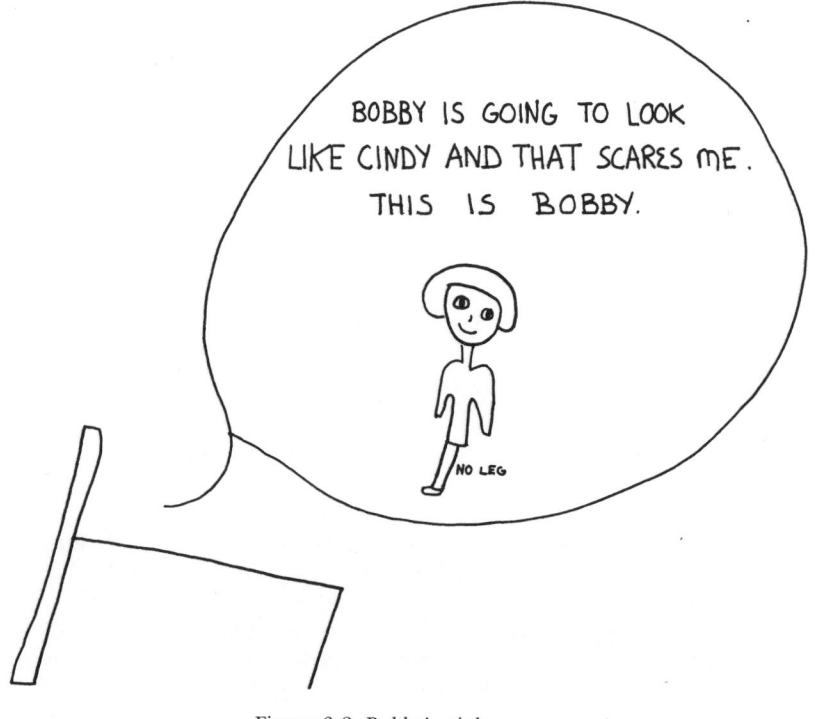

Figure 3-2. Bobby's nightmare.

The siblings' guilt can be stirred up from another source: their sense of shame. Rarely mentioned, but often lurking, is the siblings' shame at having a child in the family who is ill, disfigured, dying. The patient marks the family as "different." Siblings may attribute their shame either to themselves or to the patient; in both cases, the unacceptable feeling only increases the preexistent guilt.

The following statements illustrate siblings' sense of guilt:

Why didn't I get sick instead of Cindy. I wish it had been me. I don't like to see her hurt.

(Bobby, ten; brother of Cindy, fourteen, osteogenic sarcoma)

It's not fair that she had the amputation. She was a star athlete. I was never involved in athletics. I should have gotten it.

(Irene, seventeen; sister of Debbie, fifteen, osteogenic sarcoma)

These vignettes illustrate aspects of the shame:

Ken went through a period of hiding from people saying: "I don't want people to look at me. They will laugh at me." His explanation was somewhat garbled, but it did involve Brad.

(Ken, four; brother of Brad, two, leukemia)

Bobby had originally written his story about Cindy and himself at school (see *Visibility of the Illness and the Treatment Process*). He reported: "I threw it out because another kid read it." Bobby often talked about how embarrassed Cindy would be to go swimming, "because everyone would say things about her because of the amputation."

(Bobby, ten; brother of Cindy, fourteen, osteogenic sarcoma)

The siblings need the opportunity to discuss feelings of guilt or shame privately with their parents or another adult close to them. It is also important to ensure that siblings do not constrict their activities out of guilt that the patient cannot participate with them.

Siblings and Their Parents

The mother of a hospitalized patient reported having seen a car bumpersticker which read: "Have you hugged your child today?" She said that the slogan jolted her into realizing how little time she had spent with the siblings at home.

This vignette illustrates a critical issue between siblings of a patient and their parents: attention and nurturance. A pervasive complaint of the siblings is the diminished attention from their parents, especially when the patient is in the hospital. At these times, the parents may be both physically and emotionally unavailable to the children at home. Older siblings, who themselves are feeling deprived, may resent stepping in as "surrogate parents" for the younger children. The issue is often symbolized in siblings' concern about food, in physical symptoms, and in their need for reassurance about being loved.

Three well siblings in one family all complained that whenever the patient was in the hospital, their mother didn't have time to cook. All they ate were T.V. dinners.

Bobby was overheard talking to himself: "Maybe if I catch a cold, Mom will stay home with me more."

(Bobby, ten; brother of Cindy, fourteen, osteogenic sarcoma)

Ken's parents had been at the hospital with Brad since early morning. When they called home that evening, Ken reported matter-of-factly: "I have something bad to tell you. Carl (the other well sibling) is bald and you had better come home right away."

(Ken, four; brother of Brad, two, leukemia)

An eight-year-old sibling of a leukemia patient has appeared to be coping well throughout the four years of her sister's illness. However, she constantly leaves notes for her parents that say "I love you."

When the patient is home, whether ill or in remission, the siblings' complaint shifts slightly from that of "too little attention" to "preferential treatment of the patient." The parents are struggling concurrently: how to maintain equality and normality when, in fact, there is a distinctly "abnormal" factor in the family constellation. Parents may, at least initially, find it difficult to punish the patient, whereas disciplinary measures for the well siblings remain in effect.

Bobby drew a picture showing how his mother treated him differently from Cindy. Both children are reaching for the bowl of fruit. Mother yells at Bobby: "You'd better not touch that fruit." To Cindy, she says: "Please do not touch." After Bobby drew the picture, he smiled, seemingly in relief, and asked if he could draw the picture again — bigger this time! (see Figure 3-3)

   (Bobby, ten; brother of Cindy, fourteen, osteogenic sarcoma)

A painful issue is the siblings' anger at the parents for not having been able to protect the patient from the illness. Parents may be perceived as having played a role in the occurrence of the illness. Young siblings may come to this conclusion through a magical juxtaposition of events. Older siblings may wonder why the parents did not check the patient's symptoms earlier, echoing the parents' own self-questioning. The siblings are shaken by having a life-threatening illness strike so close, and insecure in the parents' ability to protect them.

"Brad is sick in the hospital. My mother drove him in there."
   (Ken, four; brother of Brad, two, leukemia)

Just before Brad's diagnosis of leukemia, the family dog had been given away. While Brad was in the hospital, Ken accused his mother of "lying" to him: "The dog is really dead."

It is important that the siblings express their concerns about the relationship with their parents. While some siblings may mention only the general decrease in attention (if even that), others may indicate

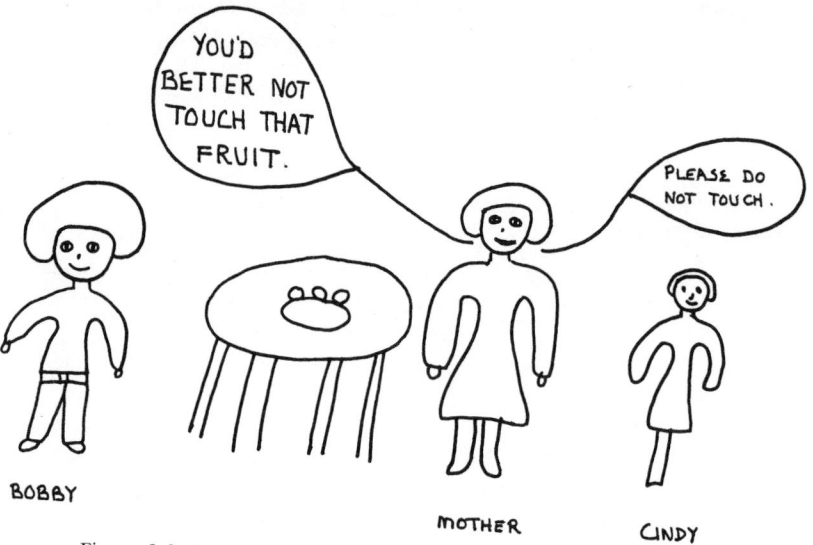

Figure 3-3. How Bobby's mother treats him differently from Cindy.

specific complaints such as disorganized meals, or missing favorite activities. Their concerns may change over time and circumstance. Once informed, the parents can mobilize their own priorities and commitments more effectively. Siblings need regular times alone with one or both parents for sharing feelings and thoughts, and for reassurance that they will be "protected" to the parents' optimum capacity. Older siblings should not be pushed into a "surrogate parent" role, even if they have assumed such responsibility in the past. During the patient's illness, other caregivers' support should be enlisted for the younger siblings. However, it is important to recognize that for some children, their "parenting" duties can be a means of assuaging their own sense of helplessness.

Academic and Social Functioning

The siblings' concern with the patient's illness often affects two areas of daily functioning: school and peer relationships. Siblings' academic performance may be impaired because of their preoccupation, or they may focus on school to assure a sense of competence in the face of stress and helplessness.

When asked whether he worries during the day about having his leg cut off, Bobby responded solemnly: "I think about it so much. Sometimes the teacher is giving out papers and I don't hear what she tells us to do because I'm so busy thinking and then she yells at me." During this same period, Bobby insistently requested tutoring in certain subjects, saying that his poor schoolwork was his worst problem.

(Bobby, ten; brother of Cindy, fourteen, osteogenic sarcoma)

Ken had a temper tantrum upon arrival at nursery school. Once calm, he explained that he didn't want to come to school that day because: "I had to go to work to take care of a very sick baby."

(Ken, four; brother of Brad, two, leukemia)

With regard to peer relationships, siblings may curtail contact in their need for a family focus, or they may turn increasingly to their friends for support.

Ken had all the children in his class write their names on a card to Brad, so that: "All my friends will know Brad and Brad will know all my friends."

(Ken, four; brother of Brad, two, leukemia)

When Cindy was sick, I was evil with all my friends. I knew they were just trying to cheer me up. I don't know what happened to me.

(Joanne, seventeen; sister of Cindy, fourteen, osteogenic sarcoma)

School and peer relationships represent the ongoing "normal" part of the siblings' lives. They are areas which provide opportunity for mastery, support, and distance from the illness experience. Teachers must be made aware of the family situation, and consultation must be available to them should siblings manifest problems in the classroom. Parents must maintain and encourage the siblings' peer activities.

Somatic Reactions

Somatic reactions, whether they be actual physical symptoms, sleep problems, or accident proneness, are commonly found within a sibling group. The symptoms may develop as a means of getting parental attention. Or, the siblings' preoccupation with the patient can lead to carelessness about themselves. In other instances, the symptoms represent symbolically a psychological process which the sibling is experiencing at the time.

> Cliff began to bedwet nightly during Susan's prolonged hospitalization. The mother thought that the enuresis was his means of delaying her daily departures to the hospital, since she would wash and change his linen before leaving (Sourkes, 1977).
>
> (Cliff, six; brother of Susan, thirteen, osteogenic sarcoma)
>
> I think about Cindy whenever I'm alone. I haven't slept well in two years.
>
> (Joanne, seventeen; sister of Cindy, fourteen, osteogenic sarcoma)
>
> Joanne fell on the stairs at school and split her lip open the day before Cindy's amputation. Her explanation: "I was walking in flat heels on the stairs. I thought of Cindy's operation. That's why I fell."
>
> (Joanne, seventeen; sister of Cindy, fourteen, osteogenic sarcoma)
>
> As Susan became more emaciated, Jane gained more and more weight. Jane articulated that "getting skinny means that you are dying," and so she kept eating.
>
> (Jane, eleven; sister of Susan, thirteen, osteogenic sarcoma)

Helping siblings to understand the psychological meaning behind the somatic concerns may relieve them of the necessity for psychosomatic expression.

Bidirectionality of the Sibling-Patient Relationship

A bidirectional focus on the sibling-patient relationship is critical within a systems view of the family. The relationship is always a two-way process, regardless of how skewed the balance may be because of one child's illness. Within the reciprocal system of well sibling and patient, the predominant themes of mutual anger/resentment and mutual protectiveness/caring emerge.

Siblings may resent the extra attention and privileges accorded the patient, while simultaneously feeling guilty about being healthy. The patient, angry to be sick, resents the siblings for escaping the illness. The patient's anger at the siblings, rarely mentioned in the literature, can be quite devastating for the other children.

> Katy asked her mother: "Why is Frank always so healthy and I'm so sick all the time?" Frank overheard her question, and when he couldn't sleep that night, called his mother into his room to "have a talk." In exact reverse, he asked: "Why am I so healthy and Katy so sick?" Katy's resentment was graphically expressed in her family drawing. She drew only her parents and Frank, saying upon questioning that she "forgot" to put herself into the picture. When asked to add herself, she, with forethought, drew herself on top of Frank's head.
>
> (Frank, four; brother of Katy, eight, leukemia)

Susan resented that when she was home, Jane spent much time out with friends. Jane was angry that during periods of Susan's hospitalization, she hardly saw her peers because of babysitting responsibilities at home. Susan felt guilty for making demands on Jane's time; Jane for not abiding more by her sister's wishes.

(Jane, eleven; sister of Susan, thirteen, osteogenic sarcoma)

Given the problem-oriented perspective of the clinical literature, it is not surprising that the positive caring between the patient and siblings has been overlooked. To ignore this reciprocity is to neglect the children's most adaptive means of coping.

Ken was proud to bring a candy to Brad in the hospital. In his therapy sessions, Ken would pretend to be a doctor taking care of baby Brad. When Brad was home again and the family was at a restaurant, Ken overheard another child laughing at Brad's baldness. Ken immediately went up to the child and said: "If you say anything bad about my baby brother I'll punch you. He is bald because he is sick."

(Ken, four; brother of Brad, two, leukemia)

Karen (patient) said to the therapist: "Please could you go and talk to my sister *alone*. She needs someone to talk to. Please do it as a favor to me."

(Karen, thirteen, leukemia)

Susan's explanation for her sister's infrequent visits to the hospital was: "Jane is afraid to see me without any hair and looking so sick, although I wish she would come more often." Jane thought that Susan was ashamed to be seen, and in fact wanted to visit more (Sourkes, 1977).

(Jane, eleven; sister of Susan, thirteen, osteogenic sarcoma)

The most critical task for the therapist is to facilitate communication between the patient and siblings. It is important to know what the relationship was like before the illness, as a baseline for understanding change. Parents can be encouraged to observe the sibling relationship and to help the children broach problems as they arise. If necessary, focused joint sessions with the patient and sibling can be helpful at times of crisis.

DEATH OF THE PATIENT AND BEREAVEMENT OF THE SIBLINGS

With the death of the patient, the siblings suffer multiple losses: the patient himself or herself, and then all the roles which were inherent in the relationship. While the patient is alive, a huge amount of time and energy is invested in that person, as the center of the family constellation. When the person dies, much reordering must occur as part of the family's readaptation process.

A controversy exists in the literature over children's capacity for mourning. Wolfenstein (1966) and Nagera (1970) have both stated that children are not capable of mourning until they have gone through a normal passage of adolescent object loss. Adolescence is a trial period to prepare for the autonomous decathecting of lost love objects at a later time. They consider children incapable of the sustained, prolonged experiencing of sad or angry feelings which adults undergo in

normal mourning. Feinberg (1970) points out that childhood mourning may be distinct in form from the adult process. Children try to
relive the lost relationship in real life rather than through conscious
remembering. They manifest painful affect only if it is induced by an
adult, and not through spontaneous expression.

Furman (1973) takes issue with this view. He states:

> The child's lack of an externally visible grief reaction similar to that of an adult has
> to my mind no more bearing on his internal capacity for mourning than his
> apparent sexual innocence would indicate the absence of his sexual feelings and
> fantasy life (p. 226).

Furman believes that if a child is presented with the reality of the
finality of death, and if object constancy has been attained (usually by
the age of four), then true mourning can occur.

Children's mode of expression varies from adults' in many life situations. Thus, it is not surprising that their grieving may be different,
although no less valid, than the adult process. In psychotherapeutic
work with bereaved siblings, the aim is to make the covert overt in their
mourning. Verbal interaction, drawing and dollhouse play are all
means of inducing expression.

At home, there are two central issues during the acute bereavement
period. First is the question of the siblings' attendance at the funeral. If
parents discuss the issue directly with the siblings, then they can often
make a decision based upon the children's direct or indirect cues. No
child should ever be forced to attend. Secondly, while it is important to
talk about the deceased child, the here-and-now life focus of the well
siblings should also be stressed. This is a critical period to ensure
prevention of insidious comparison with the idealized dead child, or
the beginning of a replacement child process.

In the following examples of siblings' mourning, note the interplay
of conventional verbal reminiscence with the more concrete working
through of younger children. The description of Frank's reactions (age
4) to Katy's death (age eight, leukemia) was obtained from the parents
in follow-up interviews and phone calls.

> When Frank was told of Katy's death, he immediately said that he wished he had
> had the chance to say goodbye. Over the next few days, he asked many questions:
> Why was Katy dead; what does dead mean; what does she look like now? The
> parents told Frank that although Katy could no longer talk to him, he could still
> tell her things if it would make him feel better. During the first month after Katy's
> death, Frank asked to go to the cemetery several times. At the grave, he would
> pose questions to Katy through his mother; for example, "Ask Katy if she really
> loved me." He would recount anecdotes to Katy about his life, such as his first day
> of nursery school. When the family dog was found after being lost for a day, Frank
> insisted on going to the cemetery with the dog so that Katy would know about his
> return! In school, Frank immediately attached himself to a little girl in his class,
> and would panic on days she was absent.
>
> About a month after Katy died, while Frank was in the bathtub, he suddenly
> burst into sobs about how much he missed taking a bath with Katy. Evidently

bathtime continued to be difficult for about six months, after which it became a time for happy recollection about the bath games he and Katy used to play together. Almost a year later, Frank still wakes up some mornings and says that he feels sad because he misses his sister.

What are the instructive points to be garnered from the description of Frank's mourning process? First, in Frank's wish to say goodbye to Katy can be seen a child's understanding of the finality of death, of termination. His intellectualized questions about death are an adaptive form of cognitive mastery of a highly abstract concept. Through his "talking to Katy," Frank could begin to understand that although she was no longer alive, he could continue to remember her. Frank's immediate attachment to the girl at school represents the concrete replacement so often seen in young siblings, along with their heightened sensitivity to the threat of loss. Frank's bathtime reminiscences are similar to adult grieving, when memories are stirred up by activities once shared. Frank's expressed sadness on waking some mornings is a spontaneous form of grieving, in no way induced by adult probing.

An older child's concerns are illustrated in two therapeutic sessions with Bobby (ten years), following the death of Cindy (fourteen years).

> When asked about the funeral, Bobby responded that it had been "scary" to see Cindy's body. He noted that she looked "cold and bigger." On the therapist's suggestion, he drew a picture of her in the casket, carefully adding a necklace charm which said "I love you." He had given her this necklace for Christmas. It was suggested that Bobby write a letter to Cindy, telling her anything that felt "unfinished." He wrote: "To Cindy. I wish you would be here to see how I feel. Cindy, I wish you could come home to stay with me forever and ever. I miss going bowling with you. Love, Bobby." After he had read the letter aloud, the therapist asked him if he could further specify how he feels, using the sentence cue: "I feel . . . Bobby wrote: "I feel like a bug is just eating me up." He then drew a picture of a boy with bugs "in the leg and chest only" — the sites of Cindy's cancer (see Figure 3-4).

The expression of Bobby's grieving was induced through talking, writing, and drawing. Bobby's initial comment about his fright at seeing Cindy's body set the stage for candor throughout the sessions. Like many children, his focus on the sense impressions of seeing Cindy ("cold and bigger") was interwoven with the fear. Bobby's continuing feeling for Cindy was represented in the "I love you" necklace she wore. He expressed his missing Cindy both in general terms, and with specific reference to a favorite shared activity. In Bobby's drawing of the bug eating him up is illustrated the identification with Cindy through the illness sites, and the power of his grief. The drawing of the child after death, the letter stating "unfinished" concerns, and the "I feel . . . " sentence cue, are all valuable techniques in working with bereaved siblings.

Joanne, Bobby's seventeen-year-old sister, requested the chance to talk to the therapist. Her expression of grief took on an adult form. She

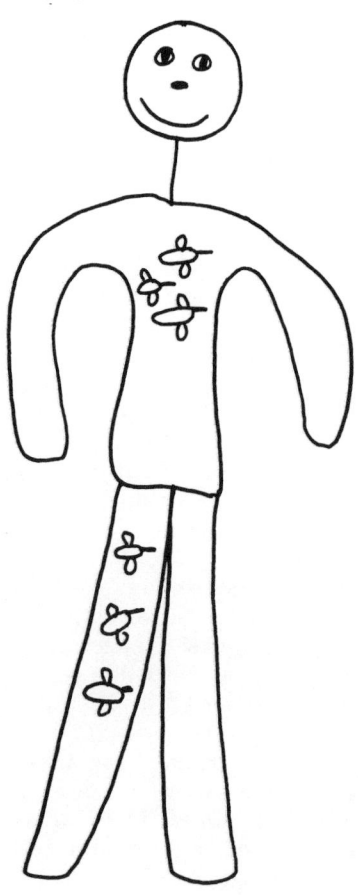

IT FEELS LIKE A BUG JUST
EATING ME UP. THE BUGS
ARE ONLY IN MY LEG AND
CHEST.

Figure 3-4. How Bobby feels after Cindy's death.

reviewed the process of Cindy's illness and death, and reminisced about their relationship. During the next few months, Joanne chose an intellectualized means of coping with her grief. She did a school project on the cancer center, and explained in the prologue:

> This project is dedicated to my beloved little sister Cindy. At the age of fourteen, my little sister and closest friend departed, leaving me and her brother Bobby and Mother behind. . . . Because of my very personal involvement, I chose the cancer institute as my assignment for Urban Studies.

All these children are unusually expressive, with parents who facilitated their openness throughout the illness-death process. However, these siblings articulate what all children are thinking, and the opportunity for their mourning must be provided.

IMPLICATIONS FOR FUTURE RESEARCH AND INTERVENTION

Clinical and research data on siblings of the pediatric cancer patient have been presented in this chapter. The siblings' experience may be seen at the juncture of three perspectives: the family system; a focus on life rather than on death; and a view to positive adaptation instead of psychopathological adjustment. What are the implications of the existing knowledge for future research and intervention?

In any life stress, certain individuals are at higher risk than others for maladaptive coping. The development of a predictive risk profile for siblings is crucial in the view toward prevention. Are there sibling characteristics, in existence prior to the patient's illness, which predict later difficulty? Should all siblings be seen for diagnostic assessment early in the patient's illness?

It must be ascertained whether siblings' coping patterns change with their level of emotional and cognitive development. Are there stages of adaptation which are invariant in sequence, although variant in actual time of emergence during the patient's illness? The possibility of using specific methods, especially of a cognitive nature, to facilitate siblings' optimal coping must be explored.

The nature of the illness itself may have differential impact on the siblings. A distinction may exist between the experience of siblings of leukemic and solid tumor patients. The course of the illness — its emergence and the quality and length of remission — is also important.

The most critical focus is on the sibling-patient relationship itself. The strengths inherent and unique to this relationship are enriching, and can facilitate the adaptation of the entire family.

REFERENCES

Binger, C.: Childhood leukemia-emotional impact on siblings. In Anthony, E. J., and Koupernik, C. *The Child in His Family: The Impact of Disease and Death.* New York, John Wiley & Sons, 1973.

Binder, C., Ablin, A., Feuerstein, R., Kushner, J., Zoger, S., and Mikkelsen, C.: Childhood leukemia: Emotional impact on patient and family. *N Engl J Med,* 280, 1969.

Cain, A., Fast, I., and Erickson, M.: Children's disturbed reactions to the death of a sibling. *Am J Orthopsychiatry, 34,* 1964.

Feinberg, D.: Preventive therapy with siblings of a dying child. *J Am Acad Child Psychiatry, 9,* 1970.

Furman, R.: A child's capacity for mourning. In Anthony, E. J. and Koupernik, C. *The Child in His Family: The Impact of Disease and Death.* New York, John Wiley & Sons, 1973, pp. 225-232.

Gogan, J., Koocher, G., Foster, D., and O'Malley, J.: Impact of childhood cancer on siblings. *Health and Social Work, 2:*1, 1977.

Hendin, D.: *Death as a Fact of Life.* New York, Warner Paperback Library Edition, 1973.

Kagen-Goodheart, L.: Reentry: Living with childhood cancer. *Am J Orthopsychiatry, 47:4,* 1977.

Koch, C., Hermann, J., and Donaldson, M.: Supportive care of the child with cancer and his family. *Semin Oncol, 1:1,* 1974.

Lindsay, M. and MacCarthy, D.: Caring for the brothers and sisters of a dying child. In Burton, L. *Care of the Child Facing Death.* London and Boston, Routledge and Kegan Paul, 1974, pp. 189-206.

Nagera, H.: Children's reactions to the death of important objects. *The Psychoanalytic Study of the Child, 25.* New York, International Universities Press, 1970.

Rosenblatt, B.: A young boy's reaction to the death of his sister. *J Am Acad Child Psychiatry, 8:*1969.

Share, L.: Family communication in the crisis of a child's fatal illness: A literature review and analysis. *Omega, 3:3,* 1972.

Sourkes, B.: Facilitating family coping with childhood cancer. *J Pediatr Psychol, 2:2,* 1977.

Spinetta, J., Spinetta, P., Kung, F., and Schwartz, D.: *Emotional Aspects of Childhood Cancer and Leukemia: A Handbook for Parents.* San Diego, Leukemia Society of America, 1976.

Townes, B. and Wold, D.: Childhood Leukemia. In Pattison, E. *The Experience of Dying.* Englewood Cliffs, Prentice-Hall, 1977. pp. 138-143.

Wiener, J.: Reaction of the family to the fatal illness of a child. In Schoenberg, B., Carr, A., Peretz, D., and Kutscher, A. Loss and Grief: *Psychological Management in Medical Practice.* New York and London, Columbia University Press, 1970, pp. 87-101.

Willis, D.: The families of terminally ill children: Symptomatology and management. *J Clin Child Psychol* III:2, 1974.

Wolfenstein, M.: How is mourning possible? *The Psychoanalytic Study of the Child, 21.* New York, International Universities Press, 1966.

Chapter Four

THE ADOLESCENT WITH CANCER

Lonnie K. Zeltzer

INTRODUCTION

A DOLESCENCE CAN BE a time of elation and depression, hyperactivity and lethargy, verbosity and muteness, happiness and pain. Above all, it is a developmental period characterized by change. It is the very nature of this change that makes adolescents such an exciting group of individuals to care for or have in one's family (albeit difficult at times).

The adolescent usually perceives himself or herself as immortal. Death is seen as something in the far, far unforeseeable future. Despite the marked recent oncological advances, the diagnosis of cancer is still often connoted with death. Thus, the placement of this emotionally laden label on an adolescent who seems so full of life often creates stress, anger, and sadness in family, friends, and medical staff (particularly house staff who identify with the adolescent patient).

I am painting a depressing picture because emotional collapse is often expected of the adolescent subsequent to the diagnosis. However, to the surprise of all, most adolescents cope remarkably well. It is the very nature of the resiliency during this period that gives the adolescent the tools to spring back and function despite sometimes adverse situations. The limited expectations of others, in fact, may be more disabling to the adolescent than the disease itself.

I will focus this chapter on the adolescence of the teenage oncology patient and how an understanding of this psychosocial developmental process can facilitate promotion of healthy adaptation in these youth. As Sir William Osler once said, "It is more important to know what sort of patient has a disease than what sort of disease a patient has."

Physicians caring for teenage oncology patients may find that sometimes treating the adolescent is more difficult than treating the disease. Remission may be induced only to have the adolescent noncomply with his maintenance chemotherapy. Bargaining around the time-intervals of chemotherapy may ensue ("why can't I come every five weeks instead of every four?"). It is often all too easy for the physician unknowingly to get caught up in battles with the adolescent, with the latter perceived by the physician as "manipulative."

To clarify the puzzling and sometimes difficult behavior of the adolescent, I will outline the psychological developmental work of this age period and describe how this emotional work may present some

70

special problems for young oncology patients. A variety of common coping responses to deal with these problems will be presented, including the troublesome issue of noncompliance. Since nausea and vomiting associated with chemotherapy and procedure-related pain and anxiety appear to be the greatest problems affecting the adolescent's quality of life, the following section will focus on some forms of self-help to mitigate these symptoms, with two cases presented to illustrate these modalities. Although the subject of the dying patient is discussed elsewhere in this book, aspects that deal specifically with adolescents and their physicians will be explored. Next, the relationship between physican and adolescent patient will be examined to see how the physician may influence the behaviors of his or her patients. Finally, behavioral research pertaining to adolescents with cancer will be discussed, with ideas offered for future investigations.

DEVELOPMENTAL TASKS OF ADOLESCENCE

Successful maturation includes progression through a specific physiological sequence called pubescence and accomplishment of five psychosocial tasks, including (Zeltzer, 1978a):

1. Development of a comfortable body-image and self-esteem.
2. Creation of identity through socialization.
3. Establishment of emotional and economic independence.
4. Sexual identity formation.
5. Future goal-orientation and career-development or employment.

Body-Image and Self-Esteem

With the changes of pubescence, the adolescent begins to notice his or her own physical development and compares it with that of the peer group to determine its normalcy. With the influence of the advertising media, magazines, television, movies, and the hero worship of athletes, adolescents often hold as an ideal the concept of the "beautiful body" and degrade the "deviant body," i.e. theirs. These feelings of self-consciousness and abnormality are supported by the study of Schonfeld (1963) who found that 60 percent of healthy adolescents are dissatisfied with their bodies. As the adolescent becomes increasingly reliant upon peer approval, especially in mid-adolescence, he or she becomes even more vulnerable to what the peer group says or thinks about him or her and tends to accept their comments as real. However, young and mid-adolescents are not especially altruistic, and often take competitive advantage of the shortcomings of their rivals in the race for status in the group and for favor in the eyes of the opposite sex.

The adolescent with cancer is in long-term contact with physicians and his or her body is repeatedly examined, reinforcing this focus on "body." So that no matter how well he feels, long-term chemotherapy, radiotherapy, and repeated clinic visits continue to remind the adolescent that he is different. He is no longer a person but has become a patient. This label then accentuates his differences and his potential feelings of inadequacy. Side effects of therapy may further emphasize these differences. For example, alopecia from cyclophosphamide or other anti-neoplastic agents may mean loss of attractiveness and femininity to females, while it may mean loss of sex appeal and virility to males (Meissner, 1967). Disfigurement may not only produce current anxieties but may reactivate childhood conflicts (Adsett, 1963). The amount of stress depends on the meaning of the organ or body part to the patient. For example, an eighteen-year-old girl with metastatic rabdomyosarcoma coped with removal of parts of her pelvis and extremity but decompensated and wanted to die when a lump was noted in her breast.

Many adolescents may have a distorted body image, even when they outwardly appear normal to others. Their own fantasies about their disease and their body may distort any factual information which they are given (Kaufman, 1971, 1972; Nathan, 1973). Poor body images, then, may lead to feelings of inferiority, low self-concept, low self-esteem, incompetence, and worthlessness (Swift, 1967; Raimbault, 1967; Beard, 1969). Furthermore, adolescents who come from families which value the "beautiful body" and the athlete tend to blame their problems on their "defective bodies" (Cruickshank, 1951). Thus, it is important for physicians to give their adolescent patients ample opportunities to discuss the adolescents' feelings about their bodies and to help correct distorted perceptions of self.

Socialization

It is often difficult to separate the effects of illness on socialization from the effects on body image. The illness may limit participation in peer-related activities. The adolescent may miss school because of clinic appointments, chemotherapy, or hospitalizations. Physical limitations from amputations may prevent the adolescent from participating in driving, athletics, or dancing (activities which provide social status and feelings of competence). The adolescent may not only be removed from normal socialization because of the disease and its treatment, he may also isolate himself through his own distorted self-image and self-consciousness. These feelings may then lead to school phobia, with resultant further isolation (Lansky, 1975; Futterman, 1970; Katz, 1977). However, it should be mentioned that, in fact, most adolescents, when they are feeling well and during the weeks they are not receiving intravenous chemotherapy, do have friends and do attend school. For those adolescents who have difficulty "re-entering" the normal school activities, the physician or designee could greatly facilitate the process by contacting the school and the student's school counselor for assistance.

Emotional and Economic Independence

Adolescents with cancer may have difficulty gaining autonomy. Their illness perpetuates dependence on their parents for emotional support during medical crises and hospitalizations, for transportation to clinics and for economic support to pay for the therapy. There are further barriers to independence as the care of the adolescent gradually shifts from himself or herself to reliance upon the hospital and its staff. The adolescent is placed in a situation where things are constantly being done to him, as expressed by a sixteen-year-old young man with Stage IV B Hodgkins disease who wanted to sign himself out of the hospital "AMA" because he was "tired of being a guinea pig." Treatments may produce side effects which necessitate a parent transporting the adolescent to and from clinic. A seventeen-year-old young man who had previously transported himself to clinic via motorcycle was devastated when vomiting associated with a new chemotherapy protocol forced him to allow his mother to drive him to the hospital on treatment days. The hospital role itself provides support for regression and dependence. Meals are served in bed; the focus is on bodily intake and output; and there is marked loss of privacy. The frustration over this enforced dependency is illustrated by a fifteen-year-old young man with osteogenic sarcoma who, bedridden because of his recent amputation, was found in tears after he had urinated in bed after the nurse did not answer his call for a urinal. He exclaimed, "As if wetting my bed wasn't embarrassing enough, when the nurse came into my room she yelled at me for being such a baby!" As will be discussed in a later section, the physician's encouragement and allowance of patient participation in most, if not all, aspects of care enhance the adolescent's maturation.

Sexuality

Forming a comfortable sexual identity is one of the developmental tasks of adolescence. In accomplishing this task, the adolescent usually moves through three stages (Figure 4-1). The first stage is that of curiosity and self-exploration. With the onset of puberty, the adolescent becomes aware of his or her changing body and new feelings and drives. The young adolescent usually has few outlets for these feelings except through his or her own body, and sexual exploration is through masturbation. The second stage in mid-adolescence is characterized by much experimentation and exploration of self, same sex peers, and those of the opposite sex. This is the stage where the adolescent focuses on "trying out" some of these new body parts to achieve a sense of identity through his body. This stage is characterized by physical activity or talk of such in order to belong to and achieve status in the peer group. The final stage is that of "expressive sexuality" where sexuality becomes a form of sharing and intimacy and is "other" directed. The adolescent begins to move away from the peer group and toward a significant other individual.

Moving comfortably through these stages can be difficult for any adolescent but may be especially difficult for the adolescent with a malignancy. Most adolescents can escape prying eyes to experiment and explore, but the adolescent with cancer may be deprived of

CONCEPTUAL MODEL OF ADOLESCENT SEXUALITY

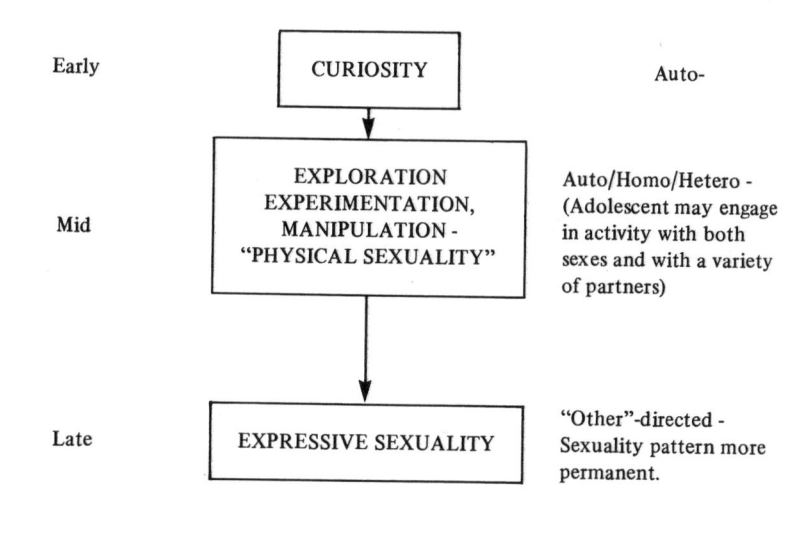

Stage of Adolescence   *Type of Sexual Activity*

Early   CURIOSITY   Auto-

Mid   EXPLORATION
EXPERIMENTATION,
MANIPULATION -
"PHYSICAL SEXUALITY"   Auto/Homo/Hetero -
(Adolescent may engage
in activity with both
sexes and with a variety
of partners)

Late   EXPRESSIVE SEXUALITY   "Other"-directed -
Sexuality pattern more
permanent.

After R. G. MacKenzie

Figure 4-1

adequate privacy to begin his sexual exploration. Overprotective parents may unconsciously set up situations that leave the adolescent little time away from them. In school, adolescents with a diagnosis of cancer may be spotlighted and continuously focused upon by teachers. Additionally, multiple clinic visits for chemotherapy or radiotherapy further remove the adolescent from his peer group and therefore from normal outlets for sexual activity. Also, if the adolescent spends one week out of every four weeks with nausea and vomiting, he or she may be less likely to want to socialize and make peer contact. A seventeen-year-old young man with acute myelogenous leukemia said that after his friends found out about his diagnosis, girls tended to stay away from him "almost as if they were afraid of catching something." The avoidance of his peers then made it uncomfortable for him to engage in normal social activities. He began to be treated by school mates as delicate. He said that, initially, this reaction produced a paranoid state in him where he thought classmates were talking about him behind his back. This discomfort around peers then enhanced his withdrawal from them.

There is some evidence that parents and physicians may see the adolescent with cancer as asexual (Zeltzer, 1978a). There may be an expectation on the part of the adults that the adolescent is not concerned with his or her own sexuality and therefore there is no need to talk about such matters. A fourteen-year-old girl whose leg was recently amputated following diagnosis of an osteogenic sarcoma explained, "The doctors talk to me all about my tumor and about the treatment but they never answered the questions that I really want to know . . . Am I still a woman? . . . Will I still have periods? . . . How do I wear a sanitary napkin if I don't have two legs to hold it in place?"

Generally, in the adolescent with cancer, there is intensification of normal adolescent anxieties related to secondary sexual development and changes in body size and shape. This intensified anxiety may be produced by some of the physical changes that accompany the disease and its treatment, including obesity, emaciation, nausea and vomiting, stunted growth, alopecia, radiation dermatitis, mutilative surgery, and changes in sexual functioning relating to gonadal radiation (Kellerman, 1977a). These changes may then impact on the adolescent's already poor self-image, further removing the adolescent from his or her peer group and retarding the development of a comfortable sexual identity.

Career Planning and Life Goals

The final task of adolescence has to do with future planning, which involves choosing a career or a job and establishing one's own belief system. How the adolescent feels about him or herself, physical limitations produced by disease and its treatment, and socialization experiences all influence completion of this task. Realistic self-assessment for the adolescent with cancer may be difficult because of unrealistic or limited expectations of parents, teachers, and perhaps physicians. Teachers may overgrade the adolescent with cancer out of a sense of pity. On the other hand, while trying to treat the adolescent with cancer as a "normal child," parents may place unrealistic demands and create unrealistic expectations. These adolescents are then "set up" to fail, with resultant poor attitudes and nonfuture orientation. Multiple school absences because of illness and/or treatments may further enhance the feelings of failure for these adolescents. The adolescent may dread returning to school to face questions from peers and the load of missed school work. Competency needs may be frustrated in adolescents who are always "catching-up" in school. These feelings of failure may then produce in the adolescent a "what's the use" attitude, especially if medical setbacks recur (Boyle, 1976).

Physicians may be unwilling to discuss prognosis and future medical problems because of their own discomforts. The adolescent's direct questions may be answered with mixed messages and clouded answers which intensify the adolescent's anxiety and place him at further disadvantage for future planning. It is helpful for physicians to be as clear as possible in their discussions of prognosis with adolescents and to encourage resumption of future-oriented activities whenever medically possible.

Reproduction capabilities and parenthood need to be discussed with the young oncology patient when helping the adolescent realistically plan for his or her future. With improved survival rates for childhood cancer, questions are being asked about future reproductive ability and adult quality of life. For the adolescent whose treatments have included direct irradiation or removal of gonads, implications for future reproduction are clear and need to be explained to the patient, allowing the adolescent ample opportunity to discuss his or her feelings about the situation. For other adolescents, the data needed for giving information in such discussions is less clear. A questionnaire survey of 142 survivors of childhood cancer (aged eighteen years or older) showed no clear evidence of psychosocial disturbances related to disease (Li, 1976). They had no increased difficulties in establishing close interpersonal relationships, and the proportion married did not differ by age and sex from figures for the general population. A study of progeny of these patients demonstrated no increase in frequency of birth defects, infant morbidity, stillbirths, or miscarriages (Li, 1974). However, a recent study of postpubertal females treated for leukemia demonstrated an increased proportion of reproductive abnormalities in those treated during pubescence than in those treated prior to the onset of puberty (Siris, 1976). Thus, further studies are needed to clarify the issues pertinent to the future planning of adolescents treated for malignancies.

COPING RESPONSES

How adolescents adapt to the diagnosis of cancer, the disease itself, and the medical therapy depends upon the adolescent's general pre-illness emotional functioning, family support, medical staff support, disease course, and types and side effects of treatments. This section will focus on some of the problem areas for adolescent oncology patients and some of the common adolescent responses to these problems, including the difficult issue of noncompliance.

The first problem faced by these adolescents is the crisis of diagnosis. Usually, the longer the prediagnosis evaluation period is, the more anxious the adolescent becomes by the time the diagnosis is discussed with him or her. In fact, that waiting period is a high-anxiety time not only for the patient and his or her family but also for the hospital staff (house staff, nurses, etc.). The staff often do not know what to say to the patient and react by saying very little of anything, often avoiding eye contact with the adolescent. The staff hold on to the myth that the patient does not know what the illness is until "all the tests are in and the attending physician has explained the diagnosis." Most often the staff want to believe this myth to ease their anxiety over patient-interaction. Most adolescents sense the staff's anxiety, and this "chain of secrecy" further intensifies the adolescent's feelings that he has "something bad." The following case illustrates this point.

Mike, a thirteen-year-old boy, was admitted to the hospital for evaluation of an "anemia with blast-like cells in the peripheral smear." By the second hospital day his diagnosis of acute lymphocytic leukemia was confirmed by the bone marrow smears. The house staff, on rounds outside Mike's room and looking at him through the glass in the closed door, remarked how convinced they were that Mike did not know his diagnosis. They felt certain that Mike suspected nothing because "he is so calm and always watching television." Just following rounds that day, Mike left his room for the first time and entered the recreation room where I was conducting a "rap" session with some of the adolescents from the unit. Oblivious to the eight other adolescents in the room, Mike slammed the door behind him and shouted at me, "You were there this morning . . . well, I have leukemia, don't I!"

Thus, even if adolescents don't show it, most know "the category" into which their illness fits and become angry and anxious when no one lets them in on the secret. As many adolescents have said, "after all, it's my body! I should be the first to know!"

Even the physician who discusses each test result with the patient is often surprised to find that the adolescent may continue to watch television and act nonchalant when the final diagnosis is explained. How many times has the experienced physician heard the frustrated intern, trying to be open and honest, saying to the adolescent, " . . . but you're not listening to me! For the fifth time, I just said you have leukemia!" with the nonsequitur patient response, "okay . . . but hurry because 'Donny and Marie' comes on soon." Thus, following the waiting period of anxiety and anger comes the response of *denial*. The patient hears what is being said but chooses to not let it register until he is ready to deal with it. The physician may expect emotional breakdown upon explaining the diagnosis to the adolescent and instead may be confused by the lack of patient response. It is often helpful for the physician to inform the adolescent during this denial phase that "we can talk some more tonight or tomorrow or when you are ready. I will be back." The physician may have to repeat everything on the return visit.

Fairly soon (hours or days) the diagnosis registers and the adolescent usually reacts with anger — "Why me?" This is the time when the adolescent may project his anger onto the medical staff and overreact to medical procedures. He may complain that his doctor keeps things from him; the house staff are butchers and don't know what they're doing; the nurses are stupid; the laboratory technicians practice on him; and the hospital food is awful. It is important for the staff to not allow themselves to get caught up in the patient's anger by reacting defensively and becoming hostile to the adolescent. It is much more helpful for the staff members to inform the adolescent that they understand how angry and upset he or she must be and that they are willing to listen to him talk about his anger.

Given an adequate period of time for the adolescent to work through his anger and given a certain amount of family support, most adolescents will then reequilibrate back to the coping response of denial.

However, this time there is intellectual understanding of the disease and its treatment, but seriousness or potential consequences of malignancy are selectively ignored. This healthy coping mechanism allows most adolescents with cancer to progress through their normal psychosocial development when they are feeling well.

Once in remission, most adolescents forget about their disease until "chemotherapy time" comes around. Nausea and vomiting associated with chemotherapy and procedure-related pain and anxiety appear to be the worst problems for adolescents with cancer. A study comparing adolescents with cancer to adolescents with other chronic illnesses on an "impact of illness" questionnaire found that the former group significantly differed from all other groups on the items that stated "my treatments are worse than my disease" (Zeltzer, 1979a). In another study (Zeltzer, 1979b) adolescents with cancer were asked to perform three tasks: (1) draw a whole person; (2) draw your illness as it presently is; and (3) draw how the treatment for your illness is working in your body (Figures 4-2–4-5). Figures 4-2A–4-2D each represent the adolescent's body image. As Figures 4-3A–4-3D show, the adolescents had a fairly realistic assessment of their disease. However, in response to the third task, 95 percent of the group (N=15) drew something that focused on nausea and/or vomiting with the description "the medicines make me sick" (Figures 4-4A–4-4D). The fifteen-year-old young woman who drew the Figure A series had acute lymphocytic leukemia in first remission for three years at the time of the drawing. The physicians were discussing the possibility of discontinuing chemotherapy but the patient saw a "big question mark" when she thought about the presence of any disease in her body. The following week, she was found to have relapsed with central nervous system leukemia and was placed on a new chemotherapy protocol. The Figure C series represent a fifteen-year-old young man whose chemotherapy had been terminated that week because he showed no further evidence of his brain tumor. Even with news of eradication of his cancer, he draws "a man with sadness in his eyes." In a sixteen-month survey of patient problems encountered by the psychosocial section of the oncology division of a large children's hospital, eleven of twenty-seven adolescents were referred because of a primary complaint of treatment-related vomiting or procedure-related pain and anxiety (Kellerman, 1979).

Therefore, the adaptive patterns of adolescent oncology patients may encompass the use of denial between treatments with maladaptive behaviors surfacing during treatment or procedure times, hospitalizations, and relapses. All of these events remind the adolescent of his role as "patient." To play this role "well," i.e., to be favored by the medical staff, the adolescent must be cooperative, have a sense of humor, allow all procedures to be performed on him with a minimum of fuss, be prompt for appointments, and be grateful to the staff for their care (Visotsky, 1961). In other words, he must act as an obedient child. This process is foreign to the adolescent who is struggling for independence and autonomy.

The adolescent may then react to this enforced dependency in several ways (Zeltzer, 1978b):

1. *Regression.* e.g. The adolescent who cries and wants his mother during clinic visits.
2. *Increased anxiety* expressed through physical and emotional symptoms. e.g. The adolescent who vomits on his way *to* chemotherapy or who screams with each intravenous infusion.
3. *High risk-taking behaviors.* e.g. The adolescent who tries to compensate for feelings of inferiority and dependency by acting "super-macho." The adolescent might drive his car or motorcycle too fast or get into fights at school.
4. *Withdrawal from peers.* e.g. The adolescent who does not want to attend school during "chemotherapy week" even if he or she feels well.
5. *Noncompliance* with medical therapy as a way of maintaining control. There are a number of reasons for noncompliance in adolescents (Zeltzer, 1978a; Moore, 1969; Becker, 1972; Hofmann, 1973). As previously discussed, the role of "patient" is often primarily a dependent one where things are being done *to* the child. The adolescent "person" within "patientdom" is often working diligently on the struggle for autonomy within the confines of this role. For those adolescents whose families allow for growth outside the confines of medical care and whose doctors encourage the adolescents' participation in this care, compliance is usually not a problem. For these adolescents, an active patient decision to terminate therapy might come about after repeated therapies fail to reinduce remission, and the exhausted adolescent may want "no more." This situation always brings up the bioethical decision of "when to consider the patient's rights versus the doctor's needs" (Schowalter, 1973). However, for adolescents who are in active battle with parents over autonomy, a struggle may take place as the adolescent tries to assert himself regarding the type and manner of treatment he receives. Lesser issues, such as bargaining over chemotherapy schedules ("can't I come every five weeks instead of every four?"), may lead to total noncompliance, if the adolescent feels he is "losing ground." The only thing that the adolescent feels he "owns" and is totally "his" may be his body and the adolescent may use it as a weapon in the final rebellion. This situation may lead to direct confrontation between the adolescent, his parents, and his physician (Himmelhock, 1970). Unfortunately, there have usually been an escalating number of flags waved by the adolescent and missed by family and physician prior to this big step. Thus, for the family and phy-

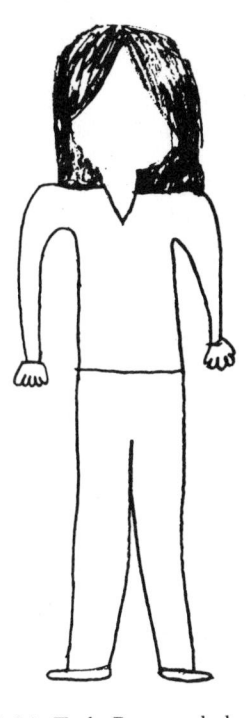

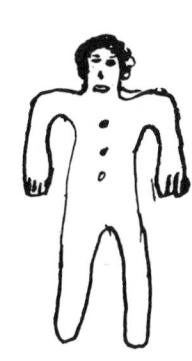

Figure 4-2A. Task: Draw a whole person. (How come she doesn't have a face?) "I didn't know whether to draw it happy or sad."

Figure 4-2B. Task: Draw a whole person. «Es una persona, es un hombre que, este hombre tiene . . . , ta malo, ta enfermo, de un enfermedad qu es canser.» "It's a person, it's a man who, this man has . . . , he is ill, he is sick, with a sickness that is cancer."

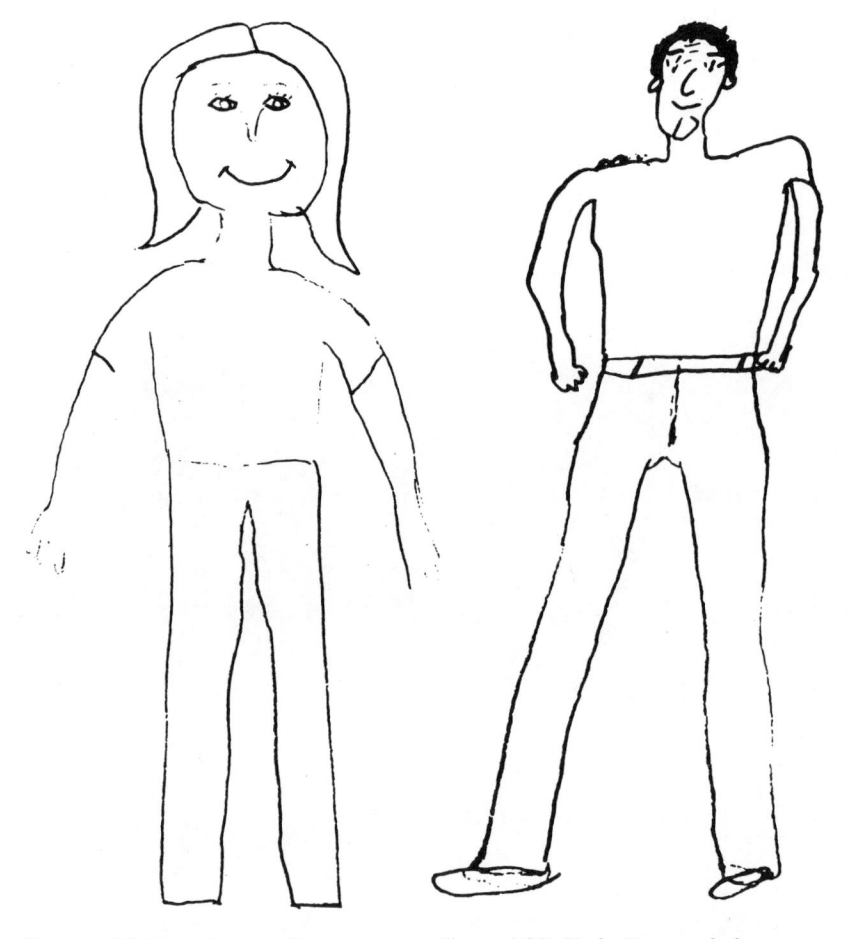

Figure 4-2C. Task: Draw a whole person.   Figure 4-2D. Task: Draw a whole person.

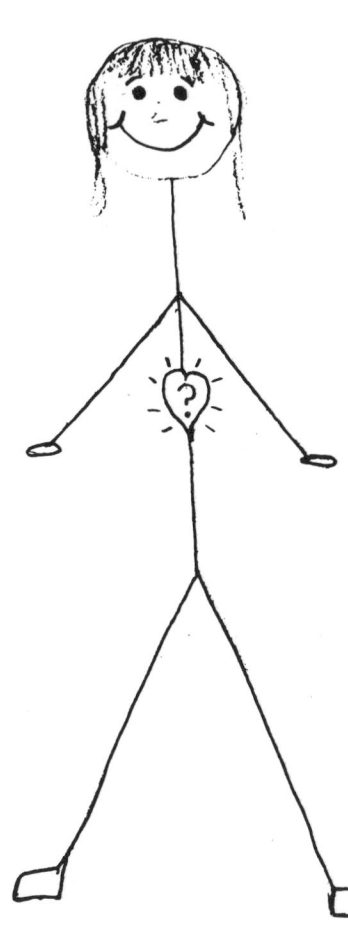

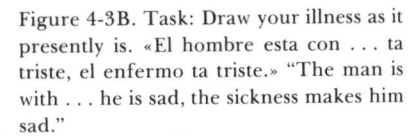

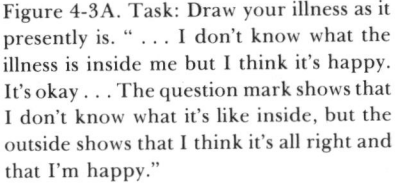

Figure 4-3A. Task: Draw your illness as it presently is. " . . . I don't know what the illness is inside me but I think it's happy. It's okay . . . The question mark shows that I don't know what it's like inside, but the outside shows that I think it's all right and that I'm happy."

Figure 4-3B. Task: Draw your illness as it presently is. «El hombre esta con . . . ta triste, el enfermo ta triste.» "The man is with . . . he is sad, the sickness makes him sad."

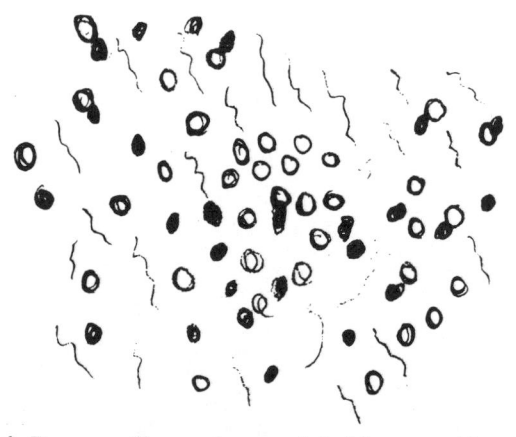

Figure 4-3C. Task: Draw your illness as it presently is. "there are white cells and red cells, and the white cells eat the red cells or the red cells eat the white cells, and they have to be balanced . . . if you have too many white cells you have cancer, I think . . . "

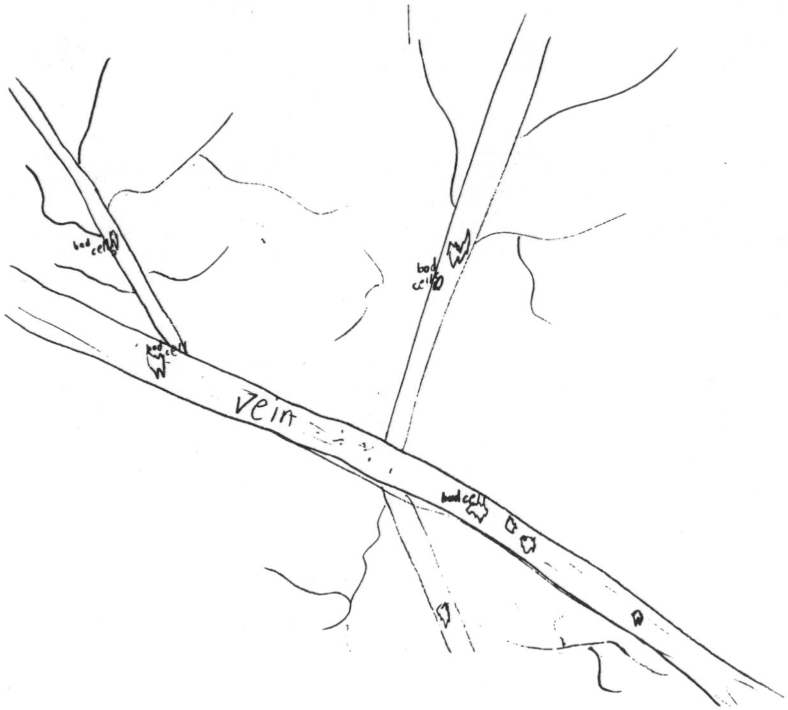

Figure 4-3D. Task: Draw your illness as it presently is. " . . . I just figure that leukemia is the bad cells in your blood that's just killing off the other cells like, and . . . "

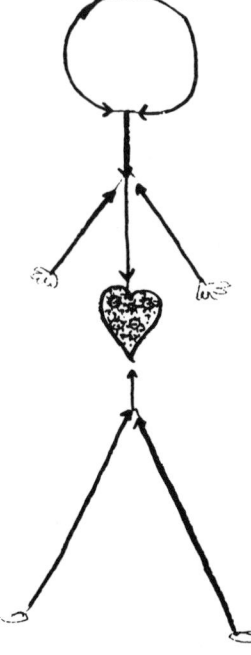

Figure 4-4A. Task: Draw how the treatment for your illness is working in your body. " . . . The arrows represent like all the medicines going through my body and these are supposed to be bugs and then there's little question marks in there where, um, the medicines have made these bugs disappear right around here . . . They're going through the body searching for these that they're going to kill. And then the heart again shows that I'm happy on the outside but on the inside are these bugs."

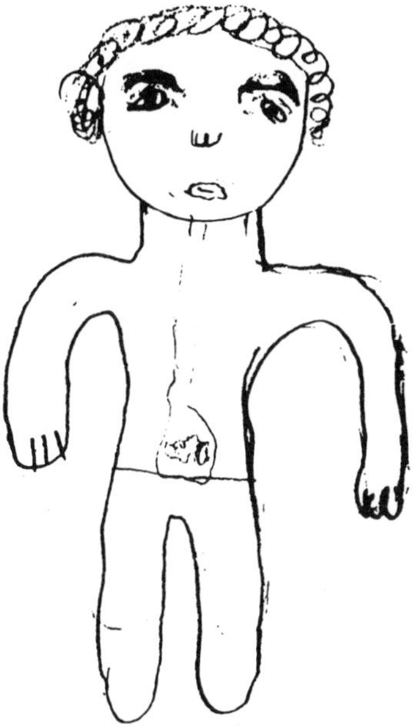

Figure 4-4B. Task: Draw how the treatment for your illness is working in your body. «Tiene, esta, tiene asco, digo, tiene revelto el estómago y esta triste de los ojos.» "He has, this, he has nausea. I say, he has churning in his stomach and has sadness in his eyes."

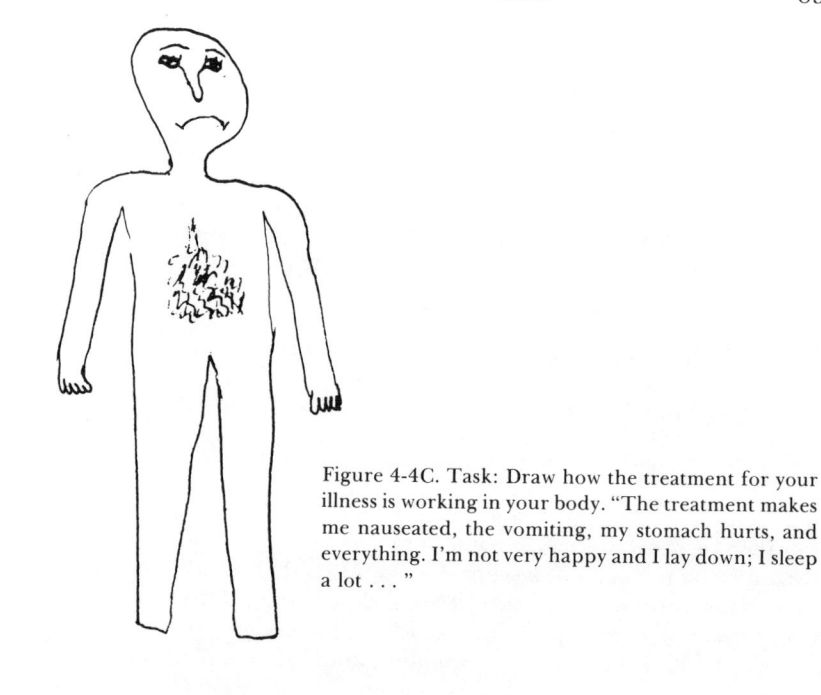

Figure 4-4C. Task: Draw how the treatment for your illness is working in your body. "The treatment makes me nauseated, the vomiting, my stomach hurts, and everything. I'm not very happy and I lay down; I sleep a lot . . . "

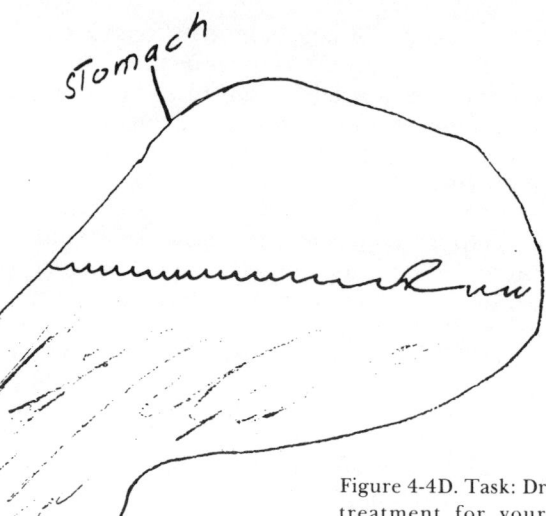

Figure 4-4D. Task: Draw how the treatment for your illness is working in your body. "it's . . . my stomach feels like an ocean . . . the waves in it make me nauseous."

sician to act surprised and angered and to try to "talk the adolescent into complying" are not the answers. To constructively work through this problem, the physician will need to be an active listener in several meetings with the adolescent and his family, especially in one or two with the adolescent alone. The purpose of these meetings would be to hear the adolescent's feelings and frustrations and work together to allow for enhancement of the adolescent's self-esteem and return of his sense of control without the treatments having to be the target of that control. The less authoritative and the more caring the physician has been all along, and the more the physician has encouraged adolescent self-responsibility and active participation in multiple aspects of treatment, the less likely will occur noncompliance as a mode of adolescent rebellion.

SELF-HELP

I have already suggested increased adolescent participation in his or her own medical management as a means of encouraging progression through the normal adolescent developmental tasks and as a means of increasing patient compliance. However, if the adolescent with cancer is to repeatedly experience invasive procedures and physical discomforts, encouraging active participation alone may not be enough. Because of the adolescent's need for mastery and independence, it may be highly desirable for the adolescent to be offered some tools for enhancing feelings of bodily control. Learned modalities exist for this purpose that are noninvasive, are capable of decreasing unpleasant or uncomfortable symptomatology, and may decrease reliance on drugs for control of these symptoms. Among the more prominent behavioral methods that have been used for this purpose are hypnosis, biofeedback, relaxation, meditation, and yoga, among others (Zeltzer, 1979c; Edmeads, 1973; LaBaw, 1974; Shafer, 1975; Carron, 1975; Crasilneck, 1973; Sargent, 1973; Peper, 1974; Andreychuk, 1975; Melzack, 1975; Bergin, 1975; Weber, 1974; Knox, 1974; Graham, 1975). These behavioral self-help modalities may assist the adolescent in experiencing a sense of increased mastery and autonomy. With increased control of bodily experiences and enhanced feelings of wellness, i.e., less life interference from disease, these teenagers then have more freedom to progress with their normal adolescent development.

To be effective with adolescents, these behavioral self-help modalities should have the following properties:

1. Reducing stress and enhancing relaxation.
2. Increasing the tolerance to procedures.
3. Decreasing or removing unnecessary symptoms, thereby reducing reliance upon symptomatic medications.
4. Easily learned.
5. Usable alone.

For the remainder of this section I will illustrate and elaborate on self-hypnosis as one type of self-help skill useful for adolescents with malignancies.

I will focus on hypnosis because it is the therapeutic modality with which I have had the most clinical and research experience (see "Adolescent Self-Help Project" in research section). A detailed discussion of self-hypnosis is covered in another chapter (J. Dash) and provides the theoretical rationale for this approach. In that chapter and in this one, hypnosis is defined as "a heightened state of attention and responsiveness to a set of ideas" (Erickson, 1959). Several hypnotic techniques are described in the chapter on hypnosis. We have found that adolescents learn hypnosis readily; and, after learning several techniques, they will create, choose, and use their favorite methods (Zeltzer, 1978c).

In the following section, two case histories of patients with whom I have worked will be presented to illustrate some uses of self-hypnosis in adolescents with cancer for reduction of disease- or treatment-related symptoms.

Case One: The Use of Self-Hypnosis for Anxiety Reduction in an Adolescent with Progressive Disease.

P. C. is a sixteen-year-old young man with metastatic osteogenic sarcoma who, during the three years since his diagnosis, has undergone leg amputation and two thoracotomies. He was inititally treated with high-dose methotrexate and citrovorum "rescue." However, after pulmonary metastases were noted, his treatment was changed to Cis-Platinum.

It was at this point in time that I was asked to see P. C. to assist him with the severe nausea and vomiting he was experiencing with his chemotherapy. In each of our two hypnosis sessions which occurred during Cis-Platinum administration, I suggested an imagery theme of "going to your special planet where you can feel comfortable and do anything you want to do." During the first session, he easily went into hypnosis and described, "how good it feels to run with two legs and to ride my bicycle really fast." He interrupted the hypnosis to vomit once and immediately went back into hypnosis. Later he said, "I remember vomiting once but it didn't bother me." Several weeks after the second session, P. C. commented that, for three years since his amputation, he had been having nightly dreams in which he had two legs and had been bothered by his inability to "feel" both legs when awake. However, he was excited that, for the first time, he had only one leg in his nightly dreams and could "feel" both legs in hypnosis whenever he wanted to do that.

After several courses of Cis-Platinum, the therapy was discontinued because of abnormal renal studies, and P. C. was begun on a course of radiotherapy. At this point it should be mentioned that, through healthy use of denial, P. C. had been coping very well with his illness for three years. He had been attending school regularly, had engaged in peer-related activities, and had needed only intermittent support. However, he became highly anxious after he developed hemoptysis and was told that a metastatic lesion was eroding into one of his pulmonary blood vessels. He again came to my office to seek further hypnosis training for relief of severe chest pain. He had just come from oncology clinic where he recalled being told that he would "have to learn to live with the pain because there was nothing they (the doctors) could do . . . they just gave me pain pills which aren't working."

Tearfully, he said "I just can't stand it any longer." When asked what "it" referred to, he paused and said " . . . cancer, the treatments, living . . . " He felt therapy was not working and wanted to stop his treatments. He knew his disease was progressing and he was mostly afraid of "dying in pain." I reminded P. C. that he had learned some special skills that he could use whenever he needed them. At this point I helped P. C. achieve a deep state of hypnosis during which he imagined going to his "special planet." This time, however, I asked P. C. if he could visualize a huge mountain. After he nodded affirmatively, I said, "can you find a pathway leading to the top? . . . do you think you can climb that mountain and let me know when you've reached the top?" P. C. nodded affirmatively and, after several minutes had passed, he smiled. When I asked what was happening, he said that he had reached the top and could see all the other mountain tops below him. He said, "man, is it beautiful out here! I can see out around me for miles and miles." I asked P. C. if he would like to spend some time there "feeling good." When he came out of hypnosis, his chest pain was gone and he was feeling more relaxed and comfortable. Five months later he reports that, although his disease is progressing, he has been able to go to "his mountain" whenever he has needed to go there "to feel good."

In this case, an adolescent with a progressive malignancy was able to use the self-hypnosis to reduce pain and anxiety and to feel "in control" at a time when he felt the doctors had "given up" on him.

Case Two: The Use of Self-Hypnosis to Reduce Nausea and Vomiting

E. J. is a six foot, five inch, seventeen-year-old young man with acute myelogenous leukemia diagnosed two years prior to the time of referral. He had achieved initial and continued remission after treatment with D-ZAPO, followed by intrathecal methotrexate and cranial axis irradiation and has subsequently received intravenous chemotherapy daily for four days monthly to maintain his remission.

E. J. experienced more anxiety associated with his therapy than with his disease. His behavioral reaction to chemotherapy began as nausea and vomiting immediately following insertion of the intravenous needle before medication was begun. The onset of vomiting gradually preceded the chemotherapy by progressively greater time intervals until, at the time of referral, symptoms began twelve hours prior to chemotherapy. The vomiting continued throughout the first day of chemotherapy and recurred at half-hourly intervals, uninterrupted, for four days and nights.

E. J. described his nausea as "a large bulldozer coming towards me . . . and I would be the brick wall trying to hold up against the bulldozer . . . but it would keep coming towards me and eventually crash right through the wall and I would vomit and feel as if I had lost the battle." He described chemotherapy as "four days of battle and losing." His vomiting was so severe that dehydration necessitated three separate hospitalizations for intravenous fluid replacement.

I first met E. J. when he was referred to our "Adolescent Self-Help" project after he had walked out of hematology clinic, refusing to have any more chemotherapy and preferring "to take 'his' chances with the disease." He was very depressed and said he could no longer tolerate the nausea and vomiting and "had enough of feeling miserable." He was informed about our project from the Patient Activities Specialist on the adolescent inpatient ward when he stopped by the unit to say goodbye. The Activities Specialist knew that we were just beginning a research project investigating the use of self-hypnosis for control of pain, nausea, and vomiting in adolescent oncology patients and asked E. J. to talk with me about his problem before terminating therapy.

E. J. met with me the same day he had planned to stop therapy and agreed to try hypnosis. He began his first self-hypnosis session by learning "finger fixation" and "confusion" induction techniques to go into a hypnotic state (see J. Dash chapter). In the former method E. J. would fixate his vision on my finger or on his own finger, which would then rise above his line of vision and he would be instructed to allow his eyes to close when he could no longer see the finger. In the latter induction method, E. J. was given a series of mathematical progressions to compute mentally. He was told that he could picture the numbers or think about them and that it did not matter whether his eyes were opened or closed. After a brief period of time during which E. J. would calculate the mathematical progressions and during which time I might change the rules or the numbers, E. J. would then be told that, if he wanted to become even more comfortable and relaxed, he could "just let the numbers float away and not have to think about anything." To deepen the hypnotic state and dissociate, he was then told, "if you want to go even deeper into hypnosis, you could take three deep breaths and feel yourself go deeper and deeper with each breath . . . and when you are ready, you could begin to descend your favorite stairs . . . with each step down, going deeper and deeper . . . so that, by the time you reach the bottom step, you will be completely relaxed and comfortable . . . and you can signal me with your index finger when you notice across the room a heavy carved door . . . when you reach there, and open the door, you will find yourself in your favorite place . . . would you please let me know when you are there?" E. J. then visualized himself skiing and was given a suggestion that he could feel cool air in his nostrils with each inspiration to replace any feelings of nausea. He left my office and went to hematology clinic where he experienced his first course of chemotherapy without vomiting. He told the nurse, who had seen him coming and promptly produced the emesis basin, that he felt the basin would not be needed that day.

Following several more heterohypnosis sessions, E. J. evolved a "favorite place" fantasy that he could use to dissociate his mind from his body during chemotherapy administration. When in hypnosis, E. J. would envision himself in the middle of the desert at night, standing on a platform preparing to climb the steps to his private spaceship. He would enter the ship and guide it "safely and *in control*" to his private planet, carefully choosing a landing location. He would then leave his spaceship and walk or run to the base of his favorite mountain. He would find ski clothes to wear and would put on his "warm, thick leather socks so that the skin on the feet would take on the texture of thick, tough leather." He would then put his "thick leather ski boots" over these special socks. (This latter image was used for foot anesthesia for the intravenous needle insertion. A previous hypnoanesthetic suggestion of "the foot feeling numb as if it had just been in a bucket of ice water" was so effective that his foot became cold and blue from vasoconstriction and the nurse was unable to start the intravenous infusion.) In this fantasy he would ride the chairlift to the top of the mountain. In his imagery, snow might be falling and E. J. would stick out his tongue to taste it. During heterohypnosis, I might suggest that E. J. feel the cool, brisk air in his nostrils, back of his throat, and his lungs. His cheeks would often become visibly flushed and he would describe feeling cold wind blowing across his face. He usually used the insertion of the intravenous needle as the signal to leave the chair and ski "rapidly and *in control*" down the mountain during the remainder of the chemotherapy. Upon completion of the chemotherapy, before he came out of the hypnosis, he gave himself the posthypnotic suggestion of being pleased with his control and feeling comfortable with the knowledge that the evening will be a relaxing and pleasant one. Although E. J. usually used the self-hypnosis without my presence, I used the contacts with him as opportunities to reinforce his "being *in control*."

Before experiencing nausea and vomiting, E. J. knew of the association between these symptoms and chemotherapy from the informed consent for the medication and from inadvertent clues given by physicians and nurses. Thus, even after E. J. learned that he no longer had to experience nausea and vomiting during chemotherapy, he believed that, in some ways, these symptoms were still necessary. He said that a nurse once told him that by-products of the medication accumulated in his system and it was important to "get rid of these." He said he had the impression from the physicians that his vomiting meant that the medications "were working." Thus, even though he had been successful in eliminating all nausea and vomiting during chemotherapy administration, he was unable to eradicate these symptoms at home. Because of the misinformation he had accumulated, E. J. tied his vomiting behavior to his remission, thereby developing a belief system in which he needed to vomit in order to maintain his remission. Even after discussions about this belief system and correction of the misinformation, E. J. "still felt the need to vomit" even though he "saw it (the vomiting) as an enemy and hated every minute of it." It appeared that E. J. was in conflict over complete elimination of these dreaded symptoms and was resisting the posthypnotic suggestions of "having a comfortable and pleasant evening" following chemotherapy administration. Having recently returned from training with Dr. Milton Erickson, I decided to try an alternative posthypnotic suggestion that worked with the symptom rather than against it (Erickson, 1970; 1976). Just before E. J. came out of the hypnotic state, I suggested that "soon after you arrive home you might want to choose your time and place and vomit for five minutes . . . you can time the vomiting on your watch to insure that you vomit for five whole minutes . . . and don't just vomit . . . really do it well . . . so that you get in all of the vomiting you need to have in five minutes . . . so that you can enjoy the remainder of the evening." The following day E. J. arrived at my office with a grin saying "you are not going to believe what happened last night! My dad and I were watching television, when I remembered that I was supposed to vomit. When I told my dad that Dr. Zeltzer suggested I do this, he thought you and I were both crazy! Well, it is really hard to vomit when you try to! I worked and worked at it . . . man, five minutes can sure be a long time! But, later that night I not only had no vomiting but no nausea either . . . I felt as if I had won a battle!"

E. J.'s outlook seemed to change during the eight months we worked together. He seemed to feel better about himself. He appeared more assured and self-confident. He described feelings of being "in control" and felt the hypnosis had helped him deal with family problems. Despite a parental divorce, ongoing family conflict, and his not feeling very wanted in either parental household, E. J. felt strong and good about himself. Since his initial diagnosis two and one-half years earlier, neither parent had participated in his treatment, and he had always come to the clinic alone. E. J. felt that his skill with self-hypnosis gave him the extra strength and self-confidence to handle his treatments and to comply with his chemotherapy, and felt that the hypnosis helped him believe in himself. He is now looking forward to the promised completion of his chemotherapy, celebrating the third year of his remission.

THE DYING ADOLESCENT

Because the terms "cancer" or "leukemia" are emotionally laden and to some synonomous with "early death," the adolescent with such a diagnosis is often well aware of his own potential premature demise. In fact, chronically ill adolescents, in general, are more preoccupied with death and dying in themselves and in others than are adolescents without illness (Raimbault, 1969). For most adolescents with cancer, in order to be able to function, the "modus operandi" is the use of the defense mechanism of denial. They receive further support for denial from their well-being during remissions and between courses of chemotherapy. However, the anxieties and fears around dying often resurface during relapses or with the occurrence of some unexpected event or upon learning of the death of a sick peer, especially one with the same disease. Normal coping may temporarily break down and anxieties may be expressed through a variety of behaviors (Abrams, 1966). These adolescents may become irritable without obvious reason. They may become over-cooperative so that the staff will not abandon them. Their symptoms may intensify and become unbearable. Hospitalized adolescents may ring repeatedly for the nurse with numerous complaints or with concerns for their roommates, as the following case illustrates.

> A hospitalized fourteen-year-old boy with Stage IV Hodgkin's disease, who had been fairly quiet and withdrawn, startled a nurse who had entered the room to answer his roommate's buzzer by screaming profanities at her. He accused the nurse of taking "too long" to answer the call and shouted that his roommate "could have died" waiting for the nurse to come.

As in the above case, fears of dying may be manifest in concerns for a peer and in worries over abandonment. The young man above may have wanted reassurance from the nurse that if *he* needed her, she would be there and he would not be left alone, i.e., when he dies.

Most adolescents (probably all) who are in fact dying know that they are dying whether or not they verbalize their feelings. Physicians often have difficulty acknowledging this shared knowledge with their patients because of the doctor's defenses of denial or detachment or perhaps because the doctors just do not quite know what to say. However, the physician's directness may be important for the adolescent to feel understood and to be able to trust the medical staff. The following case demonstrates the importance of being clear and not circuitous in response to the adolescent's question, "am I going to die from this disease?"

> A thirteen-year-old girl with recently diagnosed acute lymphocytic leukemia asked her doctor the above question to which he responded, "I don't know. Anybody can die from anything. I could die tomorrow from something." Two weeks later she had a nightmare in which she was back in the hospital surrounded by the doctors who were treating her, and they were telling her she was going to die. After the dream she awoke and her mother gave her a tranquilizer and told her to go back to sleep. There was no further discussion until, one week after the dream, she reported her experience to the psychologist in the hematology clinic. He responded to her by saying, "Some children die from what you have. The kind of leukemia you have is fairly easy to treat and you can live a normal, long and healthy life." She gave a sigh of relief and then said, "I'd never forgive myself if I gave leukemia to my children." (case history courtesy of J. Dash).

The dying adolescent creates a need for peer support among physicians (Krant, 1972). The dying child is often avoided, with guilt feelings in the physician escalating after the patient's death (Smith, 1969; Easson, 1968). A study of the attitudes of pediatricians toward the care of fatally ill children found that physicians with the least experience most often avoided discussions of disease and prognosis with parents and patients (Weiner, 1970). In the same study, most pediatricians believed that children should seldom or never be given accurate answers about the seriousness of the illness, even when questions were directly raised by the child. However, 70 percent believed that children knew or suspected the diagnosis even if not directly told. The physician's own anxieties about death and dying may obstruct optimal patient care (Rothenberg, 1967). In fact, compared with other professionals, physicians have increased fears of death and may choose their career as a way of dealing with these fears (Feifel, 1963; Feifel, 1967).

How the adolescent reacts to his anticipated death often depends on how he has coped with his illness, how he feels about himself, how much support he has received throughout the course of his illness, and how much support is available during the period preceding death (Zeltzer, 1978a). The dying adolescent may try to hold on to reality and maintain clarity by resisting analgesics, especially those which might affect mentation. He or she may feel helpless and fear abandonment. The adolescent needs to be with people who are important to him. He wants to know that he has contributed in some way and that his life has been worthwhile. During this time, discussions of previous praiseworthy behavior may be very supportive and may be crucial in assisting the adolescent to "die with dignity."

> A thirteen-year-old young man with Wilms' tumor, whose large pulmonary metastatic lesion was choking him by external pressure on his trachea, had been sitting up in bed in constant anxiety, with his eyes wide open and unable to speak. Most of the comments and questions to him from the medical staff centered on his level of comfort and need for analgesics. A curious thing happened after I visited J. B. and expressed my appreciation for the significant contributions he had made during previous "rap groups" on the adolescent ward. I described to him the valuable ways in which he had helped various patients feel better. He smiled and for the first time seemed truly relaxed. He squeezed my hand, then closed his eyes and fell asleep. He died that night.

The dying adolescent needs a positive sense of self-worth and connectedness with those around him.

THE PHYSICIAN/ADOLESCENT PATIENT RELATIONSHIP

It is important to realize that the way in which physicians, families, peers, and others perceive the adolescent with cancer may determine the extent of the disability which the adolescent experiences (Zeltzer, 1978a). Hyman (1971) found that experienced preferential treatment by others may produce more disability than that which is produced by the illness. The onset of illness triggers a social process which shapes the adolescent's response to his ailment. The more severe the ailment, the more likely it is that the adolescent will begin to receive preferential treatment from physician, family, and peers. Certainly, a diagnosis of "cancer" elicits anxiety and may set this process into action. In turn, this special treatment affects the adolescent's self-concept as a limited, disabled person. The perception of the adolescent becomes a self-fulfilling prophecy for how that adolescent then sees himself or herself and acts.

The goal of a good physician/patient relationship then is to provide optimal medical care while promoting normal, healthy growth and development in the adolescent and reducing iatrogenic disability. The physician's ability to help the patient depends on knowledge of the disease process, the adolescent psychosocial process, and their inter-relationships.

Physicians who care for adolescents may face some difficulties. Specific patients and their parents may reactivate unresolved conflicts persisting from the physician's own adolescence, thereby influencing the physician's behavior with those patients (Zeltzer, 1975). For example, a physician whose own mother was overprotective might react in a hostile manner to a similar mother of an adolescent patient and then push the patient into more independent activities than those which the adolescent might be ready to assume. The older physician's adolescent patients may remind him of his own teenage sons or daughters. The young physician may strongly identify with the adolescent patient, especially in instances where the latter is working on developmental issues not yet completed by the former. For example, a young rebellious house officer might overidentify with and "take the side of" an adolescent patient who is refusing treatment as a control issue. The house officer might then become angry with the patient's attending physician who is seen as the "bad parent." These older and younger physicians may become angry and easily frustrated in caring for the testing, confrontive, rebellious adolescent or the depressed and withdrawn patient because they would not like to see these traits in their own sons or daughters or in themselves (Zeltzer, 1975).

Training of physicians may further hinder successful physician/patient interaction (Rothenberg, 1974). The medical model often promotes an authoritarian/dependent relationship where the doctor makes a diagnosis, prescribes a treatment plan, and expects the patient to carry out this plan. As discussed in a previous section, the adolescent process does not allow for such rigid roles for doctor and patient. If the adolescent does not follow the doctor's orders, the physician may react to the noncompliance as an affront to his effort and care and become frustrated and angry with his patient. The physician can easily get caught in a power struggle with the adolescent in which the latter is seen as manipulative with the former becoming punitive in response. Ultimately, both the physician and the adolescent "lose" this type of battle. The physician's energies are sapped and the adolescent either "loses" the struggle with further feelings of loss of control and inferiority or "wins" the struggle and dies.

A physician caring for adolescents with cancer must be willing to examine his/her own behaviors and feelings so that these do not interfere with optimal patient care. Physicians may become uncomfortable when patients ask sex-related questions and have been shown to use many avoidance techniques, such as ignoring the question, changing the subject, or actually leaving the patient's bedside under the pretext of "being busy" (Withersty, 1976).

Most ill adolescents want a physician who is open, honest, and non-judgmental. They want their doctors to show respect for them, listen to what they have to say, and enlist their aid in formulating the treatment plans. Even when treatment involves fixed protocols, there are areas in which the adolescent can make decisions, e.g., what day to start, what time to come to clinic, etc. They want a doctor who empathizes rather than sympathizes with them, encourages a responsibility for self, and cares not only for their bodies but also for their feelings (Zeltzer, 1977). As a fourteen-year-old young lady with ALL explained, " . . . I know my doctor cares about my leukemia, but I don't think he really cares about me."

RESEARCH

There is little objective data on psychosocial aspects of adolescents with cancer. The few reports focusing on the adolescent are descriptive in nature (Brown, 1977; Kagen, 1976; "Case Conference," 1976). Several authors have focused their studies on the psychological effects of children and adolescents in protected environments (Kellerman, 1976a, b; 1977b; Kohle, 1971). As in the latter studies, most authors include a few adolescents in their studies of children with cancer. Objective investigation of issues specific to the adolescent with a malignancy are few and only recently begun (Zeltzer, 1978b, 1979a, b).

If there is to be increased research focus on the adolescent, the question is one of direction of that research effort. Several studies have suggested that physical symptoms in the adolescent may be prime deterrents to adolescent development (Adsett, 1963; Meissner, 1967; Vernik, 1965; Moore, 1969; Easson, 1968; Zeltzer, 1978b, 1979a, b) and may even be a cause for suicide (Weinberg, 1970). As the adolescent is struggling for control over himself and his environment, continued discomfort may cause the adolescent to feel that he is losing control. This feeling may then lead to a chronic anxiety state and produce behaviors that are countertherapeutic. Treatment regimens may not be followed, pain may be experienced as intolerable, and vomiting may occur before the chemotherapeutic agent is even administered. Even the most understanding and psychotherapeutically oriented physician may be unable to assist the adolescent with cancer to cope with anxiety, pain, nausea, or vomiting after medical management has failed to alleviate these symptoms. In a study comparing the rated responses of thirty randomly selected adolescent oncology patients to that of thirty adolescents each in five different chronic illness subspecialty categories on an "impact of illness" questionnaire, the first group reported more intensely (p <.01) than any other group on all items that related to treatments for illness interfering with life and being worse than the disease (Zeltzer, 1979a).

Therefore, the research problem is one of evaluating ways of overcoming the limitations of the existing medical therapy for discomfort in adolescents with cancer. Additionally, the adolescent process, involving self-determination and independence, calls for researchers to investigate behavioral methods that allow the adolescent to feel a sense of control and mastery over these discomforts rather than finding new and better antiemetics, tranquilizers, and analgesics. There are studies of behavior control of acute and chronic pain (see self-help section) including LaBaw's (1975) clinical report of hypnosis with children and adolescents, although none investigates general discomfort control specifically in adolescents. J. Hilgard (1978) is completing an investigation of the use of hypnosis for pain-relief during bone marrow aspirations in children and adolescents, and K. Olness (1978) is gathering clinical observations on her use of hypnosis in young oncology patients. This dearth of objective information on hypnosis as a self-help modality specifically for adolescent oncology patients led us to our own research program.

The "Adolescent Self-Help Project" at Childrens Hospital of Los Angeles is a three-year study of the effectiveness of self-hypnosis on pain, nausea, and vomiting in adolescents with malignant disease (Kellerman, J.; Zeltzer, L.; Dash, J.; Ellenberg, L.; Rigler, D.: Effectiveness of self-hypnosis for control of pain, nausea, and vomiting in adolescents with cancer. American Cancer Society, California Division (Macomber Foundation) #C-141.) The project goal is to teach adolescents with cancer self-help skills to become more comfortable during procedures and chemotherapy. In operational terms, the goals are as follows:

1. Reduction in amounts and frequency of analgesics, antiemetics, and tranquilizers.
2. Reduction of noncompliance as a result of intolerable symptoms or as an adolescent control issue.
3. Reduction in illness- and treatment-related anxiety.
4. Enhancement of feelings of self-control and facilitation of normal adolescent development.

The subjects in the study are adolescents with cancer, ages twelve–twenty-one years, who are referred to the project by their physicians or by self-referral for problems of nausea, vomiting, chronic pain, or acute pain or anxiety related to treatments or procedures. Each subject is given a pretest battery of measurements of trait-anxiety, self-esteem, health locus of control, and impact of illness. This latter test was devised by us to evaluate the adolescent's perception of the impact of his or her illness on the developmental tasks of adolescence. We have standardized this test with other adolescent chronic illness groups and with healthy adolescents. This test is also administered to the adolescent's parents to evaluate differences between parental and adolescent perceptions of health/disease-related issues. The adolescent is asked to self-record his or her symptoms and medications through one course of chemotherapy as a baseline before hypnosis training is begun. We are using each adolescent as his or her own control and are following self-ratings, nurse-observer ratings, medications, and changes in the four objective measurements in relation to hypnosis training, disease process, and medical therapy over time. We are following each adolescent for at least a one-year period, using an analysis of variance to analyze the data for within-subject comparisons. After one year of the operation of the study, the clinical progress of the sixteen adolescents involved in the study to date has been very promising, with preliminary review of data demonstrating reduction of symptoms during procedures and chemotherapy.

A move of the study's principal investigator to Texas allowed for the same study to be undertaken collaboratively at the Children's Cancer Center in The University of Texas Health Science Center at San Antonio. This latter study has accrued fifteen adolescents during the four months since its conception and has found preliminarily the same changes during treatments as that in the Los Angeles study, allowing for more generalizability of the results. A longitudinal five-year study of self-hypnosis for adolescents with cancer is presently planned in San Antonio with an "equal support time but no hypnosis training" control group.

The projects in Los Angeles and San Antonio represent a beginning in objective measurements of behavioral methods for self-control of disabling symptoms in adolescents with cancer. Objective data is still needed in the areas of adolescent and family adaptation to the disease and its treatments and in the area of the effects of cancer and its therapy on pubescence and future reproductivity.

SUMMARY

Teenagers with cancer are faced with the same crises of puberty and adolescence as are their healthy peers. However, their disease and its treatments may impose special problems that affect their body image, self-esteem, socialization, sexuality, and future-planning. Despite the label of "cancer," most adolescents with this diagnosis cope remarkably well. A variety of adaptive and maladaptive responses of the adolescent with cancer has been presented. The issue of self-help has been a focus of this chapter because it is a pathway for adolescents to grow despite continued need for reliance upon hospitals and doctors. Even during the dying process, adolescents need to feel a sense of self-worth and respect from others. Because physicians are trained to focus on pathology, the adolescent person inside the "sick body" may be overlooked.

Behavioral research thus must include objective studies of methods that enhance adolescent adaptation to treatments and promote self-growth. If the adolescent with cancer feels trusted and valued by significant others, he or she will be able to utilize both the experiences surrounding the disease and the physician/patient relationship as building blocks in the path toward adulthood.

REFERENCES

Abrams, R. D.: The patient with cancer — his changing pattern of communication. *N Engl J Med, 274:*317, 1966.

Adsett, C. A.: Emotional reactions to disfigurement from cancer therapy. *Can Med Assoc J, 89:*385, 1963.

Andreychuk, T. and Skriver, C.: Hypnosis and biofeedback in the treatment of migraine headache. *Int J Clin Exp Hypn, 23:*172, 1975.

Beard, B. H.: Fear of death and fear of life: The dilemma in chronic renal failure, hemodialysis, and kidney transplantation. *Arch Gen Psychiatry, 21:*373, 1969.

Becker, R. D.: Therapeutic approaches to psychopathological reactions to hospitalization. *Int J Child Psychotherapy, 1:*65, 1972.

Bergin, A. E. and Suinn, R. M.: Individual psychotherapy and behavior therapy. *Ann Rev Psychology, 26:*509, 1975.

Boyle, I. R.; di Sant' Agnese, P. A.; Sack, S.; et al.: Emotional adjustment of adolescents and young adults with cystic fibrosis. *J Pediatr, 88:*318, 1976.

Brown, A. and Bjelic, J.: Coping strategies of two adolescents with malignancy. *Matern Child Nurs, 6:*77, 1977.

Carron, H.: The management of cancer pain. *Va Med Mon, 104:*643, 1975.

Crasilneck, H. B. and Hall, J. A.: Clinical hypnosis in problems of pain. *Am J Clin Hypn, 15:*161, 1973.

Cruickshank, W. M.: The effect of physical disability on personal aspiration. *Q J Child Behav, 3:*323, 1951.

Easson, W. M.: Care of the young patient who is dying. *JAMA, 205:*203, 1968.

Edmeads, J.: Management of the acute attack of migraine. *Headache, 13:*91, 1973.

Erickson, M. H.: Hypnosis: Its renascence as a treatment modality. *Am J Clin Hypn, 13:*71, 1970.

Erickson, M. H.: Hypnosis in painful terminal illness. *Am J Clin Hypn, 1:*117, 1959.

Erickson, M. H.; Rossi, E. L.; and Rossi, S. I.: *Hypnotic Realities.* New York, Irvington Publishers, 1976.

Feifel, H.: in Faberow, N. L.: *Death in Taboo Topics.* New York, Atherton Press, 1963.

Feifel, H.; Hanson, S.; Jones, R.; and Edwards, L.: Physicians consider death. Proceedings, 75th Annual Convention, Am. Psychol. Assoc., 201, 1967.

Futterman, E. H. and Hoffman, I.: Transient school phobia in a leukemic child. *J Am Acad Child Psychiatry, 9:*477, 1970.

Graham, G. W.: Hypnotic treatment for migraine headaches. *Int J Clin Hypn, 23:*165, 1975.

Hilgard, J.: Manuscript in preparation, 1978.

Himmelhoch, J. M.; Davies, R. K.; Tucker, G. J.; and Alderman, D.: Butting heads: Patients who refuse necessary procedures. *Psychiatry Med, 1:*241, 1970.

Hofmann, A. D. and Becker, R. D.: Psychotherapeutic approaches to the physically ill adolescent. *Int J Child Psychotherapy, 2:*492, 1973.

Hyman M. D.: Disability and patients' perceptions of preferential treatment: Some preliminary findings. *J Chronic Dis, 24:*329, 1971.

Kagen, L. B.: Use of denial in adolescents with bone cancer. *Health Soc Work, 1:*70, 1976.

Katz, E. R.; Kellerman, J.; Rigler, D.; Williams, K. O.; and Siegel, S. E.: School intervention with pediatric cancer patients. *J Pediatr Psychology, 2:*72, 1977.

Kaufman, R. V.: Body-image changes in physically ill teen-agers. *J Am Acad Child Psychiatry, 11:*157, 1972.

Kaufman, R. V. and Hersher, B.: Body-image changes in teen-age diabetics. *Pediatr, 48:*123, 1971.

Kellerman, J. and Katz, E. R.: The adolescent with cancer: Theoretical, clinical and research issues. *J Pediatr Psychology, 2:*127, 1977a.

Kellerman, J.; Katz, E. R.; and Siegel, S. E.: Psychological problems of children with cancer, unpublished manuscript, 1979.

Kellerman, J.; Rigler, D.; and Siegel, S. E.: The psychological effects of isolation in protected environments. *Am J Psychiatry, 134:*563, 1977b.

Kellerman, J.; Rigler, D.; Siegel, S. E.; McCue, K.; Pospisil, J.; and Uno, R.: Pediatric cancer patients in reverse isolation utilizing protected environments. *J Pediatr Psychology, 1:*21, 1976a.

Kellerman, J.; Rigler, D.; Siegel, S. E.; McCue, K.; Pospisil, J.; and Uno, R.: Psychological evaluation and management of pediatric oncology patients in protected environments. *Med Pediatr Oncol, 2:*353, 1976b.

Knox, V. J.; Morgan, A. H.; and Hilgard, E. R.: Pain and suffering in ischemia. *Arch Gen Psychiatry, 30:*840, 1974.

Kohle, K.; Simons, C.; Weidlich, S.; Dietrich, M.; and Durner, A.: Psychological aspects in the treatment of leukemia patients in the isolated-bed system "life island." *Psychother Psychosom, 19:*85, 1971.

Krant, M. J.: The organized care of the dying patient. *Hosp Practice, 7:*101, 1972.

LaBaw, W.; Holton, C.; Tewell, K.; and Eccles, D.: The use of self-hypnosis by children with cancer. *Am J Clin Hypn, 17:*233, 1974.

Lansky, S. B.; Lowman, J. T.; Vats, T.; and Gyulay, J.: School phobia in children with malignant neoplasms. *Am J Dis Child, 129:*42, 1975.

Li, F. P. and Jaffe, N.: Progeny of childhood-cancer survivors. *Lancet, 2:*707, 1974.

Li, F. P. and Stone, R.: Survivors of cancer in childhood. *Ann Intern Med, 84:*551, 1976.

Meissner, A. L.; Thoreson, R. W.; and Butler, A. J.: Relation of self-concept to impact and obviousness of disability among male and female adolescents. *Percept Mot Skills, 24:*1099, 1967.

Melzack, R. and Perry, C.: Self-regulation of pain: The use of alphafeedback and hypnotic training for the control of chronic pain. *Experimental Neurology, 46:*452, 1975.

Moore, D.; Holton, C.; and Marten, G.: Psychologic problems in the management of adolescents with malignancy. *Clin Pediatr, 8:*464, 1969.

Nathan, S.: Body-image in chronically obese children as reflected in figure drawings. *J Pers Assess, 37:*456, 1973.

Olness, K.: Personal communication, 1978.

Peper, E. and Grossman, E. R.: Thermal biofeedback training in children with headache. Presented in part at the Biofeedback Research Society Meetings, Colorado Springs, Colorado, February 15-20, 1974.

Raimbault, G. and Royer, P.: L'enfant et son image de la maladie. *Arch Fr Pediatr, 24:*445, 1967.

Raimbault, G. and Royer, P.: Thématique de la mort chez l'enfant atteint de maladie chronique. *Arch Fr Pediatr, 26:*1041, 1969.

Retreat from death? Case Conference, *J Med Ethics, 2:*200, 1976.

Rothenberg, M. B.: Reactions of those who treat children with cancer. *Pediatr, 40:*507, 1967.

Rothenberg, M. B.: The unholy trinity — activity, authority, and magic. *Clin Pediatr, 13:*870, 1974.

Sargent, J. D.; Walters, E. D.; and Green, E. E.: Psychosomatic self-regulations of migraine headaches. *Seminars in Psychiatry, 5:*415, 1973.

Schafer, D. W.: Hypnosis use on a burn unit. *Inter J Clin Exp Hypn, 23:*1, 1975.

Schonfeld, W. A.: Body-image in adolescents: A psychiatric concept for the pediatrician. *Pediatr, 31:*845, 1963.

Schowalter, J. E.; Ferholt, J. B.; and Mann, N. M.: The adolescent patient's decision to die. *Pediatr, 51:*97, 1973.

Siris, E. S.; Leventhal, B. C.; and Vaitukaitis, J. L.: Effects of childhood leukemia and chemotherapy on puberty and reproductive function in girls. *N Engl J Med, 294:*1143, 1976.

Smith, A. G. and Schneider, L. T.: The dying child. *Clin Pediatr, 8:*131, 1969.

Swift, C. R.; Seidman, F.; and Stein, H.: Adjustment problems in juvenile diabetes. *Psychosom Med, 29:*555, 1967.

Vernik, J. and Karon, M.: Who's afraid of death on a leukemia ward? *Am J Dis Child, 105:*393, 1965.

Visotsky, H. M.; Hamburg, D. A.; Gross, M. E.; and Lebovits, B. Z.: Coping behavior under extreme stress. *Arch Gen Psychiatry, 5:*27, 1961.

Weber, E. S. P.: Autogenic training and EEG biofeedback training in coronary heart disease. *J Med Soc N J, 71:*927, 1974.

Weinberg, S.: Suicidal intent in adolescence: A hypothesis about the role of physical illness. *J Pediatr, 77:*579, 1970.

Weiner, J. M.: Attitudes of pediatricians toward the care of fatally ill children. *J Pediatr, 76:*700, 1970.

Withersty, D. J.: Sexual attitudes of hospital personnel: A model for continuing education. *Am J Psychiatry, 133:*573, 1976.

Zeltzer, L.: Crisis-intervention groups on an adolescent medical inpatient unit. Unpublished data, 1977.

Zeltzer, L.; Zeltzer, P.; and Comerci, G.: An audio-visual technique for self-instruction of principles of adolescent medicine. Abstract, *Acta Paediatr Scan, Suppl, 256:*266, 1975.

Zeltzer, L.: Chronic illness in the adolescent. *in:* Shenker, I. R.: *Topics in Adolescent Medicine.* New York, Stratton Intercontinental Medical Book Corp., 1978a.

Zeltzer, L. K.; Kellerman, J.; Ellenberg, L.; Dash, J.; and Rigler, D.: Self-help training for chronically ill adolescents. Presented at the Society for Adolescent Medicine — American College Health Association Spring Meeting. New Orleans, Louisiana. March, 1978b.

Zeltzer, L. K.: Hypnosis with adolescents. Workshop for Society for Adolescent Medicine — American Academy of Pediatrics, Fall Meeting, Chicago, October, 1978c.

Zeltzer, L.; Kellerman, J.; Ellenberg, L.; Dash, J.; and Rigler, D.: Objective identification of illness impact, experienced disease control, and self-concept in adolescents with cancer and other chronic diseases: Implications for health care delivery. Presented at Southern Society for Pediatric Research, January, 1979, New Orleans, Louisiana.

Zeltzer, L. K.; Kalmowitz, J.; and Barbour, J.: Adolescents with cancer: Perceptions of disease and treatment through drawings. Unpublished data, 1979b.

Zeltzer, L. K.; Dash, J.; and Holland, J. P.: Hypnotically-induced pain control in sickle cell anemia. *Pediatrics, 64:*533-536, 1979c.

Chapter Five

TWO FAMILIES: AN INTENSIVE OBSERVATIONAL STUDY*

HELEN DESMOND

IN THE STUDY of the psychological impact of childhood cancer upon the family research is necessarily a complex process which must accommodate many individual and interactive factors. Binger (1973a) lists: personality structure; past experiences; current adjustments; and the special meaning that the threatened loss has for the individual in particular, as relevant considerations in understanding each person's reaction to loss. In addition, he underscores the necessity of viewing the individual within the family context. Such a perspective includes the added dimension of viewing the individual as acting upon, and acted upon by other persons living within the compelling forces of a family system.

Such complexity presents an imposing challenge to clinicians and researchers. The existing literature on the psychological impact of childhood cancer on the family contains confusing and contradictory findings. Many authors report that the death of a child has long-lasting pathological effects on the family, especially the siblings (Bender, 1954; Binger, 1973a, 1973b; Binger, Ablin, Feuerstein, Kushner, Zoger, & Mikkelsen, 1969; Cain & Cain, 1964; Cain, Fast, & Erickson, 1964; Kaplan, Smith, & Grobstein, 1972, 1973; Kliman, 1969; Lansky & Lowman, 1974; O'Malley, 1977; Moriarity, 1967; Rosenblatt, 1967, 1969; and Tooley, 1974). Others (Chodoff, Friedman, & Hamburg, 1964; Fergusson, 1976; Futterman & Hoffman, 1970, 1973; Futterman, Hoffman, & Sabshin, 1972; and Stehbens & Lascari, 1974) have challenged this position, and Santostefano (1967) holds that the stress of early loss in childhood, if mastered, may be growth fostering. It was

*This chapter is based upon portions of a dissertation submitted by the author to the California School of Professional Psychology at Los Angeles. The research was supported in part by a doctoral training fellowship awarded through the Division of Hematology-Oncology, Childrens Hospital of Los Angeles (Clinical Cancer Training Grant 5T12 CA 08128-08, National Cancer Institute, National Institutes of Health).

The author wishes to thank: the medical and clinical staff of Childrens Hospital of Los Angeles for their support of the original research project; Gregg Furth, William Partridge, and Glen Roberts for their assistance with portions of the data analysis; and David Rigler, Zanwil Sperber, John Spinetta, and Alastair Stunden for their encouragement and very helpful suggestions throughout the original project.

my belief that many apparently discrepant findings in the existing literature might be discovered to have explanations consistent with one another if the impact of the illness was studied in conjunction with individual and family character and coping styles. The resulting intensive study of two families was exploratory in nature and as such its emphasis was discovery rather than proof.

In 1957 when Bruno Bettelheim asked Jules Henry to study families of some psychotic children by living in their homes, Henry welcomed the opportunity because, in his words:

> For many years it had been my conviction that the etiology of emotional illness required more profound study than had heretofore been possible and that the best way to new discoveries in the field was through study of the disease-bearing vector, the family, in its natural habitat, pursuing its usual life routines — eating, loving, fighting, talking, taking amusements, treating sickness, and so on — in other words, following the usual course of its life . . . (1967, p. 31).

Likewise, Anthony (1970) and Bermann (1973) found the study of families in their own homes particularly revealing.

Because I wished to acquire as complete an understanding as was possible of the impact of childhood cancer on each member of the family, like Henry (1965, 1967), Anthony (1970), and Bermann (1973), I chose naturalistic observation as my method of study. While Henry (1967) effectively answers objections about the distorting effects of the observer on family interaction, to my knowledge there is not a research methodology developed which yields all there is to know about a phenomenon and does not in some way change the phenomenon under study. Consequently, I relied upon the convergence of information from several methodological sources in attempting to understand this problem. Naturalistic observation in the home was augmented by projective and objective assessments, formal and informal interviews, and a review of the medical records.

BOWLBY'S ATTACHMENT THEORY

Childhood cancer is a potentially fatal disease and diagnosis of the child forces upon the parents a profound confrontation with death. In those cultures with highly advanced medical technologies and low child mortality rates this confrontation is all the more unexpected and incomprehensible. Further, the threatened loss of the child is often accompanied by many actual separations and losses.

The physical limitations imposed on the sick child by the illness force upon siblings the loss of a playmate and companion. If the sick child is hospitalized as is often necessary, this loss is intensified. The mother's and father's physical presence to the siblings is greatly reduced by the demands of caring for the ill child, transporting the child for medical care, and/or visiting in the hospital. But perhaps most important is the emotional loss that each member of the family undergoes. The parents, while suddenly confronted with the catastrophic awareness that the life of one of their children is gravely endangered, and faced with greatly increased physical demands upon them, have fewer emotional resources to devote to their well children. The knowledge that one of their children has a fatal illness relentlessly erodes the parents' own feelings of immortality and their role as protectors of their child (Wallace, 1967). Such awareness places an immense stress on their relationships to each other and to their children.

Because the diagnosis of cancer in a child threatens to disrupt the established relational bonds within the family, Bowlby's attachment theory, a comprehensive treatment of relational bonds, was chosen as the theoretical foundation of this study. According to Bowlby human beings display a propensity toward establishing strong affectional bonds with particular others. An important feature of attachment theory is its contention that many of the most intense emotions arise during the formation, maintenance, disruption, and renewal of attachment relationships. Unwilling separation and loss give rise to many forms of emotional distress and disturbance, including anxiety, anger, and despair (Bowlby, 1969, 1973, 1975). Bowlby defines attachment behavior as any form of behavior that results in a person attaining or retaining proximity to some other differentiated and preferred individual. Clinging, crying, calling, greeting, smiling, protests over separations, and anger over an attachment figure's failure to meet an individual's demands are all examples of attachment behavior.

Bowlby and Parkes (1970) state that attachment behavior is elicited whenever a person (child or adult) is sick or in trouble, and is elicited at high intensity during fright or during times when the attachment figure cannot be found. Attachment behavior is regarded as a normal and healthy part of human instinctive makeup. The authors hold that anger at unwilling separation can serve adaptive purposes, and they state that the frequency with which anger occurs as part of normal mourning has been habitually underestimated. They further state that strong affectional bonds can be relinquished only gradually and after the expression of much yearning, anger, and sadness. These theoretical speculations provided a general frame of reference for me as I observed the people in the two families of this study. While I tried to remain open to observation of all aspects of their lives and interactions, this theory led me to be particularly attentive to manifestations of attachment behavior and expressions (direct or indirect) of anger and anxiety. Naturally I was also interested in any family conversations and communications about illness, loss, or death.

METHOD

The Families

The individuals who took part in this research were the members of two families of children with cancer under treatment at Childrens Hospital of Los Angeles. Families meeting the following criteria were approached for participation in the study:

1. A child under sixteen years of age had been diagnosed with cancer within the preceding two or three weeks
2. Both parents were living in the home
3. One or more siblings over six years of age were present in the home
4. English was spoken in the home

Initially, three families meeting the above criteria were approached for participation. They were informed that I was studying families in which a child had cancer, that participation in the study was voluntary, and that refusal had no effect on the child's treatment. Two of the first three families approached agreed to participate.

The patient in one family was a fifteen-year-old boy with two younger brothers ages ten and five years. The patient in the other family was an eight-year-old girl with a seven-year-old brother. These families will be pseudonymously referred to as the Deacon and Tandem families respectively (see Chart A). In each of these families the ill child was diagnosed with acute lymphocytic leukemia. Teresa Tandem died five months after her diagnosis and Brian Deacon was in his first remission at the time of the last research visit.

CHART A
COMPOSITION OF RESEARCH FAMILIES

Deacon Family		
Father:	Patrick	38 yrs.
Mother:	Mary	38 yrs.
Patient:	Brian	15 yrs.
Sibling:	Timothy	10 yrs.
Sibling:	Robert	6 yrs.
Tandem Family		
Father:	Charles	41 yrs.
Mother:	Carol	33 yrs.
Patient:	Teresa	8 yrs.
Sibling:	Tom	7 yrs.

Procedure

Home observation visits of about one and one-half hours in duration took place on a weekly basis for approximately ten weeks. Most of these visits were scheduled around the dinner hour, but samplings of other times during the day were also included. Family members were requested to behave as they would if I were not present. Audiotape recordings of family conversation and written behavioral observations were made during these visits.

Individual and conjoint family history interviews were conducted with the parents. Assessments were administered to each person in the family shortly after the initial diagnosis and again approximately eight weeks later. On both occasions the same instruments were administered to each person in the family. The Spinetta three dimensional doll test, the Roberts' Apperception Test, and Kinetic Family Drawings.

In order to measure indirectly concern about death and the seriousness of the illness, Spinetta designed a three-dimensional replica of a hospital room with a steel floor marked off in squares (Spinetta, Rigler, & Karon, 1973, 1974; Spinetta & Maloney, 1975). In this test individuals are presented with magnetized dolls representing meaningful persons in their environment, e.g. family members, medical staff, and minister, and told to place the dolls in the room as they tell a story about a child who is sick and in the hospital. The distance of the placement of each of the dolls from the sick child in the hospital bed is recorded on a special page marked off in grids identical to the grids on the floor of the hospital room replica. The stories are recorded on tape and later transcribed and scored. The content of the stories is scored for themes of: (1) separation, loneliness or isolation imagery; (2) imagery relating to intrusion into body integrity and functioning, or mutilation; (3) death imagery; (4) present negative affective state; (5) negative anticipatory goal state; and (6) denial or wish fulfillment.

Like the Thematic Apperception Test (TAT), the Roberts' Apperception Test (RAT) consists of presenting an individual with cards containing sketches and requesting that the person make up a story about what is seen in the picture. In discussing the TAT, Cronbach (1970) states that the responses are dictated by the constructs, experiences, conflicts, and wishes of the individual telling the story. This type of test then, is a good source of information about an individual's intrapsychic functioning. The sketches on the RAT cards represent family scenes and consequently also pull for information on how individuals see their position within the family.

The first fifteen cards from the RAT were presented to all family members on two occasions. An exception was made to the usual presentation of the card portraying a child sitting up in bed. Rather than present a card portraying a child of the same sex as the individual taking the test, I presented family members with the card portraying a child of the same sex as the patient in the family. This was done in order to pull for any thoughts and feelings about the ill child.

The transcribed story to each card was read for the purpose of identifying three types of general responses: clinical indicators, support statements, and resolution statements. In most cases there was more than one clinical indicator in the story to the individual card. An example of such a story is one in which the individual might say that the boy is afraid (anxiety) because the father is mad (aggression), and the boy gets spanked (punishment) which makes the mother sad (depression). Responses were also scored in terms of the relationship portrayed in the response. For example, the statement "His father hugged him" would be scored support-father. A detailed account of how this test was scored can be found in the original report of this study (Desmond, 1977).

The Kinetic Family Drawing test was included in this research because family drawings have been identified as a useful source of information about how the individual perceives his family and his interaction with the members of his family (Hulse, 1951, 1952). Burns and Kaufman (1970, 1972) developed a method of asking children to draw the members of their family doing something. They felt that the addition of movement to the drawings would help mobilize feelings, both in regard to self-concept and in regard to interpersonal relations.

The guidelines of Bach (1969, 1974) for the somatic and psychological interpretation of drawings were followed in the analysis of the drawings. Bach's method was developed in conjunction with an interdisciplinary research study group at the University Neurosurgical Clinic, Zurich. Since 1951 this study group has analyzed 3500 drawings of 600 patients. Their procedure is to study the drawing, knowing only the age and sex of the drawer and whether the drawer is left-handed or right-handed or color-blind. The study group's findings regarding diagnosis, prognosis, and psychological and somatic condition of the patient are then compared to the extensive medical records available on the patient. Unfortunately, in spite of this extensive data base, in her monograph, Bach makes no reference to formal validation studies of her research.

Analysis of the Data

Results were presented in the form of core reports for each of the two families. These reports included: (1) a description of the family based upon interview material and observational notes; (2) results of the projective assessments; (3) analysis of the observational data.

Expert opinions were obtained for the analysis of the projective assessments. For the Spinetta Three Dimensional Doll test and the Roberts' Apperception test the originator of the test was consulted regarding scoring and interpretation of test results. A third expert, a psychologist nationally and internationally known for his work on the somatic and psychological interpretation of drawings of children with cancer, interpreted the Kinetic Family Drawings. He was presented all at once with the complete set of drawings from one family. The only information with which he was provided was the age and sex of the subject. The format for the presentation of the results of the projective assessments was a separate psychological report for each of the three procedures for each member of the family.

The typed transcripts of four tape recordings of family conversation for each family were analyzed in detail. This sample included the following home visits: two dinners; one Sunday lunch; and one weekday morning. The behavioral notes and tape transcript of the weekday morning visit included family conversation and activities from the time the children were awakened from sleep until they left for school.

Family conversation was examined from the perspective of rationally occurring units, or conversations, among people in the family rather than discrete communications between individuals (Chapple, 1970). An interactional unit, or event, was defined as a communication between two or more members of the family which began with an initiation and continued until the direction, or topic of conversation, was changed or until the conversation was terminated. Interactional units varied in length from two segments (an initiation and one response) to fifty-one segments (an initiation and fifty responses).

Each interactional unit was analyzed for the following information: initiator; object of initiation; participating personnel; intensity of interactional unit (total number of segments); and subject matter. The tallies of each of these categories were examined for patterns. Patterns as well as changes in patterns were the basis of statements made about family interaction.

"Normal" Families under Stress

Before embarking upon a discussion of the results of this study, it is important to stress that these families were "normal" families under severe stress. Further, they had the courage to allow a stranger equipped with a tape recorder and note pad to come into their homes and scrutinize their every behavior during the very difficult days and weeks shortly after learning of their child's diagnosis.

It is important to remember that the relationships and interactions which will be presented in the following pages with documentation to support the interpretation being made actually emerged after months of data analysis. The subjectivity of my own perceptions and emotional reactions was repeatedly brought home to me as I slowly worked my way through all the data. On the occasion of the observations those aspects of family interaction which touched personal issues for me evoked much stronger reactions on my part than others. With the analysis of the transcripts of the tape recordings it became apparent that there had been a precipitating event behind the interchange that so vividly impressed me at the time of the home visit. There were also many less obvious relationships that emerged with the analysis of the tapes. If it took a trained observer months of data analysis to uncover some of the relationships to be discussed, it should not be too difficult to imagine how far hidden they were from the participants.

Impact of the Observations on the Observer

Prior to initiating this study, I had had considerable experience visiting the homes of families with an ill member — frequently a terminally ill person. However, in these instances I had entered the home in a service capacity, as a representative of a home medical care team. It was a very different matter to enter the homes of these stressed families for the purpose of gathering the data for my doctoral thesis. Initially I experienced considerable conflict over feelings of "using" the suffering of the individuals in these families to get my degree. This conflict increased my concerns about creating additional burdens for these people.

As time passed and I saw how much the families wanted me to come more frequently, to stay longer, and to become more personally involved with them, my conflict had a different focus. I found myself struggling against urges to abandon research and professional restraints. I began to try to figure out ways "to help" the individuals in these families and at one point even considered extending the routine observation visits over a much longer time — perhaps a year or two. It was only with the insistent direction of advisers that I was able to keep some perspective on my involvement with these families.

The individuals in these two families had a profound impact on me. At times, blinded by the forgotten memories of my own past hurts and struggles and consequently unable to admit to the similarities between these individuals and myself, I left their homes angered and even enraged at what I had witnessed. I became very frustrated with the research restraints and desperately wanted to do something about what I perceived to be happening in the family. When I was able to admit to the similarity between my own vulnerability and foibles and those of the individuals in these families, I left their homes exhausted and deeply saddened by their pain. During these times it was no longer quite so clear what was most needed by these people. At those times when I was able to accept the loneliness and isolation in my own life I could recognize the love, caring, and humor in the lives of these families. While I sought throughout the course of this study to remain true to my scientific role, I am very aware that what I perceived, recorded, and reported has been colored by my own perspective on life and, most especially, on my own life.

Distorting Effect of the Observer's Presence Upon Family Interaction

Once I entered the homes of these families, I became incorporated at least to some degree into the family system. As a perceiving and feeling person my every action, reaction, nonaction, and nonreaction spoke in some way to the family members. Further, the individuals in both of these families formed relationships to me. After a couple of visits different family members, parents as well as children, wanted me to visit, eat, swim, camp, and stay overnight with them. Some addressed me as "Miss Desmond," some as "Helen" and some never directly addressed me. The person who transcribed the interview tapes commented on the "openly flirtatious" quality of one of the father's conversation during the family history interview.

While there is no question in my mind that my presence had a distorting effect on family interaction, I believe Henry's arguments regarding the relative importance of this distorting effect are quite germane (1967). Citing such factors as fixed action patterns, the inflexibility of personality structure, and the pressures toward habitual behavior exerted by the children in the home, he argues in essence that these effects will be minimal. He further adds that the assumption that the persons being observed will have the same understanding of the implications of their behavior as the observer is often not grounded in reality. In such cases the person being observed will not know which behaviors should be inhibited or concealed.

When asked whether or not my presence had any effect on family behavior Mrs. Deacon answered that her children did not "fuss" (argue and fight) as much when I was in the home. After the first dinner observation, when Mr. Tandem informed me that he would not be home on the day I was suggesting for my return, Mrs. Tandem, who was apparently unaware of his work schedule, started to angrily object, then looked at me and laughed self-consciously and never finished her sentence. Only a week before during the combined family history interview, Mrs. Tandem said: "Gee, by the time you observe us we'll know you really well and we won't hide anything — we'll even fight in front of you." Mr. and Mrs. Tandem never did fight in the observer's presence. Further, in each family, an incident occurred which indicated that, as the parents in these families readily admitted, during the research visits they were considerably curtailing their punishment of the children. Each of these incidents involved a situation where one of the children was given a single loud slap as a means of discipline.

Because both families curtailed their expression of anger in my presence, I am not confident that I obtained a clear understanding of the actual amount of anger and aggression, or the degree to which physical punishment as discipline, may have existed in these families as a relatively specific response to the diagnosis. Nonetheless, I also feel that the family's need to keep their expression of anger outside the observation periods is in itself information bearing on their ability to allow free expression of anger and aggression in response to the threatened disruption of an attachment bond. The projective protocols and interview transcripts are available sources of information on this subject. Consequently I hold that there is sufficient information to support the statements made in the following discussion.

MAJOR FINDINGS

One of the most important findings of this study was a clear demonstration of the necessity of understanding the particular character of a family prior to trying to understand the adaptation of that family to the crisis of childhood cancer. Understanding the individual family character is essential to research on stressed families, because defenses are frequently exacerbated during times of stress and the use of defense often includes distortions in perception and memory. While all four parents in the two families reported that their family was at least as "close" and as "happy" as most other families they knew, the initial projective assessments of all family members in both families contained considerable evidence of emotional isolation. Three of the four adults reported that the illness brought them and their spouse "closer together"; however, the second projective assessment of seven of the nine family members in the study evidenced markedly increased feelings of isolation. When the parents' statements about the illness drawing the family closer together are examined within the context of individual and family character the apparent contradiction between these findings disappears.

The Tandem Family

"Never too far away, but never too close" is the phrase which best describes the nature of the attachments in the Tandem family. The Tandems kept in close physical proximity to one another. They always ate dinner together, most of the time very crowded around a small kitchen table even though a larger table was available in the dining room. All family members participated in 40 percent of the interactional units during the two meals for which tapes were analyzed. They participated in several activities as a family. They went camping and to baseball games together. Both children were in a soccer league and the entire family attended all games. The evening Mr. Tandem was away on a bus trip Tom incessantly demanded his mother's attention.

In spite of this evidence of attachment behavior, relational bonds within the Tandem family were characterized by emotional isolation. Tom's attempts to engage his mother in play the evening Mr. Tandem was away were largely ignored by her. Only after he had persisted in calling her several times would she respond. Even though all family members frequently participated in the interactional units, the particular quality of the Tandem family interaction gave evidence of emotional isolation.

The television was continuously on during all of the research visits and, with the exception of conversation during those dinners the family ate in the kitchen, communication between family members either competed with, or was a commentary on, the programs on the television. Statements were frequently made to no one in particular. Questions and directions were frequently repeated, often more than once or twice, and a second person often began to respond before the first had finished talking. Sometimes both individuals repeated exactly what they had originally said, overlapping the second time as well. In one instance Mrs. Tandem told Tom to "go wash" ten times in rapid succession before he made a move to do it. Often I had the feeling that interactional segments were more like near-simultaneous parallel actions than interactions.

This combination of physical proximity and emotional isolation corresponded with the responses of both Mr. and Mrs. Tandem to the questions regarding their marriage relationship. Both stated that they were quite satisfied with the companionship they received from one another; both were not satisfied with the love and affection they received.

Themes of emotional isolation were pronounced in the projective assessments of all family members. Mr. Tandem's RAT stories contained few themes of support or resolution of the problem presented in the story. In spite of considerable improvement in his daughter's health, at the time of the second assessment, themes of separation and abandonment were markedly increased in Mr. Tandem's 3-D story. His spatial placement of the dolls representing family members indicated a growing sense of isolation. Compartmentalization, absent in his first KFD, appeared in his second KFD.

Mrs. Tandem's RAT stories portray the husband as minimally involved with the family. Her stories present the children as having no interaction with each other. One of her stories at the time of the second assessment is a poignant description of feelings of isolation. She ended this story about a family in which a child has died by saying: "Everybody is feeling bad, and they are all in their own feelings." "Hopefully they will come closer together in their feelings and comfort each other." Interestingly her first story (seven weeks earlier) to this card had been very similar with the exception of a slight but telling change in the ending. In that first story even though family members "are all kind of looking away from each other" in the end "they all comfort each other." Themes of isolation were also increased in Mrs. Tandem's second 3-D story. On both occasions Mrs. Tandem drew KFD's in which none of the figures were portrayed looking at or touching one another or participating in any kind of cooperative activity.

While Teresa's second series of RAT stories portray increased support from brother and friends, only one story portrayed the father giving support and no stories portray the mother as supportive. By the end of her second 3-D story she had moved the family dolls to the edge of the room — as far away as possible from the sick child. The compartmentalized figures of her first KFD were impersonally labeled "mom," "dad," "sister," and "brother."

At the time of the second testing Teresa drew: "Dad" eating an apple; "me" standing next to a swing; "Tom" riding his bike; and "mom" looking at birds. A swing separates Teresa from her father. Tom is next to Teresa, but he has his back to her and is riding away from her. Teresa's mother is far away in the corner of the page "looking at the birds." While the individuals in this drawing are no longer impersonally named, Teresa is isolated from everyone else in the family.

Both times only one of Tom's 15 RAT stories contained a theme scored for support. The content of his stories graphically portrays a perception of parents as inadequate sources of emotional support. One of the cards presented to Tom showed a woman hugging a girl. During the first testing Tom told a story about a mother who comforted a girl. At the time of the second testing his story made no mention of the mother. He told about a girl who fell down and hurt her knee. When he was asked to give his story an ending, he said: "Then it felt better."

Perception of the mother as inaccessible came through again when he told a story in response to a card showing a young girl watching a woman holding an infant. He said: "The lady is playing with the baby. And the girl is trying to tell her something (sixteen-second pause)." When asked to provide an ending for the story he replied: "Can't think of anything." When pressed for an ending, he repeated that he couldn't think of anything. Finally he said: "She just likes the baby." Tom's next story was about a girl who was frightened by the wind. He said: "Then she gets home and goes to her mother . . . (twelve-second pause) . . . I don't have anything else." The last card shown to Tom was a picture of a boy talking to a man. This card has been found to ordinarily elicit a story about the father-son relationship. Tom's change in his story to this card was particularly revealing. He said:

> The boy was asking his father a question . . . (nine seconds) . . . Oh, the boy has a surprise for his dad, and he is telling his dad, "here is a surprise." The boy gives the present to his dad.

This story reveals both wishes for a father to whom a son can turn with questions and feelings that it is up to the son to take care of the father.

Although the second projective assessments of each of the Tandems evidenced markedly increased themes of isolation, when the Tandem family character is taken into consideration, it is not difficult to understand how Mr. Tandem would report that the illness brought his family closer together.

Once Teresa became ill, the Tandem family characteristic of expressing "closeness" through efforts to retain close physical proximity with one another was heightened. Teresa was never left alone in the hospital. Mrs. Tandem spent weekdays at the hospital and Mr. Tandem spent weekends. When Teresa complained about not having her father with her on weekday nights, in order to help her feel her father's presence during the week, her father's church choir made a special tape recording for her. She frequently listened to this tape, particularly at night when she went to bed.

When Teresa was at home both she and her brother demanded that one of their parents sleep with them. Although Teresa and Tom shared a bedroom, frequently one of the parents would sleep with Teresa in the children's room and Tom would sleep with the other parent in the adults' bedroom. When Mr. Tandem was away on business, Mrs. Tandem crowded into the children's room and slept with both of them. The day after Teresa was found to be in a state of relapse, Mr. Tandem displayed markedly increased physical expression of affection with both of his children.

Neither parent expressed any awareness of the growing emotional isolation in the family. Mr. Tandem repeatedly stated that his method of dealing with conflict was to "tune out" people "because if I didn't — there is a lot of people — if you listen to them they'd drive you up a wall." Of his wife specifically he said: "She says a lot of things to me and

I don't pay any attention." Mr. Tandem's habit of "tuning out" his wife enabled him to remain unconcerned about her dissatisfaction with their marriage.

While Mrs. Tandem was the one adult in the study who did not report that the illness had strengthened her marriage, she specifically denied that her marriage relationship was in more trouble as a result of the illness. She stated that it's coming to a point where it has been coming for a long time but that now she and her husband could no longer so easily avoid the problems and they had to work them out. She expressed confidence that their marriage would survive the present stress.

The Deacon Family

In the Deacon family also a contrast existed between what the parents reported to be the effect of the illness on family relationships and what analysis of the data indicated was the effect. Both Mr. and Mrs. Deacon stated that Brian's illness brought the members of their family closer together, but the data analysis revealed that these statements were an inadequate description of this family's experience.

Deacon family interaction was characterized by an absence of direct expression of affect, however, anger and attachment were indirectly expressed. Overt manifestations of angry behavior in this family were few, but an underlying mood of tension and conflict permeated all interaction. While family members seldom manifested attachment behavior, they incorporated into their family structure compensation for the lack of strong affective bonds.

The Deacon family's religious orientation provided them with a means of feeling that they were a close family. They were a family united in the Lord. Sundays were a day of worship. On this day the children did not visit friends and the family stayed together throughout the day. The people in this family always ate dinner together. This structural conceptualization of their family as close and united obscured from the Deacons awareness of the fact that when they were together at home they in actuality were frequently isolated from one another.

Reading and watching TV together were in the minds of Mr. and Mrs. Deacon family activities which indicated their closeness. These activities meant that they were all home together. Though the Deacons always ate dinner together, they didn't talk very much to each other during the meal. Only 7 percent of the analyzed interactional units contained participation by all family members.

While this structural compensation for the lack of close affective bonds in the Deacon family kept the family intact, the projective materials and analysis of tape recordings indicate emotional isolation among the family members. Mr. Deacon's family drawings contain faceless people. Brian's stories had repeated themes of the boy going off to his room alone. Timothy's stories described the child running away from

home. Few of the drawings of any of the Deacons portrayed related-
ness between any family members. Although Mr. and Mrs.
Deacon felt that their family was about as "close" as most families they knew, the
analysis of the data reveals that the attachment bonds of this family
were characterized by feelings of isolation.

Both Mr. and Mrs. Deacon repeatedly stated that they felt that
Brian's illness brought their family "closer together." The analysis of
the tape recordings of family conversation provides important clarifi-
cation of this parental report.

In a detailed analysis of the transcripts of family conversation on two
occasions when all the Deacons were present, segments in the interactional units (see p. 9) were rated as collaborative, oppositional, or
neutral. Collaborative segments were defined as follows: addressing
the person with a term of affection; giving support; praising; assisting;
asking for permission; giving permission; being solicitous; attachment
behavior; making personal statements about one's activities, thoughts,
or feelings; expressing appreciation; or relating an occurrence with
"human interest." Oppositional segments were defined as: ignoring;
complaining; correcting another; interfering with another; inter-
rupting an on-going interactional unit; addressing another with a
depreciating nickname; criticizing; refusing to comply with directions;
teasing; withholding an object or information; infantalizing another;
responding with defeat or defensiveness; or making a depreciating
assumption about another. The following behaviors were judged neutral in quality: asking questions or making statements with no personal
content or "human interest"; giving and following directions in a
perfunctory manner; or asking for food.

The qualitative rating for each interactional unit was obtained by
determining the specific category with the greatest number of segments in that particular unit. For example, if an interactional unit
contained five collaborative segments, two oppositional segments, and
four neutral segments, it would be scored as a collaborative unit. In the
event that no one category contained a greater number of segments
than the other two, no score was given that unit. Initiations and segments directed toward the observer were not scored; however, interactional segments among family members during that unit were scored.

The qualitative scores for the Deacon family interaction during the
two analyzed tape recordings of conversation are summarized in Ta-
bles 5-I and 5-II. The columns of Table 5-I contain the following

TABLE 5-I
DEACON FAMILY INTERACTIONS

Tape	Coll	Opp	Neut	No Dom Cat	Unclear	Total
1	15	18	12	11	10	66
2	13	24	8	6	3	54

TABLE 5-II
DEACON FAMILY INTERACTIONS

Tape & To-tal Units	Collaborative		Oppositional		Neutral	
	# Units	% Total	# Units	% Total	# Units	% Total
1 — 66 units	15	23	18	27	12	18
2 — 54 units	13	24	24	44	8	15

information: the total number of units scored as primarily collaborative (COLL); oppositional (OPP); and neutral (NEUT); the total number of units without one dominant category (NO DOM CAT); the total number of units with insufficiently clear conversation to assign qualitative ratings (UNCLEAR); and the total number of interactional units in the recorded sample (TOTAL). Table 5-II presents a comparison of the qualitative analysis of the two samples of conversation.

The analysis of the tape recordings revealed that at the time that Brian appeared most ill, 27 percent of the conversational units were scored oppositional, 23 percent collaborative, and 18 percent neutral. When Brian's physical condition was markedly improved 44 percent of the conversational units were scored oppositional; 24 percent collaborative; and 15 percent neutral. In other words the amount of collaborative and neutral interaction remained relatively constant despite changes in Brian's physical condition, while oppositional interaction was significantly reduced when he was most ill.

These results support the repeated statements of Mr. and Mrs. Deacon *and* provide additional information essential for understanding the meaning of what they said. The Deacons understood "closer together" as a decrease in oppositional interaction rather than an increase in collaborative interaction among family members. Within the context of this information the apparently paradoxical effect of Brian's illness, i.e. perception of the family as "closer together" accompanied by increased feelings of emotional isolation, is readily explained.

Mr. Deacon's Kinetic Family Drawings were a graphic portrayal of this apparent paradox. In his first drawing, Mr. Deacon set his wife apart from the rest of the family. In his second drawing he placed her at his side. She was the only person in his drawing with any facial features; however, he gave her an incomplete face. She had eyes and a nose but no mouth. Though seated next to her husband, she was turned away from him — reading a book. Mr. Deacon pictured himself reading a newspaper. He and his wife are portrayed as "closer together," but they are unable to communicate with one another.

Mrs. Deacon stated that after Brian's diagnosis, she and her husband got along better than they ever had. She added that she felt it was because they needed each other more than they had before. While Mrs.

Deacon's projective protocols manifested decreased feelings of isolation, the content of her RAT stories showed that these feelings of increased "closeness" were a result of greater mutual need between her and her husband rather than as a result of perceiving her husband as more understanding of her feelings or perceiving the two of them as better able to resolve any conflict between them.

Thus, when parental self-report is analyzed within the context of data collected from other sources, a common theme emerges in both the Tandem and the Deacon families. When three of these four adults reported that the illness brought their families "closer together" they were less than adequately describing the full emotional impact of the child's illness on their families. The projective assessments of seven of the nine people in these two families manifested markedly increased themes of emotional isolation at the time of the second assessment. *In each instance the parental perception of "closer together" was based upon denial and avoidance of conflict rather than upon increased resolution of conflict or increased collaborative interaction.* Unfortunately for the individuals in these families, the significance of this parental response to stress was not limited to the nature of responses to research interview questions. The ramifications of this parental defense will be discussed in a later section of this chapter. However, before proceeding to this topic, it is important to put the issue of the parental perception of the family experience into the perspective of what is already known within the field of psychology and personality.

In his article on the limits for the conventional science of personality, Fiske (1974) points out that this field is severely handicapped by its reliance on words and by its dependence on complex observer judgements arrived at by processing diverse perceptions. He writes: "any statement about a person is a function not only of that person's behavior but also of the observer, and the interaction between the observer and the observed" (1974, p. 2). In another article (1975) he points out that very high agreement, close to true consensus, will not be obtained among sources who are using different material for their judgements. He gives the example of a therapist, a spouse, and a coworker, seeing the same individual in different environments, and adds that the relationships that these people have with the individual under study will inevitably affect their judgement on all but minor factual matters. He states that the difference in perceptions from varied sources are important to understand and recommends that instead of seeking to minimize them, researchers should seek to identify the unique components of the perceptions and judgements from each source.

An earlier work by Fiske (1971) emphasized that a person's answers about previous experience are always largely determined by his present perceptions, his present outlook, and his current mood. Even with so-called objective and standardized measuring instruments there are problems. Using multitrait-multimethod matrices as the method of analysis, Campbell and Fiske (1959) show how poor the evidence for validity of many psychological tests actually is. In many instances, results from established and accepted measures designed to get at different traits, but which also happened to employ the same method, had higher correlations than results from independent, established, and accepted efforts to measure the same trait. The authors refer to this as the absence of discriminant validity. Halo effects, test form factors, and response sets are cited as some of the sources of error.

It should be apparent then that the fact that there are such differences between the perceptions of the parents and the researcher regarding the family experience is not something unique to the specific individuals referred to in this study. Rather, according to Fiske, such differences are to be expected and adequate understanding of these two families can only be reached when these differences have been identified and integrated. In summary, parental report is an essential source of information about the family experience. However, this report must be considered within the broader framework of multiple sources of information in order for its full meaning to be understood.

Parental Use of Defense to Cope With the Child's Illness

The following comments are by no means offered as a comprehensive discussion of the overall adaptive value to the individual of using denial or some other defensive response to this crisis. The purpose of these comments is simply to call attention to the need for a more exhaustive study of the full impact of an individual's use of defense before one can assess the overall adaptive value of such a coping strategy.

Chodoff, Friedman, and Hamburg (1964) and Friedman, Chodoff, Mason, and Hamburg (1963) take the position that use of the defense of denial "within an optimum range" helped the parents of leukemic children cope with the child's illness. The authors based this conclusion on data obtained from observation of the parents' ability to participate in the physical care of the ill child and from parental self-report of how these individuals fulfilled their "other responsibilities." Neither article contains discussion of the ability of the parents to meet the *emotional* needs of the ill child, nor is there discussion of assessment or observation of how the parents functioned in relationships and responsibilities beyond tending to the ill child in the hospital.

While it is unclear as to what Chodoff et al. (1964) consider to be an "optimum range" of the use of denial, I wish to stress that the parents in these two families openly confronted the reality of their child's disease. Throughout the course of the study they spoke of their fears about the child's chances for survival. Further, at the outset of the research the fathers in these families volunteered that they had "no secrets" in their families. Both families included the ill child in the initial interview. Full information regarding the diagnosis and prognosis was available to everyone in the Deacon family and everyone but Teresa (the patient) in the Tandem family (Teresa knew her diagnosis but not her prognosis).

It was my belief that how the parents coped with their fears about the child's illness would be an important source of information about the effect on the family of parental defense. Consequently, in the initial individual interviews I asked each of the parents what they most feared about their child's illness. The answers to this question in combination with the observational data of this study illustrate the serious consequences of parental use of defense on the emotional welfare of the children in the family.

Mrs. Tandem stated that she worried most about Teresa being in pain — "especially when I know that some of that pain (is) caused by something that she is worrying about and maybe she won't talk about it." During the individual family history interview it was apparent that Mrs. Tandem herself found it very difficult to talk about her own emotions. How Mrs. Tandem dealt with her painful feelings and fears can be seen from her discussion of her father's sudden death when she was thirteen years old.

After describing in great detail several of the events of "that particular evening," just at the point when she was beginning to talk of her feelings her voice faded and she never completed her thought. When questioned further regarding her feelings on that occasion Mrs. Tandem started to answer the question and then in mid-sentence began talking about how she always felt secure about having someone to take care of her. In other words, when she began to talk about her feelings associated with her father's death she spoke of feelings opposite of what might have been expected. She reversed her feelings from those of fear and loss to those of security. Mrs. Tandem responded in a similar manner to her daughter's fatal illness.

When Teresa talked about not wanting time to go so fast, Mrs. Tandem understood her daughter's statements to be related to her fear of procedures rather than a fear that her life had almost run out. She would reassure her daughter by saying: "You want it (time) to go fast to get it over with." When Teresa didn't want her mother to call the doctor because she was afraid of what he might say, Mrs. Tandem responded by telling her that the doctor was just trying to help her. Mrs. Tandem felt that her daughter was talking about her worries that the doctor would hurt her and didn't consider the possibility that Teresa was concerned that the doctor was the person who knew how bad her situation actually was. In each of these instances it was Mrs. Tandem's "reassurance" and not Teresa's reluctance which precluded further discussion of Teresa's fears.

In one instance I observed Teresa directly address her mother about her fear of death and again it was Mrs. Tandem who was apparently unable to engage in this conversation. When Teresa asked her mother about the relationship between a certain lab report and being "out like a light," Mrs. Tandem answered simply: "I don't know." Teresa then asked "Why?" After a long pause during which her mother made no reply Teresa said questionly "dead?" Mrs. Tandem answered one word: "No." There was no exploration of what may have prompted Teresa to say what she did. In order for Mrs. Tandem to have been able to allow her daughter free expression of her fears Mrs. Tandem herself would have had to be able to endure the conscious experience of her own fear. Mrs. Tandem clearly stated in the family history interview that she had never received assistance in learning how to do this and as a small child she was discouraged from talking about her own feelings and fears. Mrs. Tandem's need to defend against her own unrecognized feelings about the possibility of her daughter's death made it impossible for her to allow her daughter to talk about such fears and she in fact created the situation she most feared with regard to Teresa's illness. Just how difficult it was for Mrs. Tandem to experience her own fear in this instance can be seen from her question to me one year after Teresa's death: Mrs. Tandem wanted to know if I thought it was possible that her daughter had known she was going to die.

When Mr. Tandem was asked what worried him most about his daughter's illness he answered: "Something that doesn't bother her — that's her hair . . . because I know how cruel people can be — because I know how cruel kids can be." His concern was not so much that his daughter would be ridiculed but rather that people would stare at her or hurt her. Teresa never complained of any difficulty with the children at school or in the neighborhood. She did not hesitate to go to school or outside to play with nothing on her head. (While Teresa was in the hospital her teacher discussed with the children in the class the possibility that Teresa's medication would cause her to become temporarily bald.) I never observed Teresa to cover her head when visitors stopped by the Tandem home. Further, Teresa persistently refused to wear the expensive wig her parents purchased.

Ironically, during all of my visits, the only person I observed to call attention to Teresa's hair was Mr. Tandem. Over the course of Teresa's illness Mr. Tandem repeatedly called attention to his daughter's hair loss and on more than one occasion Teresa was clearly bothered by this. One incident graphically illustrated Mr. Tandem's attention to his daughter's baldness. At Teresa's repeated request Mr. Tandem had taken his children for their first swim of the summer. Shortly after they returned home I arrived for a visit. Within minutes of my arrival Mr. Tandem began to rub Teresa's scalp. He then pulled her head directly under a nearby lamp. For a few moments longer he rubbed her head and peered at her scalp. He then looked to me and justified his actions with the statement: "the chlorine is clearing her scalp."

Mr. Tandem never acknowledged a personal feeling of horror or urge to stare at his bald little girl. He saw his obsession with her hair and bald head as behavior motivated by concern for her welfare. He explained to me that possibly because he made such an issue out of her hair Teresa would be glad to have the wig and would begin to wear it. Because Mr. Tandem was unable to recognize his own urge to stare in horror at his bald daughter, he was unable to refrain from converting this impulse to behavior and consequently repeatedly called attention to her baldness. He never seemed to realize that it was he and not Teresa who needed the protection of having her baldness hidden from view. In the last analysis he created for his daughter the very situation that he most feared others would create.

The particular course of Brian's disease had an important bearing on the fears and reactions of both Mr. and Mrs. Deacon. Brian first became ill approximately two months before his diagnosis with leukemia. Initially he was extremely fatigued and then he developed bone pain and swelling of the joints. When he was taken to the doctor his blood test was normal and he was treated for juvenile arthritis. It was only after a period of weeks that a second blood test showed abnormal changes and he was referred to a specialist who diagnosed leukemia. By that time Brian's pain was so severe that he could barely move about.

A senior pediatric hematologist told me that leukemia accompanied by bone involvement has a much slower recovery rate than other types of leukemia. He stated that exercise can be very painful for these patients. Although he thought that he had adequately explained the nature of Brian's disease to the Deacons, they told me that Brian's joint and bone pain would not have become so severe if he had not been allowed to "sit home and do nothing" during those first weeks when he was treated for arthritis. Mr. and Mrs. Deacon liked the hematology resident who "gave Brian hell" for not exercising and they were dissatisfied with the senior hematologist who they perceived to be "too lenient." The senior hematologist told me that he had decided to become more active in Brian's treatment, because he was concerned that Brian was being pushed too hard to exercise.

A further complication in Brian's treatment was his continued weight loss even after he was in remission. At the time of his diagnosis Brian was very underweight and his eating habits had been a long-standing source of conflict between him and his parents. Brian's illness exacerbated this conflict. The physician could find no medical explanation for Brian's weight loss, and he was concerned about the danger to Brian's life if it continued.

In response to my question regarding what he most feared about his son's illness, Mr. Deacon replied: "I am really not worried about his sickness — it may sound harsh, but I am really not." Mr. Deacon's behavior, however, was not that of someone who was "not worried" about his son's sickness.

Shortly after Brian was diagnosed, both of his parents began to feel that he had "given up" and was passively accepting his disease. A poster hung in Brian's room while he was still in the hospital indicated that both of his parents feared this eventuality even before they saw any evidence that he was "not fighting." It was a large picture of a dejected football player, sitting on the bench with head bowed and helmet in his hands. In very large letters were the words "I QUIT." In the lower corner of the poster was a small picture of Jesus Christ carrying a crucifix with the words "I didn't." This poster was prominently displayed near the foot of Brian's bed.

When Brian came home from the hospital he was very weak and had a bad cough. Mr. Deacon stayed up three nights in a row spoon feeding his son lemon and honey until 1:00 a.m. when Brian finally fell asleep. Mr. Deacon closely observed how little food Brian ate, often corrected him for spoiling his appetite before the meal, and continuously urged him to eat more during meals. He checked up on Brian to make sure that he was taking his pills.

In spite of the physicians' recommendations that Brian's exercises be left to Brian and his doctors, Mr. Deacon could not restrain himself from physically "exercising" Brian's muscles. During my initial interview with him, Mr. Deacon explained that he'd given Brian a couple of days to begin doing his exercises. When Brian didn't go in the swimming pool his father "rode him" the third and fourth days, and he could see his son's spirits drop. At that point he decided to "stay off Brian's back" and let the doctor handle it with Brian. However, Mr. Deacon then added that if Brian wasn't exercising in a couple of days he would begin again to "remind" his son about exercising.

One week later Mr. Deacon told me that his son's back was so "stiff" he couldn't bend over. Mr. Deacon was concerned that radiotherapy would make Brian sick and he would not be able to bend over to vomit so he "began exercising Brian's back." Of these exercises Mr. Deacon said: "If you would come by here it would sound like someone getting murdered — yesterday morning was terrible." When I commented that this must be very hard on Mr. Deacon he agreed and said that that morning he had started to cry while exercising his son and he didn't try to hide his tears from Brian. They both cried together and Mr. Deacon felt that this helped Brian to understand that he wasn't just being mean. It was about this time that the senior pediatric hematologist decided to become more active in Brian's treatment because he was concerned that Brian was being pushed too hard to exercise.

The extent of Mr. Deacon's need to deny feelings of helplessness and anxiety was apparent in the initial interview. At that time Mr. Deacon was a man under extreme stress. He'd recently learned that his son had leukemia and he spoke of this disease as a "terminal" one which would certainly kill his son. In addition, after thirteen years of steady employment he'd been unemployed for five months. In the face of these problems Mr. Deacon said to me: "I'm not a worrier — I can't think of anything I worry about." He then tellingly added: "I'm sure I worry but I don't admit it."

Mr. Deacon took recourse to action as a means of sparing himself the conscious experience of anxiety. The preceding discussion gives some indication of how active Mr. Deacon became in his son's medical treatment. In addition, in spite of all the time he devoted to Brian's care, during a five month period he solicited thirty-seven companies for employment. Tragically, because he was unable to recognize his own anxiety about his son's illness and his consequent recourse to action as a means of relieving this anxiety, Mr. Deacon was unable to assess how helpful his behavior was for his son.

Painfully, for both Brian and himself, Mr. Deacon required his son to exercise in order to enable him to bend over the toilet to vomit when he began radiotherapy. Brian ironically did not experience nausea after undergoing radiotherapy. In spite of the physicians' recommendations to the contrary, Mr. Deacon was unable to refrain for more than a couple of days from pressuring his son to exercise. He believed that it was very important for him to encourage his son to fight his disease. Even though Mr. Deacon could tell me that he saw his son's spirits drop when he pressured him to exercise, he never recognized the impact of his continued "encouragement" on Brian, an adolescent described by his parents as a loner and a lazy child. As it turned out, Brian, in fact, never did return to school that year; spent much of his time alone in his room; and continued to lose weight well after he was in remission. In order for Mr. Deacon to have been able to evaluate the helpfulness to Brian of his actions, he would have had to have been able to recognize that in the last analysis it was his own emotional state and not Brian's physical condition that was the impetus for his "encouragement."

When asked what worried her most about her son's illness, Mrs. Deacon answered:

> I am torn between feeling that he is going to die and feeling he's not going to die. I don't see the point of all this treatment for a few months in a world that's going to pot anyway.

More than anything else, Mrs. Deacon didn't want to see her son suffer. Although she knew her husband and her son's physicians didn't agree, at first she "just prayed that the Lord would take him" but she "kind of got over that." Mrs. Deacon repeated several times that she did not see the point of putting Brian through all the suffering he was going through for a few extra months of life.

The meaning of Mrs. Deacon's comments about making Brian suffer becomes more clear when considered in the context of her statements about her own experiences of physical pain. Because of her concern about the pain of childbirth, her two eldest children were delivered while she was under general anesthesia. She told me that she had been unprepared for the pain after Brian's delivery. She "expected to be knocked out" for her third child's birth, but a different physician cared for her, and she found it upsetting to learn that she would only be given a spinal anesthetic for delivery. Mrs. Deacon, then, was a woman who found the thought of pain to be something quite frightening long before Brian became ill.

Several of her statements revealed how important it was for her to see her son as a strong person. During the initial interviews Mrs. Deacon described how once Brian fell out of a tree and broke both of his arms, but insisted on playing in the school band with casts on both arms. She referred to this accomplishment as a "status symbol" for her son. Later she told me Brian was hoping to go back to school that year "to show his friends his needle marks." (I never observed any indication that Brian was planning to return to school that year.)

Mrs. Deacon dealt with her own fears about watching her son suffering in pain by perceiving his pain as something within his control. In spite of the physician's explanations to the contrary, she believed that had it not been for "that month (when) he sat around and did nothing" his pain would not have become so severe. She stated that Brian was supposed to be exercising to strengthen his back for relief from pain. She could see no evidence that Brian was exercising and, as the following incident illustrates, become intolerant of his pain.

One evening during an exceptionally long church musical program Brian complained to his mother that his back and his head were hurting from sitting so long. After the service Mr. Deacon found Brian lying down on the car seat crying and asked why he hadn't said anything during the service. Brian answered: "I told Mom and she told me to 'shut up and listen to the show.'" Later that evening Mrs. Deacon expressed disappointment that Brian wasn't a "tough cookie" and stated: "I can't be too sympathetic with someone who won't take care of himself." Mrs. Deacon's fear of physical pain and her consequent need to defend against seeing her son in pain made it difficult for her to respond with compassion to Brian's suffering.

The preceding discussion presented several situations in which the parents' ability to meet the needs of their children was hampered by their perception of their child's experience. What was common to each situation in which either the Tandem or the Deacon parents failed to perceive the full ramifications of their child's experience was that this misperception spared the parent a very painful self-confrontation. The experience of the individuals in these two families points to the need for further investigation of the role of defense in adequate coping with this crisis.

A Different Perspective on Coping With Childhood Cancer

Chodoff et al. (1964) state that coping can be thought of as consisting of two aspects, an externally directed one judged for effectiveness in social terms and an internally directed or defensive aspect which serves to protect the individual from disruptive degrees of anxiety and which is judged for effectiveness by the degree of comfort resulting. Friedman et al. also speak of the external and internal aspects of coping with the "totality of events associated with being the parent of a child with a fatal disease" (1963, p. 616). In both these studies the externally directed aspect of coping was evaluated by observation of the parents' ability to participate in the physical care of the ill child and by parental-report of how these individuals fulfilled their "other responsibilities."

While many authors write of coping having several aspects, a careful review of their work reveals a subtle emphasis on the primacy of defense in coping. "Facts" based upon self-report are discussed and emotional behavior usually is linked with maladaptive coping. Chodoff et al. place emphasis on the ability of the parents to carry out the necessary tasks "without being overwhelmed with despair and anxiety" (1964, p. 743). A similar bias toward viewing the experience of strong and distressing emotions as maladaptive rather than adaptive behavior is present in the criteria for coping used in other studies. In evaluating the effectiveness of their program of emotional management of childhood leukemia Lascari and Stehbens (1973) chose the following criteria: satisfaction of parents with this method; few prolonged grieving reactions; and absence of significant emotional complications in the parents. Townes et al. (1974) also placed emphasis upon *absence of uncomfortable emotions rather than presence of effectiveness in meeting a variety of emotional and functional tasks* in assessing parental adjustment to childhood leukemia. By operational definition they equated minimal presence of negative affect with acceptance of the diagnosis and the prognostic implications of childhood leukemia.

For the parents in these two families assessment of the externally directed aspect of coping included assessment of impairment in their ability to function as partners to each other and as parents of their ill and well children. The preceding pages presented a discussion of how the parents' use of defense in coping with their child's illness obscured feelings of isolation among most members in their families. Several situations were discussed in which the parents' ability to meet the needs of their ill children was hampered by their need to defend against their own fears related to the child's illness. Space did not permit discussion, in this chapter, of how the parents' use of defense hampered their ability to offer emotional support to their well children during the critical weeks following the ill child's diagnosis. Such a discussion can be found in the original report of this research project (Desmond, 1977).

The findings of this study illustrate the necessity of gathering a broader base of information than has previously been compiled in evaluating the role of defense in aiding or impairing the parents of childhood cancer patients to cope with "the totality of events associated with being the parents of a child with a fatal disease" (Friedman et al., 1963, p. 616). Based upon the assumption that full experience of painful feelings and fears may lead to some kind of breakdown in ability to function, denial can be looked upon as an aid to adaptation. However, examination of the ramifications of limited parental perception of the family experience reveals the very high toll which can accompany the use of denial as a means of coping with painful situations. If coping skills are viewed as the ability to continue functioning in the face of painful emotions, adequate coping no longer need be predicated on the assumption that loss of awareness of self is an asset.

Within Bowlby's theoretical formulations, frank expression of hostility, frequently directed toward others, would be an adaptive response to threatened loss — a position radically different from that taken by Friedman et al. (1963). Other *adaptive* responses identified by Bowlby and Parkes are: "yearning for the impossible, intemperate anger, impotent weeping, horror at the prospect of loneliness, pitiful pleading for sympathy and support" (1970, p. 210).

Caplan, in his forward to the work of Glick et al. (1974), described his own growth in understanding coping. Although his comments were focused on the mourning of widows I believe they have significant applicability to the crisis of childhood cancer. He wrote:

> In our earlier formulations we had thought a widow "recovers" at the end of the four to six weeks of her bereavement crisis on condition that she manages to accomplish her "grief work" adequately. . . . We now realize that most widows continue the psychological work of mourning for their dead husbands for the rest of their lives . . . since I was applying the short time-frame of crisis to the mourning situation, I sometimes tended to evaluate continuing signs of strain or cognitive and emotional deviations of a widow a year or two after the death of her husband as either a manifestation of current pathology or a predictor of future illness. This book has led me to greater sophistication (pp. viii-ix).

Futterman and Hoffman (1970) also take the position that for families of fatally ill children the usual criteria for psychopathology are difficult to apply. They state that transitory symptom formation in these families is related to coping processes which may at times be circuitous but are nonetheless adaptive reactions.

Bowlby conceptualizes emotions as part of human perceptual or appraising process. He takes care to point out that whether or not, and if so, to what extent, feeling plays a causal role in appraising has not been established. However, he does state that the most discriminating appraisal and reappraisal processes can occur only in conditions that give rise to conscious feeling. While I do not know how Bowlby's thought will emerge in the third volume of his comprehensive work I am cognizant that he has identified the third phase of a child's response to loss, that of detachment, with the problem of defense or detachment in adult psychopathology.

The results of this study indicate that these four defended adults formed families with attachment bonds that were characterized by alienation and emotional isolation, and that when confronted with the possible death of one of their children, both their defense and their emotional isolation were exacerbated. It is my opinion that until greater attention is given to critical evaluation of the aspects of coping other than comfort, or lack of personal distress, statements about the role of defense in aiding coping with childhood cancer are premature. It is possible that the defensive needs of researchers and professionals to insulate themselves from the continuously repeated experience of feelings of absolute helplessness in the face of death have led them to emphasize the value of keeping anxiety, anger, and despair minimized, and to de-emphasize the value of "yearning for the impossible, intemperate anger, impotent weeping, horror at the prospect of loneliness, and pitiful pleading for sympathy and support" (Bowlby & Parkes, 1970, p. 210). The lack of critical evaluation of the role of defense in coping with childhood cancer may well reflect the eventuality that although death has "come out of the closet," it is no more integrated as a part of life than when it was a taboo topic.

REFERENCES

Anthony, E. J.: The mutative impact of serious mental and physical illness in a parent on family life. In E. J. Anthony & C. Koupernik (Eds.), *The Child in his Family*. Vol. 1 of the Yearbook of the International Association for Child Psychiatry and Allied Professions. New York, Wiley-Interscience, 1970.

Bach, S.: Spontaneous paintings of severely ill patients. *Documenta Geigy: Acta Psychosomatica*. Basle, J. R. Geigy, 1969.

Bach, S.: Spontaneous pictures of leukemic children as an expression of the total personality, mind and body. *Acta Paedopsychiatr* 1974/75, *41* (3), 86.

Bender, L.: *A Dynamic Psychopathology of Childhood*. Springfield, Thomas, 1954.

Bermann, E.: *Scapegoat: The Impact of Death-fear on an American Family*. Ann Arbor, University of Michigan, 1973.

Binger, C. M.: Childhood leukemia — emotional impact of siblings. In E. J. Anthony & C. Koupernik (Eds.): *The Child in His Family: The Impact of Disease and Death*. Vol. 2 of the Yearbook of the International Association for Child Psychiatry and Allied Professions. New York, Wiley, 1973a.

Binger, C. M.: Jimmy — a clinical case presentation of a child with a fatal illness. In E. J. Anthony, & C. Koupernik (Eds.): *The Child in His Family: The Impact of Disease and Death*. Vol. 2 of the Yearbook of the International Association for Child Psychiatry and Allied Professions. New York, Wiley, 1973b.

Binger, C. M., Ablin, A. R., Feuerstein, R. C., Kushner, J. H., Zoger, S., & Mikkelsen, C.: Childhood leukemia, emotional impact on patient and family. *N Engl J Med*, 1969, *280*, 414.

Bowlby, J.: *Attachment and Loss (Vol. 1)*. New York, Basic Books, 1969.

Bowlby, J.: *Attachment and Loss (Vol. II Separation: Anxiety and Anger)*. New York, Basic Books, 1973.

Bowlby, J.: Attachment theory, separation anxiety and mourning. In D. Hamburg & K. Brodie (Eds.) *The American Handbook of Psychiatry (Vol. VI)*. New York, Basic Books, 1975.

Bowlby, J., & Parkes, C. M.: Separation and loss within the family. In E. J. Anthony & C. Koupernik (Eds.): *The Child in his Family: The Impact of Disease and Death* Vol. 1 of the Yearbook of the International Association for Child Psychiatry and Allied Professions. New York, Wiley-Interscience, 1970.

Burns, R. C., & Kaufman, S. H.: *Kinetic Family Drawings (K-F-D): An Introduction to Understanding Children Through Kinetic Drawings*. New York, Brunner/Mazel, 1970.

Burns, R. C., & Kaufman, S. H.: *Actions, Styles, and Symbols in Kinetic Family Drawings (K-F-D): An Interpretive Manual.* New York, Brunner/Mazel, 1972.

Cain, A. C., & Cain, B. S.: On replacing a child. *J Am Acad Child Psychiatry,* 1964, *3,* 433.

Cain, A. C., Fast, I., & Erickson, M. E.: Children's disturbed reactions to the death of a sibling. *Am J Orthopsychiatry,* 1964, *34,* 741.

Campbell, D. T., & Fiske, D. W.: Convergent and discriminant validation by the multitrait-multimethod matrix. *Psychol Bull,* 1959, *56(2),* 81.

Chapple, E.: *Cultural and Biological Man: Explorations in Behavioral Anthropology.* San Francisco, Holt, Rinehart & Winston, 1970.

Chodoff, P., Friedman, S. B., & Hamburg, D. A.: Stress, defenses and coping behavior: observations in parents of children with malignant disease. *Am J Psychiatry,* 1964, *120,* 743.

Cronbach, L.: *Essentials of Psychological Testing.* New York, Harper & Row, 1970.

Desmond, H.: The psychological impact of childhood cancer on the family. (Doctoral dissertation, California School of Professional Psychology, Los Angeles) Ann Arbor, Mich.: University Microfilms, 1977, No 78-2822.

Fiske, D. *Measuring the Concepts of Personality.* Chicago, Aldine, 1971.

Fiske, D. W.: The limits for the conventional science of personality. *J Personality,* 1974, *42(1),* 1.

Fiske, D. W.: A source of data is not a measuring instrument. *J Abnormal Psychology,* 1975, *84(1),* 20.

Friedman, S. B., Chodoff, P., Mason, J. W., & Hamburg, D.: Behavioral observations on parents anticipating the death of a child. *Pediatrics,* 1963, *32(604),* 610.

Futterman, E. J., & Hoffman, I.: Transient school phobia in a leukemic child. *Journal of the American Academy of Child Psychiatry,* 1970, *9,* 477.

Futterman, E. H., & Hoffman, I.: Crisis and adaptation in the families of fatally ill children. In E. J. Anthony & C. Koupernik (Eds.): *The Child in His Family: The Impact of Disease and Death.* Vol II of the Yearbook of the International Association of Child Psychiatry and Allied Professions. New York, Wiley, 1973.

Futterman, E. H., Hoffman, I., & Sabshin, M.: Parental anticipatory mourning. In B. Schoenberg, A. C. Carr, B. Peretz, & A. H. Kutscher (Eds.): *Psychosocial Aspects of Terminal Care.* New York, Columbia University, 1972.

Fergusson, J. H.: Late psychologic effects of a serious illness in childhood. *Nurs Clin North Am,* 1976, *11(1),* 83.

Glick, I., Weiss, R., & Parkes, C. M.: *The First Year of Bereavement.* New York, John Wiley & Sons, 1974.

Henry, J.: *Pathways to Madness.* New York, Vintage, 1965.

Henry, J.: My life with the families of psychotic children. In G. Handel (Ed.), *The Psychosocial Interior of the Family.* Chicago, Aldine, 1967.

Hulse, W. C.: The emotionally disturbed child draws his family. *Q J Child Behavior,* 1951, *3,* 152.

Hulse, W. C.: Childhood conflict expressed through family drawings. *Journal of Projective Techniques and Personality Assessment,* 1952, *16,* 66.

Kaplan, D., Smith, A., & Grobstein, R.: The problems of siblings. Paper presented at the American Cancer Society's National Conference on Human Values and Cancer, Atlanta, Georgia, June, 1972.

Kaplan, D. M., Smith, A., Grobstein, R., & Fishman, S. E.: Family mediation of stress. *Social Work,* 1973, *18,* 60.

Kliman, G.: The child faces his own death. In A. Kutscher (Ed.): *Death and Bereavement.* Springfield, Thomas, 1969.

Lansky, S., & Lowman, J. T.: Childhood malignancy. *J Kans Med Soc,* 1964, March, 91.

Lascari, A. D., & Stehbens, J. A.: The reactions of families to childhood leukemia. *Clin Pediatrics*, 1973, *12(4)*, 210.

Moriarity, D. M.: *The Loss of Loved Ones.* Springfield, Thomas, 1967.

O'Malley, J. E.: Long-term follow-up of survivors of childhood cancer: psychiatric sequelae. Paper presented at the American Psychological Association 85th Annual Convention, San Francisco, August, 1977.

Rosenblatt, B.: Reactions of children to the death of loved ones: some notes based on psychoanalytic theory. In D. Moriarity (Ed.): *The Loss of Loved Ones.* Springfield, Thomas, 1967.

Rosenblatt, B.: A young boy's reaction to the death of his sister. *J Amer Acad Child Psychiatry*, 1969, *8*, 321.

Santostefano, S.: Children cope with the violent death of parents. In D. Moriarity (Ed.): *The Loss of Loved Ones.* Springfield, Thomas, 1967.

Spinetta, J., Rigler, D., & Karon, M.: Anxiety in the dying child. *Pediatrics*, 1973, *52(6)*, 841.

Spinetta, J., Rigler, D., & Karon, M.: Personal space as a measure of a dying child's sense of isolation. *J Consult Clin Psychology*, 1974, *42*, 751.

Spinetta, J. J., & Maloney, L. J.: Death anxiety in the outpatient leukemic child. *Pediatrics*, 1975, *56(6)*, 1034.

Stehbens, J., & Lascari, A.: Psychological follow-up of families with childhood leukemia. *J Clin Psychol*, 1974, *30(3)*, 394.

Tooley, K.: The choice of a surviving sibling as a "scapegoat" in some cases of maternal bereavement: a case report. *J Child Psychol Psychiatry*, 1975, *16*, 331.

Townes, B. D., Wold, D. A., & Holmes, T. H.: Parental adjustment to childhood leukemia. *Journal of Psychosom Res*, 1974, *18*, 9.

Wallace, J.: Family functioning in "care of the child with cancer." *Pediatrics*, 1967, *40*, 487.

Chapter Six

SPECIAL TREATMENT MODALITIES: LAMINAR AIRFLOW ROOMS*

JONATHAN KELLERMAN
STUART E. SIEGEL
DAVID RIGLER

INFECTIONS ARE A LEADING cause of death in many patients with cancer. Apart from the direct life-threat posed by infectious complications, there is also an indirect hazard resulting from impediment to the application of aggressive anti-cancer chemotherapy. Because of these concerns several studies have examined the use of protected environments (PE) as an adjunct to intensive oncologic treatment (Preisler and Bjornsson, 1975; Levine et al., 1973; Bodey et al., 1971; Schimff et al., 1975; Yates and Holland, 1973; Siegel et al., 1975).

PE techniques involve the use of physical barrier isolation mechanisms combined with chemical sterilization techniques, such as oral antibiotics, to approximate a *gnotobiotic*, or germ-free environment. Initial PE studies were conducted within the confines of life-islands (Bodey et al., 1971; Kohle et al., 1971) which consisted of plastic tents constructed over conventional-sized beds. There are early reports (Kohle et al., 1971) of psychological disturbance related to treatment in these highly restricted environments. More recently, the use of laminar airflow units has been adopted. These employ room-sized modules within which sterilization is accomplished through the use of mechanical cleansing of air blown through filters in parallel (laminar) layers. Such airflow minimizes pockets of turbulence with which bacteria tend to colonize.

Treatment of patients in PE involves elimination of skin-to-skin contact with other individuals, restriction of movement due to confinement within a relatively small space, and in general, raises the possibility of both sensory deprivation and social isolation. This is particularly true when prolonged treatment is carried out.

In October, 1974, Childrens Hospital of Los Angeles began installation of four laminar airflow units as part of a study funded by the Division of Cancer Treatment, National Cancer Institute, investigating the use of PE in treating pediatric cancer patients with advanced stage solid tumors. Due to the aforementioned psychological concerns, a behavioral component was incorporated into the study, and a psy-

---

*This study was supported by National Cancer Institute Contract No. N01-CM-53831.

128

chosocial study team was created. The goals of the adjunctive study were:

1. To screen patients in terms of psychological eligibility for treatment in PE.
2. To identify the nature and degree of psychological disturbance related to treatment in PE.
3. To ameliorate such problems.

Due to the fact that this research was the first systematic psychological investigation of childrens' response to protective isolation, there was a lack of direct behavioral data upon which to draw. Research findings from several related areas did, however, exist.

Sensory Deprivation in Adults

One major area of inquiry is that of the general effects of sensory deprivation and social isolations upon human beings. Comprehensive compilations of such research are contained in volumes by Zubek (1969) and Rasumussen (1973) and include studies conducted in laboratory (Bexton et al., 1954; Doane, 1955; Vernon et al., 1961; Wexler et al., 1958), field (Zubek et al., 1963; Haggard, 1973), and clinical (Mendelson and Foley, 1956; Mendelson et al., 1958) settings. These last studies are perhaps most directly relevant and report clinical observations of psychotic-like symptoms in poliomyelitis patients confined in tank-type respirators under perceptually sterile conditions. Concordant findings from recovery room, coronary, and general intensive care units have also been reported (McKegney, 1966; Nahum, 1965). Data from laboratory and field studies have been variable (Zuckerman, 1969) and obtained results have generally tended to concentrate upon disruptions of sensation, cognition, and affect.

Despite the voluminous nature of the sensory deprivation literature, extrapolation to a pediatric oncology setting is hampered by several factors: First, the term sensory deprivation has been used to refer to several different processes. As Corso (1967) has noted, distinctions must be drawn between attempts to absolutely reduce sensory stimulation, as represented by the experimental work of Lilly (1956) and Shurley (1960), and situations where levels of input are maintained at conventional levels but patterns of input are modified. Another important distinction that needs to be made is that between the reduction or alteration of interpersonal stimulation (social isolation), and modification of sensory input (sensory deprivation). Perhaps the most important limitation, however, is the fact that the bulk of sensory deprivation-social isolation data has been obtained from adults. An exception to this is a field study by Haggard (1973) of socially isolated children in Norway, which reported perceptual, affective, and intellectual differences between such children and matched controls.

There are obvious ethical constraints to the experimental use of sensory deprivation and social isolation with children. Pediatric data does, however, exist from several sources.

Physical Restraint in Children

Hill and Robinson (1930) reported the case of retarded development associated with restricted movement in a six-year-old boy whose hands were tied to prevent him from scratching his eczematous skin.

Sibinga and associates (Sibinga and Friedman, 1971; Sibinga et al., 1968) studied the effects of sensory and physical restraint as it effected the psychological development of children with phenyketonuria (PKU). These authors compared children with PKU who were immobilized during the first three years of life with patients who had experienced no such restriction, and found greater impairment in the restricted group of social and interpersonal behavior, language comprehension, and intelligence, as well as increased moderate to severe personality disturbance.

Schecter (1961) conducted a psychoanalytic observation of children with polio and concluded that enforced immobility lead to passivity, masochistic tendencies, poor self-image and decreased reality testing.

Levy (1944) studied two groups of patients. The first consisted of six children, two to four years old, isolated due to measles, who manifested head rolling, head banging, and rocking that stopped when toys were restored. The second was a sample of nineteen children whose hands were restrained to prevent thumbsucking. Levy felt that concomitant symptoms of tantrums, enuresis, and restlessness were related to sensory restriction. He went on to note that children who were bound as infants due to cultural prescriptions did not show any such effects (Dennis and Denms, 1935; 1940; 1951) and hypothesized that early restraint, that is, restriction which is imposed prior to the development of critical drive levels is less likely to effect psychological functioning than restraint during later periods.

Similarly, Higgins (1965) found impaired spatial development in eighteen-month-old children restricted due to treatment for both polio and congenital hip dislocation and suggested that a relationship existed between restraint occurring during critical periods of development of specific skills and subsequent disorders of these skills.

With the exception of the reports by Sibinga and associates, none of the previously cited references were controlled studies, and most consisted of post-hoc analyses, making definitive causal connections between restraint and impairment difficult to assert.

Abused and Deprived Children

Another area with possible ramifications to long-term protective isolation in children is that of pediatric deprivation, specifically those instances involving documented sensory restraint.

Barbero and Shaheen (1967) have reviewed the "failure to thrive" syndrome and have differentiated between disease-related and psychogenic instances of growth failure in human infants. The generally improved response of the latter group to hospitalization and increased nurturance points to the importance of environmental factors in their effect upon growth and development. Elmer et al. (1969) subsequently reported the long-term effects of environmental deprivation, upon physical, intellectual, and behavioral development.

Fischoff et al. (1971) and Whitten et al. (1969) discussed the psychological characteristics of depriving mothers and presented evidence that growth failure is secondary to nutritional, opposed to psychological factors. On the other hand, Rice (1977) has presented data indicating enhanced neurophysiological development in premature infants following a planned program of tactile-kinesthetic stimulation.

Rice's (1977) findings are substantiated by the work of several other researchers who have found beneficial auditory, visual, gross-motor, and weight-gain results from programs of sensory stimulation (Neal, 1967; Katz, 1971; Williams and Scarr, 1971; Scarr-Salapatek and Williams, 1972; 1973; Powell, 1974).

Koluchova (1972; 1976) described the results of a long-term psychological study of twin Czechoslovakian boys, abused and severely physically restrained from eighteen months to seven years. At the time of their discovery, these two children presented IQ scores in the forties, could barely walk, suffered from rickets, and failed to understand the meaning or function of pictures. Follow-up several years later (Koluchova, 1976) revealed dramatic gains in all areas. This casts some doubt about the essential nature of critical periods, in that the twins, despite the fact that they had passed the "crucial" three-year period of language acquisition, learned to speak quite rapidly after being exposed to adults. At age fourteen, their Wechsler Intelligence Scale for Children (WISC) IQ scores were 100 and 101, respectively. Koluchova's (1976) longitudinal intelligence data indicated progressive and uninterrupted IQ rise following stimulation. No psychopathological features were evident in either boy.

Koluchova (1976) also described the case of a ten-year-old girl subjected to similar deprivation and abuse and reported greater behavioral and intellectual difficulties in this child, as compared to the twins. Possible explanations included the twin's ability to mutually mediate the detrimental effects of deprivation and differing maternal psychological qualities.

Parental Separation

Early references regarding the detrimental effects of maternal separation upon child development are contained in the psychoanalytic works of Spitz (1945; 1946) and Bowlby (1960). Subsequent empirical studies were conducted by Klaus and associates (Klaus and Kennel, 1970; Klaus et al., 1972; Klaus et al., 1970) that indicated rehabilitative effects of increasing parent-child contact. Similar results have been reported by several others (Barnett et al., 1970; Fanaroff et al., 1972; Leifer et al., 1972).

There are indications (Corter, 1976) that distress related to separation is not inevitable if the separation is short-term but that long-term separation is inherently stressful for young children. It is worth noting that the majority of separation studies have been conducted with infants or children under the age of three.

Effects of Hospitalization Upon Children

Hospitalization represents one specific type of separation; during hospitalization, separation anxiety may be further intensified by the aversive and uncomfortable experiences that accompany illness and treatment. Many of the early studies of separation anxiety took place in hospital or institutional settings (Coleman and Provence, 1957; Oersten and Mattson, 1955; Prugh et al., 1953; Spitz, 1945; 1946; Robertson, 1958; Bowlby, 1960) making distinctions between the effects of hospitalization and separation, per se, less than clear. There is, however, ample evidence from the laboratory (Corter, 1976) that separation does elicit anxiety in the absence of medical treatment, and conversely, that hospitalization in the absence of separation is stressful (Vernon et al., 1965).

Mahaffy (1965) studied the effects of helping mothers support their children through a brief hospitalization for tonsillectomy and adenoidectomy, and found differences between support and nonsupport groups in terms of post-hospitalization fever, length of time to recovery, sleep disturbances, fears of medical settings, crying, and willingness to separate from mothers.

Schaeffer (1958) discussed the effects of perceptual monotony in the hospital upon infants under seven months of age and found behavioral improvement once children had returned home. Similar results have been reported by Prugh (1965) who discussed the possibility of interference exerted upon the parent-child relationship by disruption of familiar schedules. Levy (1945) talked about the increased difficulty for children under two years undergoing hospitalization due to their having less social contact and ability to cope with anxiety than older children. Delay of gratification, inherent in most hospitalization experiences, has been discussed (Dimock, 1960; Gellert, 1958) as an additional cause of frustrations in young children. Most authors have tended to view young children as most vulnerable to hospitalization-induced psychological detriment though there is some evidence that there are unique difficulties inherent at any age, including adolescence (Kellerman and Katz, 1977).

Special note should be made of a controlled study of sensory deprivation related to hospitalization conducted by Downs (1974) in which 180 adult volunteers were placed in a simulated hospital room under three experimental conditions: (1) Ambient room tone (no added stimulation); (2) Decoded radio stimulation (perceptually meaningful edited radio messages; and (3) Coded radio stimulation (randomly placed bits of radio messages spliced together to simulate snatches of conversation). After slightly less than three hours of bed rest under these conditions, during which the subjects received no social contact, perceptual distortions were experienced by members of all three groups, with there being significantly fewer such experiences reported by those receiving decoded stimulation. Downs (1974) emphasized that these "indeterminate stimulus experiences" were not psychotic in nature due to the fact that all the subjects knew they were not real. It is possible to speculate, however, that loss of reality testing might follow increased time under conditions of social isolation. Downs' study is particularly important because it represents a carefully manipulated simulation of the hospital environment, devoid of illness confounds and due to the fact that perceptual distortion was experienced after relatively short periods of time. Generalization from adults to children, however, cannot be made with confidence.

Animal Studies

The most highly controlled investigations of the psychological effects of separation and isolation come from animal research. Specifically, the work of Harlow and associates with rhesus monkeys (Harlow and Harlow, 1965; Harlow and Soumi, 1974; Harlow et al., 1970; Suomi et al., 1970; 1973; 1976), in which a syndrome of despair and protest was found to be related to induced early separation between infants and mothers, has formed the seminal experimental basis for much theorization regarding isolation experiences in humans. In fact, several reviewers (Kaufman and Rosenblum, 1967; McKinney and Bunney, 1969; Harlow et al., 1970; Hinde and Spencer-Booth, 1971; Harlow and Suomi, 1974) have pointed out similarities between rhesus reactions to separation and the data from studies of human anaclitic depression.

A later study (Suomi et al., 1976) imposed conditions intriguingly relevant to the laminar flow setting, in which six-month-old infant rhesus monkeys were subjected to periods of increasing social isolation under three varying conditions: separated by plastic mesh which allowed physical contact; with mothers physically, but not visually isolated from mothers but allowed access to peers; and, finally, physical separation from both mothers and peers. Clear despair reactions were recorded, particularly in the last two groups but, following reunion, the infant monkeys resumed normal behavior.

Isolation effects have also been found in animals lower on the phylogenetic scale than monkeys (Rajecki et al., 1977). Nevertheless, extrapolation from sub-human to human functioning is hampered by the finding that extensive interspecies variability exists (Suomi et al., 1976; Preston et al., 1970; Schlottman and Seay, 1972; Sackett et al., 1977). For example, certain species of primates, such as pigtail monkeys, do not manifest the separation-induced distress behavior.

Therapeutic Uses of Isolation and Deprivation

While the majority of studies have focused upon the detrimental effects of social isolation and sensory deprivation, there are reports of using these modalities to bring about positive psychological change.

With regard to children, Cohen (1963) and Charney (1963) utilized sensory deprivation in treating severely disturbed children in residential settings. Both of these authors reported favorable behavioral change but noted regressive loosening of the child's defensive process prior to subsequent personality reorganization. Schechter et al. (1969) used sensory deprivation and social isolation as a successful means of improving interpersonal functioning in autistic children.

Adams and associates have done extensive work using sensory deprivation with adult psychiatric patients (Adams et al., 1972; Cooper et al., 1975; Adams, 1964; Adams, 1965; Adams and Cooper, 1966). Similarly, Wadeson and Carpenter (1976) reported on the use of seclusion rooms with hospitalized psychotics. Therapeutic results have usually been explained in terms of reducing defensive systems.

Psychological Aspects of Protected Environments

Prior to the instigation of our clinical study, there existed four studies describing the psychological responses of human beings to protective isolation. These deserve somewhat detailed descriptions:

KOHLE ET AL.: In 1971, a group of researchers in Germany reported upon psychological responses of newly diagnosed adults with acute leukemia treated in the earliest form of PE — the life island (Bodey et al., 1968). Kohle's group studied nine patients treated over a total of 427 days. Methods of investigation included psychoanalytically oriented interviews with patient and spouse (or closest relative), documentation of socio-economic data, offer of counsel by a social worker, and a test battery including the following instruments: (1) Rorschach Test; (2) Object Relations Test (ORT); (3) Freilburg Personality Inventory (FPI); (4) Giessner Personality Inventory (GPI); (5) Cattell Anxiety Battery and (6) Beckmann-Zenz List of Complaints. Evaluation was begun prior to informing the patient of diagnosis and the decision to treat in PE.

Several of the psychological issues raised by Kohle et al. (1971) are not limited to those patients treated in PE but concern themselves with a diagnosis of serious illness and hospitalization also. These include dependency on others, confrontation with severity of illness, separation from family, isolation, and inhibition of motor activity. The last two can be said to be exacerbated by the physical restrictiveness of PE.

Kohle et al. (1971) found that the pressure towards passivity inherent in the isolated-bed system encouraged regressive behavior on the part of some adults which led to, in an unspecified number of patients, paranoid ideas about food being poisoned. Other symptoms included depersonalization, delirium, and suicidal ideation. Note was made of the fact that psychologic symptoms were often related to side effects of medical treatment, such as cytostatic medications, and not directly caused by isolation, though perhaps aggravated by it. Results from psychometric testing were not reported.

Contraindications for treatment in PE mentioned by Kohle et al. (1971) include: a history of psychiatric disorder or severe anxiety neurosis, depression, and hysterical affect. In addition, these authors state (pg. 90): "Beyond psychological considerations, the most cogent reason for disqualification of a patient appears to be his inability to cooperate (which makes support difficult), be it because of the severity of his physical condition or because the leukemia marks the end of a long sequence of illness and suffering which leaves little hope for the patient since a return to his life activities is impossible."

HOLLAND ET AL. Holland and associates (1971; 1977) studied fifty-two adult patients with relapsed acute leukemia treated in laminar airflow rooms and life islands at Roswell Park Memorial Institute in New York. Psychological assessment was based upon nurse's observations, a forced-choice patient questionnaire, clinical records and patient diaries. Psychiatric problems were found to be related either to the direct consequence of the disease process, resulting from leukemic infiltration of the brain, or due to side effects of treatment. Severe personality changes of a functional nature were rare (1971).

Holland (1971) stated (p. 294): "The onset of a functional psychosis, such as schizophrenia or manic-depressive illness, does not develop in the course of physical disease without prior history of significant psychiatric disturbance." She went on to conduct a rather useful discussion of the psychotropic effects of commonly used anti-cancer chemotherapeutic agents.

The Roswell Park study (Holland et al., 1977) found no evidence of sensory deprivation effects, such as problems with concentration or perceptual distortion. In addition, no consistent, isolation-related changes in behavioral scales measuring Anxiety-Depression, Positive Behavior, Discomfort, Isolation, or Delirium-Psychosis were obtained. Most scores showed minor fluctuations that appeared related to family or personal events.

Holland et al. (1977) divided their patients in terms of course of illness, using the following criteria: (1) Complete Remission; (2) Partial or No Remission and (3) Death While in PE, and found differences between groups only with regard to Anxiety-Depression, with increased levels of distress being positively related to degree of illness.

Data obtained from patient self-report indicated the majority of patients felt their stay in PE was better (48%) or the same (37%) as they had expected. More than three-fourths of patients spontaneously complained of not being able to touch people or of other isolation-related issues.

An additional finding was that many patients had increased difficulties during the first forty-eight to seventy-two hours of isolation and experienced increased ease of adaptation after this time period.

Holland et al. (1977) concluded that few psychological problems related to protective isolation, per se, existed in their sample and made general suggestions for psychosocial care.

It is important to note that the Roswell Park Study, though similar in many ways to the Childrens Hospital of Los Angeles investigation, differed in several important areas. First, and most obvious, Holland's patients were adults, and thus, theoretically, potentially better able to cope with isolation than children. Second, mean length of patient stay was thirty days, significantly lower than that of patients in the Childrens Hospital study. Third, all of Holland's patients were leukemics while the patients in the Childrens Hospital study suffered from a variety of solid tumors. In addition, Holland's (1977) data was published after the completion of the Childrens Hospital (CHLA) study and, thus, could not be used in planning our research. Nevertheless, as will be seen, several similar findings were independently obtained.

TELLER ET AL. In 1973 a multidisciplinary group in Germany headed by W. M. Teller published a monograph on the rearing of fraternal twin boys with lymphopenic hypogammaglobulinemia in PE from the age of six weeks. One twin was released from PE at twenty-nine months, the other at thirty-two months. PE took the form of a series of interlocking isolator modules.

Psychological study, coordinated by J. Kohle and C. Simons, was begun when the twins were fourteen months old. Methods of investigation included clinical records; nurses notes; interviews with nurses, physicians, and physiotherapists; administration of the Buhler-Hetzer Developmental Scale; and direct observation of daily play therapy sessions.

During the first fourteen months of treatment in PE, both twins had recurrent vomiting. One child displayed restless sleep as well as frequent grimacing subsequent to a convulsive seizure following tetanus inoculation. This led to suggestions of possible brain damage. Both children were friendly and eager for interaction with the nurses.

From fourteen to twenty-four months both children displayed extremely "vivid and intensive eye contact." They demonstrated impaired ability to handle play materials, which is not surprising considering the absence of such objects in their environment.

The developmental quotient (DQ) of one twin was age appropriate (100) and that of the second child (with suspected brain damage) was below the mean, and below the lower margin of the normal range (80). Five months later these scores remained the same, though skill with play materials, which had been introduced to the environment, improved. Learning ability remained below average.

The basic isolator unit employed in the Teller et al. (1973) study was similar to the life island, and thus, highly physically restricting. The authors interpreted their findings of developmental impairment as being due to physical restraint, prevention of regular, spontaneous movements, and narrowness of life experience. Placement of one twin, at twenty-seven months, in an enlarged isolator to which a play cubicle had been attached appeared related to subsequent development of effective problem-solving behavior in this child, while the other boy remaining in the small isolator unit showed no comparable improvement. The second twin's development consistently lagged behind that of his brother.

At two years of age the twins developed attachment behavior, showing preferences for specific nurses. Separation from favored caretakers was followed by thumbsucking and rhythmic rocking. Both children showed low tolerance for frustration, and one twin displayed intensive rhythmic scratching and sudden reversal of affect in response to frustration.

One twin developed aggressive behavior in the form of pinching and biting and did not like being held or cuddled. His brother, on the other hand, had a strong desire for physical contact.

Rhythmic rocking was present in both children by the time they were able to stand, but this disappeared after release from PE. The twin with suspected brain damage remained below the third percentile in height and weight and lagged behind his brother and his age group in motor and language development.

Upon release from PE, the less developed twin showed a noticeable arousal reaction. His pulse and breathing were accelerated; his temperature was elevated; his perspiration extensive; and he walked forwards and backwards rapidly and in quick succession. The authors attribute this to sudden sensory overload after over two years of relatively reduced perceptual input. They cite evidence of similar changes in animals (Newton et al., 1969). Three months later, the larger twin was released from PE and showed none of the above behaviors.

Teller et al. (1973) concluded with their impressions that "the twins when released from isolation were approaching a favorable stage of their psychological development." Despite learning disabilities, which the authors attributed to the lack of life experience in PE, no consistent pattern of hospitalism (Spitz, 1945) was observed. Rocking and self-stimulation were transitory.

Teller et al.'s (1973) study is valuable, because it indicated that extended PE treatment could be carried out with infants without causing long-term psychologically debilitating symptoms. Furthermore, the degree of restriction imposed by the use of the particular isolators employed was considerable. Also, the differences in the reactions of the two children indicates the importance of considering individual differences when evaluating the effects of prolonged isolation.

Strikingly absent from Teller et al.'s (1973) findings are reports of the degree and quality of parental involvement with the twins. While early mention was made of the mother's epilepsy and the father's alcoholism, the parents never reappear in the monograph. The authors do offer detailed descriptions or problems that arose with the nursing staff, including interactional difficulties between staff and the children. The extent that these were, or were not, mediated by parental contact, however, remains unknown. Similarly, in view of Bowlby's (1952), Spitz's (1945; 1946) and Klaus et al.'s (1970; 1972) writings, one might hypothesize that the quality of affectional bonds that develop between parents and children are important factors to consider in examining the effects of PE.

KELLERMAN ET AL. Prior to the beginnings of the Childrens Hospital of Los Angeles (CHLA) Protected Environment Study, a survey of thirteen PE installations around the U.S.A. concerning the psychological effects of protective isolation (Kellerman et al., 1977a) was conducted.

Respondents completed a checklist on which they noted the occurrence of psychiatric symptoms in adult and pediatric patients treated in PE. The majority of patients suffered from leukemia and other forms of cancer. Other diseases included immunodeficiencies, meningitis, and burns. Patient census ranged from six to two hundred and sixty, with a median of thirty-five. Range of days in isolation was two to two hundred and forty days, with a median of thirty-five.

Six of the thirteen installations reported removing patients from PE for psychological reasons. Removal criteria included destructive behavior; isolation-induced anxiety (including one instance accompanied by fears that the rapid airflow would cause pneumonia); regression that hampered medical treatment; and depression, often related to treatment failure. None of the patients removed for nonmedical reasons was a child.

Due to the lack of systematic psychological research conducted at these installations, precise behavioral data was impossible to obtain. When the respondents were queried regarding the general incidence of psychological problems, the majority reported incidences of anxiety, depression, withdrawal, and irregular sleep. A significant minority reported occurrences of a variety of hallucinations, disorientation to time and space, and regression. Less common were encopresis, nightmares, cognitive loss, and psychosomatic reactions.

Children appeared to incur fewer problems in adjusting to PE than did adults. Attempts were made (Kellerman et al., 1977a) to explain this, including the possibility that children are easier to stimulate than adults and may be more likely to elicit supportive reactions from staff, and the speculation that adults may be more assertive in their complaints and in actually removing themselves from isolation. In addition, it was suggested that staff may be more tolerant of deviant, particularly regressive, behavior in children than in adults.

METHOD

Patients

Psychological data were obtained for fourteen children with a variety of advanced-stage malignant solid tumors (non-Hodgkins lymphoma, neuroblastoma, ovarian carcinoma, recurrent Wilms' tumor, recurrent neurofibrosarcoma) treated in laminar airflow PE units. Patient age ranged from 2 years, 9 months to 16 years, 11 months, with a median of 7 years, 1 month.

The children's median length of stay in PE was 87.5 days, or almost three times that of the adult patients reported upon by Holland et al. (1977). Eight patients were female and six were male. Eleven of the children were newly diagnosed and, for them, placement in PE was part of initial oncologic treatment. The remaining three patients had been treated previously.

Racially, the children represented a not atypical mix for the catchment area served by Childrens Hospital of Los Angeles. Eight were caucasian, three were black, two were of Latin descent (one of these, exclusively Spanish-speaking), and one child was of mixed caucasian and Asian descent.

Setting

The children were treated in a single-ward laminar airflow unit consisting of four isolation units. The isolators were modules with transparent plastic walls with dimensions of 3.75m x 3.43m x 2.25m, and equipped with humidity control, cooling and heating systems, patient controls for nursing calls, electric drapery, and television. The constant and rapid cleaning of the air allows for a front doorway to the unit to be kept open. Entry of one person at a time into the modules was possible for periods of up to one hour, and visitors were dressed in a sterile "spacesuit," consisting of whole-body coverall, gloves, face mask, and head-covering. The four rooms were set up as pairs of double-modules. Each pair was separated by a transparent wall such that each room provided visual access to one other unit. Mutual visibility could be

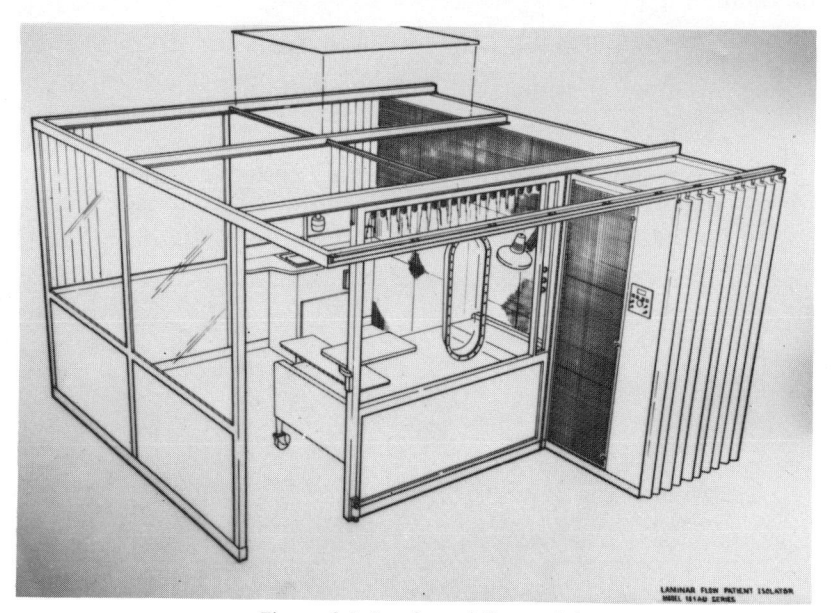

Figure 6-1. Laminar airflow unit.

terminated by the patient's operating an electric curtain control. The rooms were constructed in such a way to maximize perceptual contact with the outside world. Three of the four units had window views and all four had access to clocks.

Measures

Psychological measures included standard IQ tests (WISC, WISC-R, Binet) and a sixty-four item behavior rating form developed by the author and associates (Kellerman et al., 1976a; 1976b) entitled the Protective Environment Psychological Daily Rating (PE-PDR). The scale consisted of sixty-three behavioral items rated on a four-point Likert-type scale and one predominant mood item rated along a five-point scale accompanied by matching faces (Fig. 6-2).

The PE-PDR was completed by each child's primary nurse once at the end of each shift, leading to three daily ratings per child. Items on the PE-PDR were drawn from the literature on sensory deprivation, hospitalization, and social isolation and included ratings of appetite, sleep pattern, physical discomfort, affect, perception, activity level, social-interpersonal behaviors, and management problems (Kellerman et al., 1976b).

IQ tests were administered within the first week after admittance to PE and re-administered eight to ten weeks later, or prior to the child's leaving PE, if this took place before eight weeks.

Additional sources of information were clinical notes of nurses, physicians, psychologists, social workers, and play therapists attending on the unit.

Psychosocial Support Team

The psychosocial support team consisted of the following individuals:

1. Clinical Psychologist: The psychologist designed and coordinated an ongoing program of behavioral research on the unit, conducted initial eligibility screening of children and families, chaired weekly meetings with nursing staff, interviewed nurses for hire on the

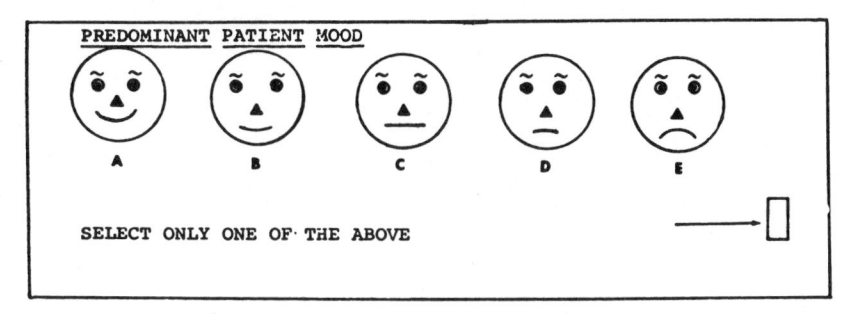

Figure 6-2. Affective rating scale.

unit, conducted orientation sessions for house staff physicians with the attending oncologist, and provided psychological consultation to the children, families, and staff.

2. Social Worker: The social worker provided counseling for parents regarding the emotional and practical problems arising from the child's stay in PE. This included counseling for extended family members and siblings as well.

3. Play Therapist: The patient activity specialist, or play therapist, helped prepare the children for medical procedures and served as a major supportive resource. Daily contact was offered to the children and included play and/or talking sessions, depending upon patient age. Such contact served both therapeutic and recreational purposes, helping patients maintain regular social interaction. This became especially important for children whose parents could not visit frequently.

In addition, a hospital-based school teacher provided daily lessons for all school-age children.

CLINICAL MANAGEMENT ISSUES

Psychological Criteria for Patient Eligibility

The development of screening criteria was difficult due to the lack of directly relevant data. The task of protecting psychologically vulnerable children from isolation-specific trauma was viewed as an important one. On the other hand, the medical protection afforded patients in PE, could, conceivably, be life-preserving or life-extending. This led us to develop rather conservative psychological criteria for *a priori* exclusion.

Conceptually, Kohle et al.'s (1971) criteria of severe premorbid psychiatric disturbance and/or conditions that made cooperation with medical procedures impossible, seemed especially useful. For children, the latter category included severe mental retardation, extreme hyperkinesis, and sensory defects. Our plan was to minimize the use of *a priori* exclusion criteria and to adopt an empirical, case-by-case approach toward evaluation of patient eligibility. By the cessation of the study, no children had been excluded from placement in PE.

Pre-entry Orientation

Teller et al.'s (1973) findings of hyperactivity, after leaving PE, in one of their two patients, raise the issue of *differential levels of stimulation* as an important construct when investigating the effects of isolation. That is, sudden shifts of perceptual input may bring about behavioral disturbance. For this reason, particular attention was paid to the two periods most likely to bring about such shifts: Entry into, and exit from, PE. In addition, the wealth of social psychological data illustrating the anxiety-reducing properties of providing prior information about stressful experiences (Janis, 1958; Cassell, 1965; Melamed and Siegel,

1975) led to the adoption of a pre-entry orientation program for the children and their families. This included:

1. Encouraging the child and family to view the unit twenty-four hours prior to entry and to ask questions.

2. When space and time permitted, allowing the child to stay, for twenty-four hours, in a "dirty" (unsterilized) laminar airflow room. This represents an attempt to create an intermediate stage between a hospital room and a sterile PE unit. The spatial and structural characteristics of the "dirty" room were identical to that of the sterile unit, but the child was free to come and go as he pleased and did not have to abide with the regulations of sterile procedure.

3. Written booklets covering both practical nursing-management and psychological issues were given to parents. Included in these pamphlets were descriptions of unit-specific procedures and restrictions and of the services provided by the psychosocial support team.

Pre-exit Counseling

Prior to the child's leaving PE, parents were customarily advised of possible changes that might occur in the child's behavior, primarily transitory changes in arousal level. (This was not begun until such changes did, empirically, occur in some of the first children treated in PE.) Counseling, with an emphasis upon keeping transition period relatively calm and avoiding major shifts in schedules and activity patterns, was offered, as was intervention aimed at helping the child return to school after prolonged absence.

Maintenance of Prior Behavioral Patterns

Just as efforts were made to minimize sudden shifts in sensory stimulation, so was attention paid to maximizing the continuation of premorbid activities while the child was in PE. Thus, when medical conditions allowed, the children were encouraged to wear street clothes, as opposed to hospital gowns, and regular entry of parents and other family members into the isolation unit was facilitated. The children were helped to maintain academic involvement by having their regular teacher send school assignments and collaborating with the hospital-based schoolteacher who made daily visits with each patient.

The children were also encouraged to bring with them familiar articles of clothing, toys, and other transitional objects that could be sterilized and placed within the unit to make it seem more home-like. In addition, attempts were made to find out from parents what their particular child-rearing pattern was and, within the medical restrictions of PE, to duplicate as much of this as possible. In line with minimizing environmental shifts, we found it useful to have the children adhere to a daily schedule, so that waking, eating, and the frequent medical procedures that were part of PE treatment (oral antibiotics three times a day, baths twice a day, intravenous chemotherapy and diagnostic tests as required) occurred on an expected, quasi-regular basis. This was done to help the children maintain a sense of time-orientation.

Compliance With Sterile Procedure

Despite the large number of regulations imposed upon the children due to sterile procedure, compliance was generally high. There was some question, initially, about the ability of young children to comprehend the concept of barrier isolation. It was found, however, that even our youngest study patient, less than three years old at time of entry to PE, quickly became familiar with the notion of "clean" vs. "dirty" and made no attempts to leave the unit. In addition the word "sterilize" became a part of her vocabulary. This made it possible to allow this patient total access to the room as opposed to confining her in a crib (which would have constituted isolation within isolation). Since the termination of the study we have treated patients as young as eleven months old and have found all of them able to grasp and comply with the spatial restrictions of PE.

Some adolescent patients made attempts to leave the unit in fits of anger. Staff reaction to this was to bodily prevent exit from the unit while offering the explanation that this was being done out of care and concern for the patient's well-being. No patient attempted to leave more than one time.

Ambivalence Toward PE

The children grasped and incorporated the concepts of sterility to such a degree that, quite apart from violating unit procedure, some of them manifested the opposite reaction — exhibiting a reluctance to leave even after their leukocyte counts had risen and it was medically safe to do so. Several of the children voiced concerns about the world outside being dirty and hazardous and needed reassurance and detailed explanations before feeling comfortable about exit. One child had to be bodily removed from PE after he refused to leave the unit for three days past the exit date.

Such ambivalence may have been increased by a reluctance on the part of the children to sever some of the emotional ties they had formed with the staff. This was particularly true in cases where parental visits were sparse. Family members were counseled about possible ambivalent reactions to leaving PE so that they would not be disappointed if the child did not gleefully leave the unit and immediately rush into their arms.

It is thus evident that children, even very young ones, can easily maintain compliance with the spatial restrictions of PE without being subjected to overly coercive procedures. It is advisable, in fact, that the importance of sterility not be overemphasized and that the temporary nature of PE treatment be specified. In any case, all the children benefited from age-appropriate medical explanations of why and how they were being treated.

Maintenance of Affective Stability

It was common for the families of the children to arrange parties around birthdays, holidays, and other occasions. In some instances, particularly when large numbers of celebrants were involved, with an accompanying increase in noise level and excitement, a "morning-after-blues" reaction was noted on the part of the patients. This transitory depression, occurring when the children were alone and the festivities had ended, was attributed to the abrupt shift in stimulation. Consequently, we began to advise parents to keep in-unit parties low-key and to postpone large-scale celebrations for when the child had returned home and become accustomed to the pre-PE activity pattern.

PSYCHOLOGICAL RESPONSES TO ISOLATION

Removal of Patients

No child had to be removed from PE due to psychological factors. Entry and exit from reverse isolation took place on the basis of medical criteria. This is congruent with the data from a previous study (Kellerman et al., 1977a) in which removal of adult patients due to behavioral disfunction was noted while removal of pediatric patients was not.

Perceptual Disturbances

Permanent alterations of the children's sensory apparatus were nonexistent. There were reports of heightened arousal immediately following discharge from PE. Some children described a temporary state during which sounds were louder and movements seemed faster. One child reported that during the trip home from the hospital automobile turns felt like a roller coaster ride. This altered state lasted, typically, for one day or less, and did not occur in all of the children.

Out of 2,910 possible ratings, done by the nurses, there were twenty-six reports of hallucinatory behavior, or less than one percent. These occurred in seven of the children, and were both visual and auditory. Follow-up interviews revealed the majority of these not to be true hallucinations, but, rather, dream-like experiences during pre-sleep or upon arousal from sleep. One child did experience bonafide visual hallucinations six times toward the end of his stay in PE, and this was believed related to febrile delirium.

Similarly, time or space disorientation was reported in less than 1 percent of rating periods, with no child exhibiting more than eight incidents. Nine children experienced transitory time disorientation, and seven were rated as being disoriented with regard to space.

Eighty-five percent of hallucinatory ratings and 67 percent of disorientation ratings occurred in children who had been in PE for six weeks or longer.

Four children, for whom rocking was a premorbid habit, maintained this form of self-stimulation throughout their stay in PE. The remainder of the children did not manifest any new signs of unusual or long-term autostimulation.

Sleep

For the sample as a whole, restless sleep was recorded during 11 percent of rating periods, with 1 percent representing restless sleep. Individual rates of restless sleep ranged from .8 percent to 24 percent. Five children experienced a total of forty-one recordable nightmares, with seven of these rated as severe. No child experienced nightmares during more than 4 percent of recording periods. All but two nightmares were recorded during or after the sixth week in PE. There was no evidence of a rate of disturbed sleep greater than what has been recorded by Hersen (1972) in the healthy pediatric population.

Sleep walking was rare, occurring in only three children and never more than three times. Talking during sleep, on the other hand, was more common, recorded 112 times in eleven children. The highest individual rate of sleep-talk was 11 percent.

Transitory or occasional enuresis was present in six children (frequency equal or less than four times) and more prolonged bedwetting was recorded in three patients, all females with metastatic neuroblastoma. One of these was two years, ten months old at the time of admission, and had been barely toilet-trained prior to diagnosis. After entry to PE, she returned to wetting herself. Reintroduction of daytime toilet training was successful, but nocturnal enuresis persisted. Such behavior cannot be considered unusual in a child of this age.

A seven-year-old girl wet her bed twenty-one times with recordings distributed throughout her stay in PE. This child suffered from severe pancreatitis during her treatment, and it was suggested by the medical staff that this may have been a factor contributing toward incontinence. The third child, a five-year-old girl exhibited fifteen instances of nocturnal enuresis.

Intellectual Functioning

IQ test-retest data indicated no consistent pattern of intellectual decrement. Two patients could not be administered complete testing due to severity of illness, one child was too young and simultaneously blind, and one did not speak English. For the remaining ten children, seven showed increased IQ scores upon retest, one patient's score remained the same, and two children showed decrements of 2 and 4 points respectively. Group means are presented in Table 6-I.

There was one Wechsler Scale subtest, Coding, for which seven out of ten patients showed decrement upon retest. This may indicate some decrease in hand-eye coordination due to prolonged reverse isolation, or may represent decreased attention span relating either to isolation or the less than optimal testing situation encountered on an often busy unit. There were no other patterns of consistent change in any other subtest.

Affect

Affective ratings were made in the form of the five-point predominant mood scale, whose faces corresponded to very positive, positive, neutral, negative, and very negative categories; and the chil-

TABLE 6-I

CHANGE IN WECHSLER IQ SCALE FUNCTIONING IN CHILDREN WITH
CANCER TREATED IN PROTECTED ENVIRONMENTS (n = 10)

	Testing 1		Testing 2		
	M	SD	M	SD	Net Change
Full Scale IQ Score	114.2	14.5	119.4	13.9	+5.2
Verbal IQ Score	109.5	14.2	111.3	12.5	+1.8
Performance IQ Score	116.7	13.2	125.0	13.7	+8.3
Subtests					
Information	10.6	2.7	11.2	2.4	+ .6
Comprehension	12.1	3.8	12.7	3.6	+ .6
Arithmetic	11.1	2.5	10.9	2.2	− .2
Similarities	13.6	2.8	13.6	2.7	-
Vocabulary	10.1	4.0	10.6	3.4	+ .5
Digit Span	11.0	2.6	11.0	5.5	-
Picture Completion	11.3	2.4	14.8	3.9	+3.5
Picture Arrangement	12.1	3.2	13.4	2.6	+1.3
Block Design	11.9	2.6	12.2	3.2	+ .3
Object Assembly	12.6	1.5	15.2	3.1	+2.6
Coding	14.8	3.3	13.3	3.0	−1.5

dren were rated on such adjectives as cheerful, friendly, withdrawn, fearful, angry, and sociable.

Rate of depression, operationally defined as the sum of negative and very negative ratings divided by total ratings, was 12 percent for the complete sample. "Severe" depression, taking into account only *very* negative ratings, was 4 percent. Individual rates of severe depression ranged from zero to 7 percent. There was no significant difference in rates of depression between on and off chemotherapy periods (On chemo = 14.5 percent; off chemo = 11 percent, x^2 = 1.1, p = 2.30). The total of positive mood ratings was 69 percent, and neutral ratings comprised 19 percent. Rates of cheerfulness, friendliness, and sociability were greater than 80 percent. The overall pattern presented is of a group of children who, despite their illness and treatment, were generally in good spirits.

The following affective pattern was found in virtually all the children: initial depression upon entry to PE, improved mood by the second week of isolation, followed by a second depressive peak between the seventh and ninth week. For patients who remained in PE past the ninth week, a period of improved mood followed, and generally low rates of depression were found until discharge. There was no correlation (−.02) between individual length of stay in PE and rate of depression.

The initial depression can be partially explained in terms of the trauma of being placed in a novel environment. In addition, for eleven of the children assignment to PE came quickly after initial diagnosis, during an inherently stressful time. For the remaining three children PE placement took place because of previous treatment failure, also stressful. There is no obvious explanation for the rise in depression at the second month, though it was noted that it became difficult to find novel forms of stimulation for the children around this time. The finding that the children rebounded after both depressive peaks is an encouraging one.

The children were divided into two groups depending upon their medical status at the end of treatment in PE. Status positive was defined as partial or complete remission of disease and status negative as recurrent or increased disease, or no improvement. Similar to Holland, et al.'s (1977) findings, no significant difference was found, in terms of depression, between these two groups. (Status positive, n = 8, % depression = 10.62, s.d. = 4.12; Status negative, n = 6, % depression = 13.55, s.d. = 5.55). No difference in severe depression was found between groups.

Management Problems

A rate of 64 percent appetite loss was obtained for the sample as a whole with *minimum* appetite loss for a given patient 22 percent. Thus, it is not surprising that getting the children to eat and drink was the predominant management problem recorded by the nursing staff (40% of recording periods). Other problems included management of oral medication (32%), toileting (18%), injections (11.4%), exercise (10.5%), and baths (10.4%). Comparison of problems relating to injections to other categories may be misleading because injections were not a daily occurrence. It is of interest to note that when injection-related difficulties did arise, there was a greater tendency for them to be severe (41%) as opposed to the other problems, where proportional severity ranged from 7 to 28%. This is in accordance with a recent study indicating conditioned anxiety related to medical procedures as a major problem among children with cancer (Kellerman et al., 1978). On a general measure of cooperativeness, the children were rated as being cooperative 77% of the time. No child was rated as uncooperative during more than 5 percent of rating periods.

Activity Pattern

As a group, the children were out of their beds 71 percent of the time. Time out of bed was greater than one and a half per eight hour shift during 34 percent of rating periods. For thirteen patients, rate of inactivity ranged from 22 to 41 percent. One seventeen-year-old girl with neurofibrosarcoma was inactive 72% of the time due to paralysis. Rates of inactivity and depression correlated .67, however, it is obviously misleading to imply causality from this relationship, as it is impossible to discern whether poor mood brought about inactivity, or vice versa. Similar to Holland et al.'s (1977) findings, it was clear that periods of lethargy, depression, withdrawal, and apathy were most often related to physical, disease-related factors, rather than to psychogenic etiology. It was observed, however, that even during periods of physical illness, encouragement of medically appropriate activity on the part of the children brought about improvement of mood.

Social Communication

As a group, the children were outgoing and sociable. They initiated conversation during 85 percent of rating periods, and did so often 34 percent of the time. On an adjectival measure of sociability, the nurses rated them as sociable 91 percent of the time.

Response to visitors was rated as positive 89 percent of the time, indifferent 9 percent, and negative 2 percent. Not surprisingly, the children were more likely to initiate conversation on days in which their predominant mood was rated as good (90%) as opposed to when they were depressed (71%).

In a previous study based upon a partial sample (Kellerman et al., 1977b) it was found that disease-related conversation on the part of the children was not linearly associated with depression. Results from the total sample confirmed this, in that there was a curvilinear relationship between the children's talking about their illness and affect. Such conversation was most likely to occur during periods of moderate happiness (25%) and least likely during extremes at both ends of the mood scale (15% of very negative mood; 16% of very positive mood). The Pearson correlations between disease-related communication and both poor mood and very poor mood were .11 and .20, respectively, indicating no strong tendency for children who talked about their illness to be either more or less depressed than those who were less communicative. Hospitalization and illness were relatively frequent topics of conversation, the former being discussed during 28% of rating periods, the latter, during 20%.

Sedation

Congruent with Holland et al.'s (1977) findings, the use of psychotropic medication was rare. Tranquilizing and/or sedating agents, primarily Chlorpromazine®, were given during 11 percent of rating periods almost always as an emetic. The rate of sedation during chemotherapy (19%) was significantly greater than during periods of no chemotherapy (9%, x^2 = 11.49, p = .001). Children who were sedated were more likely to be rated as depressed and this may have resulted from the fact that sedated children were likely to be receiving chemotherapy or feeling ill, or from the lowering of activity brought about by the medication.

STAFF ISSUES

In their study of twin boys raised under gnotobiotic conditions, Teller et al. (1973) reported several difficulties that arose in the relationship between nursing staff and patients. The nurses, not selected upon the basis of any psychological screening, initially interpreted isolation treatment as implying overprotection and restrictive handling of the children and imposed excessive rules and regulations. Excessive projective identification on the part of nurses was also noted, particularly when the children began to exhibit obstinate behavior. Conflicting styles brought about interpersonal difficulties between individual nurses, who differed in their needs to impose control upon the children. In one instance, the removal of a particularly domineering nurse was found to have beneficial results for both patients and staff.

Teller et al. (1973) took note of the fact that PE nursing is extremely demanding, in terms of the many regulations concerning sterile procedures, and the intensity of the one-to-one nurse-patient ratio. An additional factor should be mentioned: Just as PE units set up a physical barrier for patients, so do they restrict the activities of staff members. The Childrens Hospital laminar airflow rooms were set away from the general ward in a separate room. Nurses spend the lion's share of an eight hour shift within this restricted space. Compounded with this is the stress of intensively caring for seriously ill children. Subsequent heightened interpersonal tension is not surprising.

Nevertheless, though staff problems can be rationalized, strong efforts must be taken to reduce their frequency because of almost inevitable consequences upon the children. Like Teller et al. (1973) we observed a clear relationship between nursing behavior and patient mood, and like the German study, we found it necessary to remove from unit employment nurses who displayed high rates of inappropriate behavior.

Four nurses were either dismissed or encouraged not to return to the unit. A unifying characteristic of all of them was that they led unhappy lives out of work. Three were unmarried and not engaged in meaningful interpersonal relationships. One woman was experiencing marital difficulties. In two instances there was evidence of substance abuse and in one case, unbeknownst to us, there had been a previous psychiatric hospitalization. In all four cases, psychological problems of nurses led to their imposing excessive and inappropriate regulations upon patients.

These problems led to the adoption of psychological screening as a prerequisite of employment on the PE unit. Such screening was conducted by the psychologist and attempted to explore the following issues:

1. Prior experience with seriously ill children, particularly those with cancer and emotional reaction to disease-related crises.

2. Motivation for wanting to work on a PE unit. In addition to pragmatic issues, the most commonly mentioned reason given was the desire to work intensively with patients on a one-to-one basis. This led to discussion of appropriate boundaries and guidelines for such work.

3. Existence of satisfying interpersonal relationships and recreational interests off the job.

4. Understanding on the part of the nurse of the functions of the psychosocial support team and the necessity to consider treatment as part of a collaborative effort.

In addition to weeding out individuals who were not appropriate for work in PE, or helping such nurses self-select out, psychological screening was useful for apprising appropriate applicants of unit-related issues at an early stage.

In the best of circumstances, PE nursing is difficult, and it is realistic to expect that such employment should be temporary. The best prepared, most well-adjusted individuals have found it difficult to productively remain on the unit for more than two years. Thus, high turnover should be expected and, perhaps, welcomed.

In order to promote and maintain staff morale, all efforts should be made to offer psychosocial support to nurses, physicians, and psychosocial professionals. This can include educational sessions (for house staff physicians), regularly scheduled meetings to discuss patient and personal issues (for nurses and psychosocial staff), and the opportunity for nurses to float to other wards in order to experience job diversity.

SUMMARY

A psychological study was conducted of fourteen children with a variety of solid tumors treated in protective isolation in laminar airflow rooms. Consistent with similar studies of adult patients, no long-term or debilitating psychological effects were noted, contrary to what might be expected from some of the literature on sensory deprivation, social isolation, and severe illness.

Some of this may be due to the clinical efforts made at providing maximal psychosocial care. These were designed to prevent PE treatment from resembling classical deprivation or isolation situations and included physical construction that provided access to windows, clocks, and patient-patient contact; encouragement of regular daily schedules, maximal activity, and continuation of pre-illness behavior; and the use of hospital teaching, play therapy, pre-entry orientation, procedural preparation, family counseling, and careful detailed monitoring of psychological responses. Patterns of psychological reactions to PE treatment are noted as are staff responses to working in such an intensive ward. Suggestions are made for hiring criteria for nurses that minimize the likelihood of inappropriate staff-patient interactions.

The use of laminar airflow units may or may not continue as part of regular oncologic treatment, depending upon the nature of findings that accrue from medical studies of their utility. Nevertheless, it seems reasonable to predict that an increased utilization of highly technical treatment systems is probable. The psychological effects of such treatment need to be observed and managed in a systematic manner.

REFERENCES

Adams, H. B.: Therapeutic potentialities of sensory deprivation procedures. *Int Ment Health Res Newsletter*, 4:7, 1964.

Adams, H. B.: A case utilizing sensory deprivation procedures. In Krasner, L. and

Ullmann, L. (Eds.) *Case Studies in Behavior Modification.* New York, Holt, Rinehart & Winston, 1965.

Adams, H. B., and Cooper, G. D.: Sensory deprivation and personality change. *J Nerv Ment Dis, 143:*256, 1966.

Adams, H. B.; Cooper, G. D., and Carrera, R. N.: Individual differences in behavioral reactions of psychiatric patients to brief partial sensory deprivation. *Percept Mot Skills, 34:*199, 1972.

Barbero, G. J., and Shaheen, E.: Environmental failure to thrive: a clinical view. *J Pediatrics, 5:*639, 1967.

Barnett, C. R.; Leiderman, P. H., Grobstein, R., and Klaus, M.: Neonatal separation: the maternal side of interactional deprivation. *Pediatrics, 45:*197, 1970.

Bexton, W. H.; Heron, W., and Scott, T. H.: Effects of decreased variation in the sensory environment. *Can J Psychol, 8:*70, 1954.

Bodey, G. P.; Gehan, E. A., and Reireich, E. J.: Protected environment-prophylactic antibiotic program in the chemotherapy of acute leukemia. *Am J Med Sci, 262:*138, 1971.

Bowlby, J.: Separation anxiety. *Int Rev Psychoanal, 41:*89, 1960.

Cassell, S.: Effects of brief puppet therapy upon the emotional responses of children undergoing cardiac catheterization. *J Consult Clin Psychol, 29:*1, 1965.

Charney, I. W.: Regression and reorganization in the "isolation treatment" of children: A clinical contribution to sensory deprivation research. *J Child Psychol Psychiatr, 4:*47, 1963.

Cohen, R. L.: Developments in the isolation therapy of behavior disorders of children. In J. H. Masserman (Ed.) *Current psychiatric therapies,* Vol. 3. New York, Grune & Stratton, 1963.

Coleman, R. W., and Provence, S.: Environmental retardation (hospitalism) in infants living in families. *Pediatrics, 19:*285, 1957.

Cooper, G. D.; Adams, H. B., Dickinson, J. R., and York, M. W.: Interviewer's role-playing and responses to sensory deprivation: a clinical demonstration. *Percep Mot Skills, 40:*291, 1975.

Corso, J. F.: Sensory deprivation. In J. F. Corso, *The Experimental Psychology of Sensory Behavior.* New York, Holt, Rinehart, & Winston, 1967.

Dennis, W.: The effect of restricted practice upon the reaching, sitting and standing of two infants. *J Genet Psychol, 47:*17, 1935.

Dennis, W., and Dennis, M. G.: The effect of cradling practice upon the onset of walking in Hopi Children. *J Genet Psychol, 56:*77, 1940.

Dennis, W., and Dennis, M. G.: Development under controlled conditions. In W. Dennis (Ed.) *Reading in Child Psychology.* New York, Prentice-Hall, 1951.

Dimock, H.: *The Child in the Hospital: A Study of His Emotional and Social Well Being.* Philadelphia, Davis, 1960.

Doane, B. K.: *Changes in Visual Function Following Perceptual Isolation.* Unpublished Ph.D. dissertation, McGill University, 1955.

Downs, F. S.: Bed rest and sensory disturbances. *Am J Nurs, 74:*434, 1974.

Elmer, E.; Gregg, G. S., and Ellison, P.: Late results of the failure to thrive syndrome. *Clin Pediatr, 8:*584, 1969.

Fanaroff, A. A.; Kennell, J. H., and Klaus, M. H.: Follow-up of low birth weight infants — the predictive value of maternal visiting periods. *Pediatrics, 49:*287, 1972.

Fischoff, J.; Whitten, C. F., and Pettit, M. G.: A psychiatric study of mothers of infants with growth failure secondary to maternal deprivation. *J Pediatrics, 78:*209, 1971.

Gellert, E.: Reducing the emotional stresses of hospitalization for children. *Am J Occup Ther, 12:*125, 1958.

Haggard, E. A.: Some effects of geographic and social isolation in natural settings. In J. Rasumussen (Ed.): *Man in Isolation and Confinement.* Chicago, Aldine, 1973.

Harlow, H. F., and Harlow, M.K.: The affectional systems. In A. Schrier et al. (Ed.) *Behavior of Nonhuman Primates,* Vol. 2. New York, Academic Press, 1965.

Harlow, H. F.; Suomi, S. J., and McKinney, W. T.: Experimental production of depression in monkeys. *Mainly Monkeys, 1:*6, 1970.

Harlow, H. F., and Suomi, S. J.: Induced depression in monkeys. *Behav Biol, 12:*273, 1974.

Hersen, M.: Nightmare behavior: a review. *Psychol Bull, 78:*37, 1972.

Higgins, R.: Psychological effects of treating congenital disorders in hospitals. *Dev Med Child Neurol, 7:*435, 1965.

Hill, J. C., and Robinson, B. A.: A case of retarded mental development associated with restricted movements in infancy. *Br J Med Psychol, 19:*268, 1930.

Hinde, R. A., and Spencer-Booth, Y.: Effects of brief separation from mother on rhesus monkeys. *Science, 173:*111, 1966.

Holland, J.: Acute leukemia: Psychological aspects of treatment. In F. Elkerbout et al. (Eds.) *Cancer Chemotherapy.* Leyden, Leyden University, 1971.

Holland, J.; Plumb, M., Yates, J., and Harris, S.: Psychological response of patients with acute leukemia to germ-free environments. *Cancer, 40:*871, 1977.

Janis, I.: *Psychological Stress.* New York, John Wiley & Sons, 1958.

Katz, V.: Auditory stimulation and developmental behavior of the premature infant. *Nurs Res, 20:*196, 1971.

Kaufman, I. C., and Roseblum, L. A.: The reaction to separation in infant monkeys: anaclitic depression and conservation-withdrawal. *Psychosom Med, 29:*648, 1967.

Kellerman, J.; Rigler, D., Siegel, S. E., McCue, K., et al.: Pediatric cancer patients in reverse isolation utilizing protected environments. *J Pediatr Psychol, 1:*21, 1976a.

Kellerman, J.; Rigler, D., Siegel, S. E., McCue, K., et al.: Psychological evaluation and management of pediatric oncology patients in protected environments. *Med Pediatr Oncol, 2:*353, 1976b.

Kellerman, J.; Rigler, D., and Siegel, S. E.: The psychological effects of isolation in protected environments. *Am J Psychiatry, 134:*563, 1977a.

Kellerman, J.; Rigler, D., Siegel, S. E., and Katz, E. R.: Disease-related communication and depression in pediatric cancer patients. *J Pediatr Psychol, 2:*52, 1977b.

Kellerman, J., and Katz, E. R.: The adolescent with cancer: theoretical, clinical and research issues. *J Pediatr Psychol, 2:*127, 1977.

Kellerman, J.; Katz, E. R., and Siegel, S. E.: Psychological problems of children with cancer. Unpublished manuscript, 1979.

Klaus, M., and Kennel, J. H.: Mothers separated from their newborn infant. *Pediatr Clin North Am, 17:*1015, 1970.

Klaus, M.; Kennel, J. H., and Plumb, N.: Human maternal behavior at the first contact with her young. *Pediatrics, 46:*187, 1970.

Klaus, M.; Jerauld, R., Kreger, N., McAlpine, W., Steffa, M., and Kennel, J. H.: Maternal attachment — importance of first post-partum days. *N Engl J Med, 286:*460, 1972.

Kohle, K.; Simons, C., and Weidlich, S.: Psychological aspects in the treatment of leukemia patients in the isolated-bed system "life island." *Psychother, Psychosom, 19:*85, 1971.

Koluchova, J.: Severe deprivation in twins: a case study. *J Child Psychol Psychiatr, 13:*107, 1972.

Koluchova, J.: The further development of twins after severe and prolonged deprivation: a second report. *J Child Psychol Psychiatr, 17:*181, 1976.

Leifer, A. D.; Leiderman, P. H., Barnett, C. R., and Williams, J. A.: Effects of mother-infant separation of maternal attachment behavior. *Child Dev, 43:*1203, 1972.

Levine, A. S.; Siegel, S. E., and Schreiber, A. D.: Protected environments and prophylactic antibiotics: a prospective controlled study of their utility in the therapy of acute leukemia. *N Engl J Med, 288:*477, 1973.

Levitan, A. A., and Perry, S.: Infectious complications of chemotherapy in a protected environment. *N Engl J Med, 276:*881, 1967.

Levy, D. M.: On the problem of movement restraint. *Am J Orthopsychiatry, 14:*644, 1944.

Lilly, J. C.: Mental effects of reduction of ordinary levels of physical stimuli in intact, healthy persons. *Psychiatr Res Rep, 5:*1, 1956.

Mahaffy, P. R.: Effects of hospitalization on children admitted for tonsillectomy and adenoidectomy. *Nurs Res, 14:*12, 1965.

Mendelson, J. H., and Foley, J.: An abnormality of mental function affecting patients with poliomyelitis in tank type respirators. *Trans Am Neurol Assoc, 81:*134, 1956.

Mendelson, J. H.; Solomon, P., and Lindemann, E.: Hallucinations of poliomyelitis patients during treatment in a respirator. *J Nerv Ment Dis, 126:*421, 1958.

Melamed, B. G., and Siegel, L. J.: Reduction of anxiety in children facing hospitalization and surgery by use of filmed modeling. *J Consult Clin Psychol, 43:*511, 1975.

McKegney, R. P.: The intensive care syndromes — definition, treatment and prevention of a new disease of medical progress. *Conn Med, 30:*633, 1966.

McKinney, W. T., and Bunney, W. E.: Animal model of depression. *Arch Gen Psychiatry, 21:*240, 1969.

Nachum, L. H.: Madness in the recovery room from open-heart surgery. *Conn Med, 29:*771, 1965.

Neal, M. V.: *The relationship between a regimen of vestibular stimulation and the developmental behavior of the premature infant.* Unpublished doctoral dissertation, New York University, 1967.

Oersten, P. A., and Mattson, A.: Hospitalization symptoms in children. *Acta Paediatr Scand, 44:*79, 1955.

Penland, W. Z. Jr., and Perry, S.: Portable laminar-airflow isolator. *Lancet, 1:*174, 1970.

Powell, L. F.: The effect of extra stimulation and maternal involvement on the development of low-birth-weight infants and on maternal behavior. *Child Dev, 45:*106, 1974.

Preisler, H. D., and Bjornsson, S.: Protected environment units in the treatment of acute leukemia. *Semin Oncol, 2:*369, 1975.

Preston, D. G.; Baker, R. P., and Seay, B.: Mother-infant separation in the patas monkey. *Dev Psychol, 3:*298, 1970.

Prugh, D. G.; Staub, E. M., Sands, H. H., Kirschbaum, R. M., and Lenihan, E. A.: Study of the emotional reactions of children and families to hospitalization and illness. *Am J Orthopsychiatry, 23:*70, 1953.

Prugh, D.: Emotional aspects of the hospitalization of children. In M. F. Shore (Ed.) *Red Is the Color of Hurting: Planning for Children in the Hospital.* Bethesda, National Institute of Mental Health, 1965.

Rajecki, D. W.; Suomi, S. J., Scott, E. Z., and Campbell, B.: Effects of social isolation and social separation in domestic chicks. *Dev Psychol, 13:*143, 1977.

Rasumussen, J. E.: *Man in Isolation and Confinement.* Chicago, Aldine, 1973.

Rice, R. D.: Neurophysiological development in premature infants following stimulation. *Dev Psychol, 13:*69, 1977.

Robertson, J.: *Young Children in the Hospital.* London, Tavistock, 1958.

Sackett, G. P.; Holm, R. A., and Ruppenthal, G. C.: Social isolation rearing: species differences in behavior of macaque monkeys. *Dev Psychol, 12:*283, 1976.

Scarr-Salapatek, S., and Williams, M. L.: A stimulation program for low-birth-weight infants. *Am J Pub Health, 62:*662, 1972.

Schaeffer, H. R.: Objective observations of personality development in early infancy. *Br J Med Psychol, 31:*174, 1958.

Schecter, M. D.: The orthopedically handicapped child. *Arch Gen Psychiatry, 4:*247, 1961.

Schimpff, S. D.; Greene, W. H., and Young, V. M.: Infection prevention in acute non-lymphocytic leukemia: laminar airflow room reverse isolation with oral, nonabsorbable antibiotic prophylaxis. *Ann Int Med, 82:*106, 1975.

Schlottmann, R. S., and Seay, B.: Mother-infant separation in the Java monkey. *J Comp Physiol Psychol, 79:*334, 1972.

Shurley, J. T.: Profound experimental sensory isolation. *Am J Psychiatry, 117:*539, 1960.

Sibinga, M. S.; Friedman, C. J., Steisel, I. M., and Sinnamon, H. M.: The effect of immobilization and sensory restriction on children with phenylketonuria. *Pediatr Res, 2:*371, 1968.

Sibinga, M. S., and Friedman, C. J.: Restraint and speech. *Pediatrics, 48:*116, 1971.

Siegel, S. E.; Higgins, G., and Nachum, R.: Protected environments in the therapy of disseminated childhood solid tumors (abstract). Presented at the annual meeting of the *Association for Gnotobiotics,* Buffalo, N. Y., October 31 — November 1, 1976.

Solberg, C. O.; Matsen, J. M., and Vesley, D.: Laminar airflow protection in bone marrow transplantation. *Applied Microbiology, 21:*209, 1971.

Spitz, R. A.: Hospitalism. An inquiry into the genesis of psychiatric conditions in early childhood. *Psychoanalytic Study of the Child, 1:*53, 1945.

Spitz, R. A.: Hospitalism. A follow-up report. *Psychoanalytic Study of the Child, 2:*113, 1946.

Suomi, S. J.; Harlow, H. F., and Domek, C. J.: Effect of repetitive infant-infant separation of young monkeys. *J Abnorm Psychol, 76:*161, 1970.

Suomi, S. J.; Collins, M. L., and Harlow, H. F.: Effects of permanent separation from mother on infant monkeys. *Dev Psychol, 9:*376, 1973.

Suomi, S. J.; Collins, M. L., Harlow, H. F., and Ruppenthal, G. C.: Effects of maternal and peer separations on young monkeys. *J Child Psychol Psychiatry, 17:*101, 1976.

Teller, W. M. (Ed.): Rearing of non-identical twins with lymphopenic hypogammaglobulinaemia under gnotobiotic conditions. *Act Paediatr Scand Suppl,* 240, 1973.

Vernon, J.; Marton, T., and Peterson, E.: Sensory deprivation and hallucinations. *Sci, 133:*1808, 1961.

Vernon, D. T. A.; Foley, J. M., and Sipowicz, R. R.: *The Psychological Response of Children to Hospitalization and Illness: a review of the literature.* Springfield, Thomas, 1965.

Wadeson, H., and Carpenter, W. T.: Impact of the seclusion room experience. *J Nerv Ment Dis, 163:*318, 1976.

Wexler, D.; Mendelson, J., Leiderman, P. H., and Solomon, P.: Sensory deprivation: a technique of studying psychiatric aspects of stress. *Arch Neurol Psychiatry, 79:*225, 1958.

Whitten, C. F.; Pettit, M. G., and Fischoff, J.: Evidence that growth failure from maternal deprivation is secondary to undereating. *J Am Med Assoc, 209:*1675, 1969.

Williams, M. L., and Scarr, S.: Effects of short-term intervention in performance in low-birth-weight, disadvantaged children. *Pediatrics, 47:*289, 1971.

Yates, J. W., and Holland, J. F.: A controlled study of isolation and endogenous microbial suppression in acute myelocytic leukemia patients. *Cancer, 32:*1490, 1973.

Zubek, J. P.; Welch, G., and Saunders, M. G.: EEF changes during and after 14 days of perceptual deprivation. *Science, 139:*490, 1963.

Zubek, J. P.: Sensory Deprivation: *Fifteen Years of Research.* New York, Appleton-Century-Crofts, 1969.

Zuckerman, M.: Variables affecting deprivation results. In J. P. Zubek (Ed.): *Sensory Deprivation:* Fifteen Years of Research. New York, Appleton-Century-Crofts, 1969.

Chapter Seven

SEPARATION-DEPRIVATION AND CHILDHOOD CANCER: A CONCEPTUAL RE-EVALUATION

ELIZABETH J. SUSMAN
ALBERT R. HOLLENBECK
BARBARA E. STROPE
STEPHEN P. HERSH
ARTHUR S. LEVINE
PHILIP A. PIZZO

INTRODUCTION

A CONSENSUS EXISTS that prolonged institutionalization leads to changes in a child's behavior characterized by initial distress followed by a slow process of adaptation to the new environment. The distress associated with institutional care is assumed to be a response of young children to separation from the primary object of attachment, usually the child's mother. The significance of early maternal separation and subsequent deprivation on later psychological development has been consistently validated in both human and sub-human primates. Deviant maternal care plays a central role in formulations that attempt to relate deficiency conditions in early childhood to later deviant intellectual and personal-social functioning (Bowlby, 1969; Goldfarb, 1945; Spitz, 1945; Yarrow, 1961).

The effect of prolonged institutionalization on human development is an important problem for physicians, nurses, and behavioral scientists. With advances in medical treatment, children with diseases that previously meant certain death are now living an extended or normal life span, but life-sustaining treatment regimens often necessitate protracted periods of hospitalization. Childhood cancer, for example, once meant a certain and often rapid death. Recent advances in chemo- and radiotherapy have resulted in a significant improvement in survival, but often require that a child is hospitalized for multiple and extended periods of time. These multiple and extended periods of hospitalization often separate a child from family and peers, thereby changing a child's emotional support system and social-learning experiences. At one extreme, children with cancer are sometimes placed in special hospital research environments that severely restrict available sensory and emotional stimulation. Such environments, e.g. Laminar Air Flow rooms, are designed to reduce the incidence of life-threatening infection which is a common complication of cancer treatment.

The child with cancer has not been included in previous studies of the effects of hospitalization on children. The need exists to determine the consequences of prolonged hospitalization on children with cancer in order to prevent potential deleterious effects upon psychological development and to enhance their (and their families') coping with such special stresses. The purpose of this chapter is: (a) To discuss existing information on the effects of hospital separation-deprivation on children, and (b) to propose an alternative model for considering psychosocial aspects of childhood cancer. The effects of hospitalization on the child with cancer will be discussed in relation to the separation-deprivation experienced by children in Laminar Air Flow (L.A.F.) rooms. Although L.A.F. room isolation constitutes one extreme along a continuum of sensory-depriving institutional environments, it does provide the opportunity for studying prospectively the effect of separation-deprivation on humans in a systematic manner. Traditionally, prospective studies of separation-deprivation have been conducted with sub-human primates with findings generalized to humans. Studies of children in L.A.F. constitute one of the first attempts to determine empirically the effect of isolation on humans.

BACKGROUND REVIEW OF SEPARATION-DEPRIVATION

The effects of long-term separation and hospital isolation on children are well known. Spitz used the term *hospitalism* to designate "a vitiated condition of the body due to long confinement in a hospital" (p. 53, Spitz, 1945). Developmental aberrations of institutionalized children consisted of serious depressions and delayed motor and intellectual development, which Spitz attributed to the absence of perceptual stimulation as well as the absence of mother-child emotional interchanges. According to Spitz (1945), the development of emotional interaction with the mother provides the child with perceptual experiences. The child learns to grasp by nursing at the mother's breast, learns to distinguish animate from inanimate objects by an awareness of the mother's facial expressions, and learns to play through interchanges with the mother. The children in the foundling home described by Spitz were unable to speak, to feed themselves, or to acquire habits of cleanliness. Spitz concluded that it was not the lack of perceptual stimulation in general that accounted for the effects of deprivation, but the lack of stimulation by persons who could act as a maternal substitute.

There are suggestions that some of the deleterious effects of institutionalization may be irreversible. When a group of three-year-olds, institutionalized since birth, was compared with a group of matched peers with continuous foster home experience, the former group was inferior to the latter in intellectual performance requiring both verbal and nonverbal reactions (Goldfarb, 1945). After the institutional group had seven months of experience in a foster home, they were still inferior in intellectual and language performance. The notable change in the institutionalized children was an increase in friendliness to adults and an increase in social competence.

The nonhuman analog to the child isolated within a L.A.F. room is the mother-infant monkey separation paradigm. Harlow and others (Ruppenthal et al., 1976) have demonstrated that social isolation or restriction imposed early in life has devastating and sometimes irreversible effects on the social development of monkeys. Female monkey infants reared without mothers themselves became mothers who were inadequate and often abusive. Kaufman and Rosenblum (1966) found that separating infant monkeys from their mothers for four to six weeks led to an infant reaction of initial agitation followed by depression which lasted for approximately a week. Mother-infant monkey reunion was characterized by intensification of the mother-infant relationship. As in previous studies with human primates, separation occurred early in development.

In summary, existing theory and research focuses on the notion that separation and deprivation leads to deficiency states within the organism that in turn result in aberrant behaviors. Furthermore, there is evidence from both animal and human research that certain patterns of social behavior will not be triggered appropriately or may be seriously blunted if there is insufficient interpersonal stimulation during critical developmental periods. Questions remain whether critical periods exist during later stages of development that are sensitive to insufficient interpersonal stimuli, and whether the effect of deprivation is transient or irreversible.

The Meaning of Deprivation

Psychosocial deprivation is an umbrella concept used to discuss the effect of hospitalization on children, but a conceptual perspective on the meaning and nature of psychosocial deprivation is not broadly shared nor is there empirical knowledge concerning its consequences (H.E.W., 1968). Hospital environments are often assumed to be deficient in certain types of stimulation, but the exact nature of deprivation is not clearly specified. This lack of consensus on the nature of deprivation leads to major problems in considering the effects of hospitalization on children (H.E.W., 1968).

First, norms or criteria for sufficient and optimal stimulation are not available, and thus the term deprivation may refer to no more than environmental variation. Second, the hospital setting might just as significantly be considered in terms of the excess of certain stimuli. For example, children with cancer experience an excess of stress and pain associated with the life-threatening disease and treatment regimens. The excess of new people in the hospital environment can be confusing and frightening to a child. Third, a deprivation model can be misleading because it explains deprivation solely in terms of what is absent, not what is present. For example, maternal deprivation is used as an explanation for certain characteristics of infant development related to the absence of the mother, per se, rather than to the presence or absence of a specifiable set of environmental stimuli such as auditory stimulation. A fourth problem, not outlined in the H.E.W. report, is that the need for stimulation changes throughout the life-span and deprivation means different things for different age groups. Infants and young children need adults as providers of sensory and emotional stimulation, because they are not proficient at generating their own stimulation. Older children and adults are self-stimulating organisms and are less dependent on persons in the environment to provide perceptual and emotional stimulation.

Separation-Deprivation and the Child with Cancer

A number of theoretical and methodological issues limit generalization from current theory and research to the specific effects of hospitalization upon children with cancer. Effects of hospitalization have been conceptualized primarily in terms of psychoanalytic theory, which assumes that hospitalization implies maternal deprivation, and that this deprivation is an antecedent to the subsequent development of aberrant patterns of thinking and behaving. The separation imposed by hospitalization presumably deprives a child of social-emotional, as well as visual and auditory stimulation. That is, psychoanalytic theory emphasizes the deficits of a hospital environment which presumably lead to passivity and withdrawal in the hospitalized child. Deficit models that emphasize pathology may, however, reduce the likelihood that attention will be given to aspects of normal development that may be relatively independent of mother-child interactions, such as achievement, peer affiliation, and sexuality.

The models used to conceptualize psychosocial aspects of childhood cancer have similarly focused on psychopathology or coping with the problems associated with a diagnosis of cancer, while aspects of normal development have largely been ignored. Furthermore, research in this area has been conducted with varying amounts of methodological rigor. Until very recently, data consisted primarily of descriptive clinical findings derived from retrospective analysis of clinical impressions. When objective measures were employed, it was usually in the context of detecting personality aberrations that placed the individual with cancer or the family at risk. Thus, the convergence of the deficit model of the hospitalized child and the clinical psychopathology model of the child with cancer has led to a very pessimistic view of the hospitalized child cancer patient.

The utility of existing studies on effects of hospitalization are limited by an additional factor. With few exceptions, e.g., Prugh, 1953, the effect of hospitalization has been formulated in relation to infants or young children. Studies of children in late childhood and adolescence need also to be considered because of the incidence of cancer in older children. Although the incidence of cancer is relatively high in the zero to four age-group, certain specific diseases, such as lymphomas and bone tumors, are commonly found in the ten to twenty year age-group (Young, Heise, Silverberg, and Myers, 1978). The developmental level of the child is likely to influence reactions to hospitalization. Further, the nature of deprivation differs developmentally. The harmful significance of isolation for the young child is primarily related to separation from parents; while for the adolescent, separation from peers may be equally deleterious. The significance of isolation from peers may not be appreciated by medical personnel and parents, yet peers provide a source of comfort and a basis for adolescent identification.

In summary, the effects of hospitalization and psychosocial aspects of cancer have been formulated in relation to a deficit model of human behavior, limited in terms of theory, methodology, and sample. To conceptualize the effect of hospitalization on children with cancer from a more holistic perspective, aspects of normal development as well as patterns of aberrant thinking and behaving and the differences between age groups must be considered. An empirical basis for such research is essential.

METHOD

Existing theoretical frameworks of the effect of separation-deprivation place a great deal of emphasis on passivity and depression. Yet, those familiar with the behavior of children in pediatric hospitals are cognizant of the diversity and range of behaviors and emotions displayed. To determine the appropriateness of existing models, it is first necessary to describe the frequency and range of behavior exhibited by children in hospital settings.

The group chosen for study consists of children and adolescents with metastatic solid tumors and lymphomas that had failed to respond to conventional therapeutic regimens. These children and adolescents then receive experimental, highly intensive chemotherapy. Because of the severe bone marrow toxicity and an increased risk of life-threatening infection associated with this intensive therapy, the National Cancer Institute is studying the utility of protected environments in the delivery of such chemotherapy (Pizzo & Levine, 1977).

Although the isolation imposed by L.A.F. rooms is severe compared to hospitalization, in general, such isolation cannot be equated with the deprivation of children and sub-human primates in earlier studies. Deprivation in L.A.F. consists of a paucity of skin-to-skin contact and reduced visual and auditory stimulation. Persons entering a L.A.F. room are attired in a sterile gown and sterile gloves. A plastic curtain separating the L.A.F. room from the corridor allows for visual stimulation from the immediate hospital environment. Family and siblings are encouraged to enter the L.A.F. room and are allowed unrestricted visiting while outside the plastic curtain. Furthermore, each child has the same nurse (Primary Nursing) throughout the period of hospitalization.

The research was guided by the following questions: (a) What are the behaviors exhibited by children with cancer hospitalized for long periods of time, and (b) does the frequency of these behaviors change? To answer these questions, two age groups of children were observed throughout their entire stay (three to eight weeks) in L.A.F. The first group consisted of eight- to twenty-one-year-olds confined to L.A.F. (Experimental Group, N=14); these patients were observed, and their behavior was recorded for 15 minutes a day. The time of the observation was determined by random assignment. A control group (N=5) of children hospitalized on a regular pediatric oncology ward was also observed. A second group of eighteen- to forty-eight-month-old children (N=4) confined to L.A.F. was videotaped for 10 minutes every morning and afternoon, and the tapes were subsequently coded by trained observers.

Four dimensions of the child's behavior were observed: (a) Role (Nonsocial, Initiating, Reciprocating, Ignoring); (b) Behavior; (c) Communication, and (d) Affect. For the older group, the person with whom the child was interacting was also observed and scored along the same dimension as the child. This observational system allowed for determination of frequency, sequence, and qualitative aspects of interaction between the child and caregiver. A more detailed description of the observational system can be found elsewhere (Susman et al., in press).

The Behavior dimension categories consisted of the following:

1. *Play-Constructive Activities* – Behavior that is age appropriate and is not related to hospital routines or treatment regimens. These activities included reading, writing, crafts, watching TV, and schoolwork.
2. *Sleep* – Lying quietly with eyes closed and no movement.
3. *Vocal* – Audible speech not including Protest.
4. *Passive* – Lying or sitting quietly with eyes open and no gross motor movements.
5. *Physical* – Gross motor movements including walking, exercising, and taking medications.
6. *Protest* – Extreme verbal and/or physical activity associated with an emotional outburst. This includes thrashing, hitting, kicking, or crying in a tantrum-like fashion.

RESULTS

Figure 7-1 shows the mean relative frequency (the frequency of each behavior in relation to the total number of behaviors) of each behavior category for the four younger children plotted across days in L.A.F. Passive, Play, and Vocal were relatively stable throughout the period of isolation. Physical activity increased slightly after day 30. Sleep in-

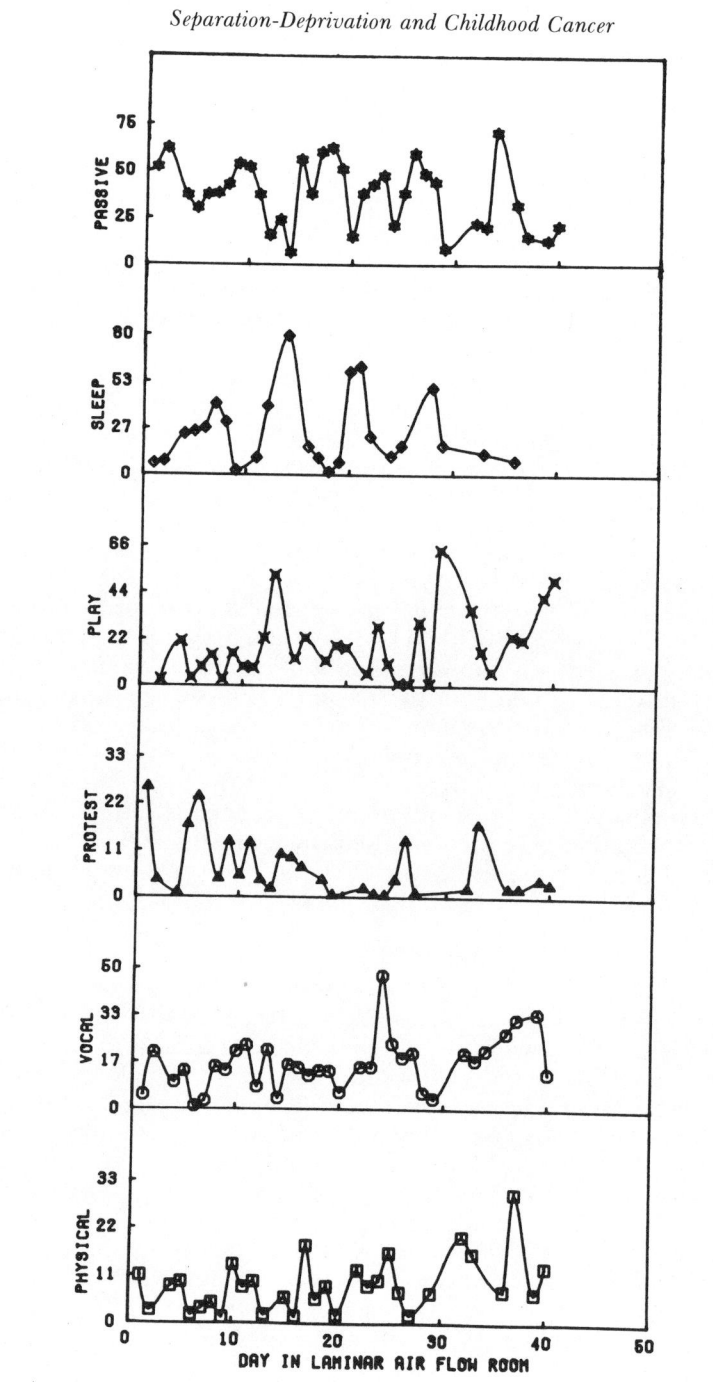

Figure 7-1. Mean relative frequency of behavior for four young children across days in L.A.F.

creased until approximately the fifteenth day and declined thereafter. The increase in Vocal, Play, and Physical between days 30 and 40 primarily reflects the behavior of one child who received a great deal of cognitive and social stimulation, nurturance, and support from his parents. Protest was high during the first days of L.A.F. isolation and declined thereafter. Thus, a sequence of initial distress followed by adaptation to the new environment described in earlier research was evidenced in these children.

In brief, the data lend some support to the psychoanalytic notion that hospitalization is accompanied by a behavioral sequence of protest, followed by inactivity that may be indicative of depression. An exclusive emphasis on these negative behaviors detracts, however, from other findings that highlight the positive behaviors that also occur. For instance, age-appropriate activities, such as Play and Vocal, were present and remained relatively stable throughout the period of hospitalization.

These young children exhibited no major psychopathology while confined to or after being released from L.A.F. None of the children had to be removed from L.A.F. because of psychological reasons. When feeling well, all of the children engaged in age-appropriate play and at no time did any of the children exhibit evidence of marked depression, such as withdrawal and lack of communication, when an interaction was initiated by a person in the environment. Although passivity was the most frequent behavior observed, it is difficult to determine the genesis or psychological meaning of passivity in this setting. Specifically, it is difficult to separate the effects of the illness and chemotherapy from the effects of prolonged isolation. Thus, it appears that although passivity is the primary response of young children to illness and separation, it does not necessarily indicate psychopathology.

Developmental Factors

Figure 7-2 shows the mean relative frequency of each behavior for the four younger children collapsed across days. Using a single-subject design, the mean for each behavior was determined. Passive behavior was the highest behavior category for all children. The lower level of Passive behavior and higher level of Play, Vocal, and Physical for child number 4 were probably related to the high level of parental involvement in this child's care. This is the same child who showed an increase in Physical, Vocal, and Play behavior between day 30 and 40 (Figure 7-1). When the parents of this patient were informed that the period of confinement to L.A.F. might be as long as three months, they expressed concerns regarding how this lengthy confinement might affect their child's cognitive and social development. These parents accurately pointed out that three months is a long time in the learning and experimental history of an eighteen-month-old and asked the staff to help them develop a cognitive and social-learning program to facilitate

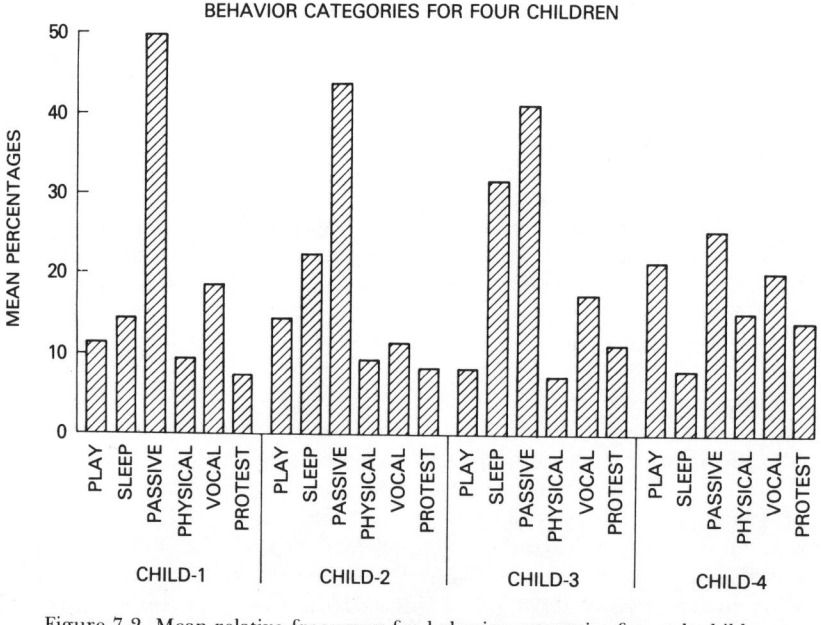

Figure 7-2. Mean relative frequency for behavior categories for each child.

their child's learning while he was in L.A.F. The parents were guided in providing materials and learning experiences to enhance the child's language development, color and shape discrimination, and physical activity. Nevertheless, passive was still the most frequently scored category for this child.

The response of older children to prolonged isolation was much more variable than for the younger children. Some children slept much of the time they were in L.A.F. The relative frequency of sleep ranged from 6 percent to 62 percent while passive ranged from 5 percent to 30 percent of total behavior. Other children spent much of their time interacting with parents, nurses, and other medical personnel. The relative frequency of social interaction ranged from 14 percent to 43 percent. Older children's reaction to isolation appeared to be related to individual differences in personality, degree of parental involvement with the child's care, and general physical condition.

The implication of these findings is that intervention must be more regular and intensive for younger than for older children if they are to maintain optimal levels of functioning. Assuming that the amount of nurse intervention is similar for all children, young children appear less able to generate their own sensory stimulation than the older children. Left to their own resources, young children become passive and uninvolved with the world around them; however, in one instance, the effects of isolation were mediated by intensive parental involvement.

Biobehavioral Relationships

The effects of hospitalization on children with cancer should be considered in relation to the nature and course of the disease. Remissions and relapses and the nature of treatment regimens bring about drastic changes in levels of adaptation. The life-threatening nature of cancer undoubtedly drastically heightens the psychological sequelae of hospitalization. The pain associated with cancer or the life-sustaining treatment regimens potentially add psychological trauma to an unknown extent. The effects of chemotherapy itself on moods and behavior may be drastic but are largely unknown. In brief, hospitalization for the pediatric cancer patient has a psychological impact far beyond that related purely to separation from mother or institutionalization in general.

Attempts to differentiate effects of illness from effects of hospitalization may have limited utility for physicians or nurses, although such precision may enhance research design. Because hospitalization occurs simultaneously with illness, a more pragmatic approach might consist of determining the covariation between changes in physiological status and changes in behavior. However, our experience with the older children in L.A.F. revealed that there is a great deal of individual variation in the way they react to similar courses of therapy. Children in the L.A.F. study all received highly experimental intensive chemotherapy and subsequently experienced a host of reactions secondary to the side effects of the drugs, including fever, stomatitis, and lethargy. There is a general consensus among hospital personnel that during the initial period of L.A.F. isolation, children are alert and interact with family and staff except during periods of nausea associated with chemotherapy. As the side effects of the drugs increase, children become febrile and lethargic and tend to withdraw and become irritable or depressed. The observational data tend to validate this notion. However, the extent to which the child withdraws from social interaction varies greatly among children. For instance, the relative frequency of vocalizations (per day) during periods of drug-induced toxicity ranged from 0 to 86 percent. One adolescent exhibited the highest frequency of vocalization (76%) during the period when stomatitis and fever were present. For this adolescent, vocalizations were emitted in response to initiations from his mother or hospital personnel.

Although there are similarities in the way that children react to L.A.F. isolation, particularly among young children, withdrawal and passivity are not inevitable concomitants of isolation and severe illness. Reactions to isolation and illness are mediated by individual differences and the degree to which persons in the environment interact with a child. The high degree of involvement of parents, nurses, and other medical personnel in L.A.F. units can prevent the deleterious effect of isolation described in earlier work. Descriptive data such as these lend credence to the notion that our conception of the ill child as necessarily depressed and withdrawn may be inaccurate. These data also support the intuitive notion that interventions in the form of social interactions are effective in engaging the child even during severe illness and prolonged isolation.

In summary, young children isolated for three to six weeks showed a behavioral sequence characterized first by protest and then by increased sleep. Passive was the most frequently observed behavior category during isolation of young children. Especially for older children, behavior was mediated by individuals in the social environment and by changing physiological status.

Theoretical Approaches to Remediation of Separation-Deprivation

Both psychoanalytic and social-learning theories have been used to formulate approaches to remedying the deleterious effects of separation. Although these theoretical models are somewhat antithetical, both approaches include the notion that aberrant behavior is not a necessary concomitant of prolonged separation or hospitalization. Robertson and Robertson (1971) proposed several factors that determine individual differences in response to separation from mother. These include level of ego maturity and object constancy, quality of mother-child relationship, nature of defenses, fantasies about illnesses and separation, and pre-separation experience with illness and separation. Robertson and Robertson (1971) demonstrated that the despair and distress generally associated with separation did not appear when stress factors that complicate institutional care were eliminated, for example, by placing children in a substitute home environment and by providing adequate substitute mothering. Earlier psychoanalytic theory and research (Bowlby, 1958; Goldfarb, 1945; Spitz, 1945) attributed the child's distress to the loss of mother as an object of attachment. The mother is not only an attachment object, Robertson and Robertson (1971) contend, but is also a buffer between her child and the environment. As such, she mediates environmental stresses and demands so that they are within the child's tolerable limits. Hence, the distress of a separated child is determined not only by the loss of mother as a loved person but also by the extent that the caretaker responds to the child's cues, keeps life running in a familiar fashion, and protects the child from stressful environmental impingements. Thus, when the criteria for adequate substitute mothering are met, the stress of separation is lessened.

Gerwitz (1978) proposes that the social behavior of institutionalized children is explainable in terms of the principles of social learning. He suggests that formulations attempting to relate deficient conditions of stimulation in early childhood to aberrations in later behavior patterns rest on the unproved assumption that if a child does not receive an adequate number of essential stimuli from the caregiving environment over a lengthy period, systematic changes occur in behavior related to this deprivation. Gerwitz (1978) further suggests that use of the deficiency model to explain the behavior of hospitalized children discourages attention being given to environmental stimuli, and to the child's behavior, at the level of detail required for an operational analysis of behavior. Therefore, he proposes a social-learning approach for studying the effect of institutionalization. Using such a model, the behavior analyst identifies the functional relationship between stimulus and response prior to their removal, as well as the child's behavior in response to stimuli in the new setting. Hence, the outcome of environmental shifts are viewed as reflecting an adjustment of the child's behavior to changed conditions, including the child's capacity for *new* learning resulting from altered reinforcement. From this perspective, it is not sufficient to focus on which or how stimuli are provided to the child to understand the development of human social motivation under conditions of deficient stimuli. One must determine the circumstances under which stimuli are made available and whether these stimuli are functional in relation to the child's repertoire.

Gerwitz (1978) further contends that with a deficiency model, the solution for dealing with inadequate conditions of stimulation is to simply increase stimulation, e.g. provide more and more attention and nurturance without regard to their influence on the behavior being exhibited by the child. In actuality, the caretaker will provide stimuli for some contingent relative to the child's behavior. For instance, if the child cries at mealtime, food will be provided. The provision of stimuli equated with the provision of attention and love may be contingent upon attention-seeking behavior, e.g. tantrums. Tantrum responses may be strengthened and other new learning thereby precluded. Unless desirable responses are specified, widely varying behavioral outcomes are possible. If, however, the caretaker consistently provides stimuli designed to evoke valued responses, e.g., the nurse is attentive when the child is doing schoolwork, these behaviors will be strengthened and the outcome will be favorable.

An Alternative Model

Because of the lack of existing theoretical frameworks, we have developed a conceptual model for understanding human development within the context of a life-threatening illness. It appears to us that previous paradigms are inadequate because of their emphasis on pathology. For example, the prevailing paradigm used in considering psychosocial aspects of cancer consists of the following:

1. Children with cancer have psychological problems.
2. Assessment of psychopathology is important and leads to:
3. Diagnosis of the problem, which allows for:
4. Intervention to remedy pathology.

Our alternative model consists of the following:

1. Children with cancer experience an atypical course of development.

2. Assessment of the nature and frequency of new behavioral contingencies is valuable, as is:
3. Client-professional mutual identification of goals/problems. This can bring about:
4. Intervention to alter or maintain the frequency of selected behaviors.

This model assumes that emotional, social, and cognitive development may be altered by a diagnosis of cancer because of its life-threatening nature and because of the nature of treatment regimens. For instance, a child with cancer is deprived of many peer group socializational experiences because of extended periods of hospitalization. Thus, it is important to assess how cancer affects psychological development. However, reactions to such an illness need not be synonymous with problems of adjustment, an assumption underlying much of the research on psychosocial aspects of cancer, and a child may be oriented to achieving goals within the context of the illness. Therefore, it is important to determine a child-client's goals or problems. Intervention may then be appropriate to increase, maintain, or decrease certain behaviors. Behavior in this context refers to both overt behavior and emotions.

In summary, an assumption of this model is that individuals progress along a developmental course, and although such a course may be altered by major medical crises, basic processes of psychological development still occur. Two corollaries of this assumption are: (a) Physiological, social, and cognitive development will proceed in spite of illness and hospitalization; and (b) the reactions to illness and hospitalization, although stressful, need not be pathological and are likely to be oriented to age-related developmental concerns. Research conducted within this conceptual framework will incorporate a wide variety of psychological dimensions not merely those dimensions designed to detect psychopathology or coping strategies.

Similarly, intervention based on this model will be less likely to focus on pathology or remediation. Rather the emphasis will be on promotion and maintenance of age-related developmental concerns and behaviors. For instance, the emphasis on psychosocial programs for the hospitalized cancer patient might focus on promoting school achievement (Katz et al., 1977) and keeping children up to grade level, which is important for children's feelings of self-esteem and status within peer groups. If this developmentally oriented viewpoint is viewed as over-optimistic, given the high mortality rate associated with childhood cancer, consider the following:

B., a twelve-year-old male in the final stages of Burkitt's Lymphoma, was determined to get two more Boy Scout badges before he died. Thus, he asked his mother to solicit coins and stamps from hospital personnel to help him with his goal. His goal was accomplished approximately a week before he died.

In summary, this model is oriented to maximizing human development and is useful even in the context of dying. Such an approach stresses an understanding of the continuing developmental needs of the whole child and the multiple roles that the child occupies — peer, sibling, student, as well as patient.

Summary and a Look to the Future

The models commonly used in discussing the effects of hospitalization on young children were developed from studies of institutionalized children or sub-human primates. Over-generalizations from these models have led to an image of the hospitalized child as one who is depressed, passive, and withdrawn. Implicit in deficit models is the notion that hospitalization leads to inevitable social and emotional dysfunctional development. This implication has reduced the incentive for considering aspects of normal growth and development which proceed in spite of hospitalization. An alternative social-learning model predicts that behavior in hospitals is governed by the same principles of reinforcement and extinction that operate in any other environment. From this perspective, the solution to conditions of deprivation is not merely to provide additional stimulation but to determine the functional relationship between the stimulation provided and the child's behavior.

Data have been presented that lend some support to the contention that hospitalization leads to a sequence of protest, denial, and despair; however, this is mainly true for children younger than five. For both younger and older groups of children, age-related developmental concerns and activities were evidenced even after long periods of hospitalization and even when the children were very ill.

The models commonly employed for conceptualizing the effects of cancer on children were developed from psychiatric or clinical psychological assessments of the child-patient or the child's family. The emphasis has been on identifying psychopathology associated with a diagnosis of cancer, and professionals have frequently discussed cancer patients and their families in the same terms as are used to discuss psychiatric patients. The mother who discusses her child's potentially fatal illness is accused of intellectualizing or obsessing about the illness. Conversely, the mother who does not discuss her child's illness is accused of denying, and not facing up to reality. Thus, focusing upon aberrant aspects of development may introduce distortion.

Rather than exclusively concentrating upon psychopathology, we believe that behavioral researchers would do well to investigate whether children with cancer and their families have hopes and concerns for the future that are similar to those of families and children in general. Preliminary analyses of our interview data indicate that children and families realize that restraints on family activities and a child's later development are imposed by a diagnosis of cancer and the necessary treatment regimens. However, the concern of most children and their families is on living as normal a life as is possible given these limitations. A mother whose son was tumor-free and was about to complete his course of chemotherapy articulated this perspective in the following manner: "Everyone looks at him and says, 'He has made it' because he looks so good. They don't realize that osteogenic (sarcoma) is slow growing and could reappear at any time."

She then went on to discuss the problems her son had experienced finding a job because he had not completed a college education. The decision was made that the son return to college to pursue "a college degree so he could compete in the job market." This was the same young man who when still an adolescent stated, "I've got to do things. What am I going to do? Sit around and think 'Oh, boy! I've got cancer.'" This family is cognizant of the ever-present threat of illness. But are their aspirations not like those of most families?

The paradigm for further research and intervention proposed earlier is a more holistic approach to psychosocial aspects of cancer and allows for inclusion of a wider and more varied range of studied phenomena. If a child hospitalized for prolonged periods of time is viewed as a changing, developing person, even while coping with a life-threatening illness, greater emphasis will be placed on research designed to ascertain those acts on the part of parents and caregivers that enhance normal development, that lessen the need for rehabilitation post-hospitalization, and that hasten re-entry into home, school, and community.

Our model for conceptualizing the effects of cancer on psychological development would also place a greater emphasis on parents as participants in the therapeutic process rather than parents as "patients." True, the parent whose child has cancer may at times be in need of psychiatric or psychological consultation. However, the parent remains the child's best advocate and the individual most concerned with the child's recovery and growth to his or her greatest developmental potential. Furthermore, parents know their child best and can almost never be replaced, from the child's perspective, by even the warmest and most nurturing parent surrogate. Therefore, it is proposed that parents not be shielded from the problems inherent in the medical and nursing management of the hospitalized child. Parents frequently feel isolated and fearful while they watch experts care for their child. Active participation in the child's care helps to reduce this sense of fear and isolation.

Finally, we propose that the term "mother-child" in relation to discussions on attachments, hospital care, and provider of emotional support be replaced by the term "parent-child." Based on psychiatric models, we continue to attribute effects of hospital separation to loss of the mother. Is loss of the father not equally important? A mother recently asked a group of psychologists: "Since when did mothering replace parenting?" Although fathers frequently have career restraints that prevent them from spending long periods of time with their hospitalized children, their involvement is very important, for it reduces the strain on the mother brought about by her being continually at the clinic or in the hospital with the child. Mothers often become more knowledgeable about the child's illness and treatment than anyone else in the family, which may lead to paternal feelings of inadequacy, isolation, and frustration. In addition, it seems clear that the presence of both parents for both the ill child and his/her siblings helps to promote optimal security and family unity.

REFERENCES

Bowlby, J.: *Attachment and Loss.* New York, Basic Books, 1969.
Bowlby, J.: The nature of the child's tie to his mother. *Int J Psychoanal, 39:*1, 1958.
Gerwitz, J.: Social learning in early human development. In A. C. Catania and T. A. Brigham (Eds.), *Handbook of Applied Behavior Analysis: Social and Instructional Processes.* New York, Irvington Pubs, 1979.
Goldfarb, W.: Effects of psychological deprivation in infancy and subsequent stimulation. *Am J Psychiatry, 102:*18, 1945.
Katz, E. R.; Kellerman, J., Rigler, D., Williams, K. O., and Siegel, S. E.: School intervention with pediatric cancer patients. *J Pediatr Psychology, 2:*72, 1976.
Kaufman, I. C.; and Rosenblum, L. A.: Depression in infant monkeys separated from their mothers. *Science, 155:*1030, 1967.
Perspectives on Human Deprivation: Biological, Psychological and Sociological. National Institute of Child Health and Human Development, Public Health Service, U.S. Department of Health, Education, and Welfare, 1968.
Pizzo, P. A.; and Levine, A. S.: The utility of protected environment regimens for the compromised host: A critical assessment. In E. B. Brown (Ed.), *Progress in Hematology.* (Vol. 10). New York: Grune & Stratton, 1977.
Prugh, D.: Toward an understanding of psychosomatic concepts in relation to illness in children. In A. J. Solnit and S. A. Provence (Eds.), *Modern Perspectives in Child Development.* New York, Intl Univs Pr, 1963.
Robertson, J.; and Robertson, J.: Young children in brief separation, *Psychoanal Study Child, 26:*264, 1971.
Ruppenthal, G. C.; Arling, G. L., Harlow, H. F., Sackett, G. P., and Suomi, S. J.: A 10-year perspective of motherless-mother monkey behavior. *J Abnorm Psychol, 85:*341, 1976.
Spitz, R.: Hospitalism: An inquiry into the genesis of psychiatric conditions in early childhood. *Psychoanal Study Child, 1:*53, 1945.
Susman, E. J.; Hollenbeck, A. H., Nannis, E. D., Strope, B. E., Hersh, S. P., Levine, A. S., and Pizzo, P. A.: Interactions between primary caregivers and children with cancer: A methodology for systematic observation in a hospital setting. In L. Bugen (Ed.), *Death and Dying: Theory, Research and Practice.* Dubuque, Iowa, W. C. Brown, in press.
Yarrow, L.: Maternal deprivation: Toward an empirical and conceptual re-evaluation, *Psychol Bull, 58:*459, 1961.
Young, J. L.; Heise, H. W., Silverberg, E., Myers, M. H.: Cancer incidence, survival, and mortality for children under 15 years of age. *American Cancer Society Professional Educational Publication,* 1978.

Chapter Eight

PSYCHOLOGICAL EFFECTS OF CENTRAL NERVOUS SYSTEM TREATMENT OF CHILDREN WITH ACUTE LYMPHOCYTIC LEUKEMIA

Howard A. Moss
Ellen D. Nannis

O VER THE PAST ten years the chances of surviving childhood leukemia have increased greatly. This change has been brought about primarily through the use of prophylactic treatment of the central nervous system in order to destroy leukemic cells in the cerebro-spinal fluid that because of the blood-brain barrier may have escaped the effects of traditional systemic treatment. This is done in order to prevent meningeal leukemia and thus to minimize the chances of relapse.

Recently, concern has been expressed as to possible deleterious effects of this CNS treatment. As a consequence, there is an increasing number of studies which attempt to evaluate the neurological problems associated with this central nervous system (CNS) treatment. Although these studies include subjects of all ages, the authors tend not to differentiate analyses and findings in terms of developmental variables. Studies on the effects of CNS treatment can be grouped into three general classes depending on the focus of the research: (1) those involving evaluation of structural changes in the brain through the use of histological or photographic techniques; (2) studies of personality or psychological changes associated with CNS irradiation; and (3) assessments to determine whether the level of intellectual, cognitive, or perceptual functioning had been affected by the treatment. The results of these studies are at best suggestive and equivocal. They are usually based on very small samples, are often anecdotal, lack adequate control groups, do not control for age, and involve research designs which do not effectively partial out confounding factors.

Studies of personality changes associated with CNS irradiation are particularly sparse and ambiguous because of poor controls and the retrospective nature of these data. Those changes which have been reported tend to be minimal considering the nature of the treatment. Frequently reported behavioral symptoms include anorexia, apathy, irritability, depression, and a slight increase in the incidence of mental disorder. About 75 percent of the children with acute lymphocytic leukemia who receive CNS irradiation develop a postirradiation syn-

172   *Psychological Aspects of Childhood Cancer*

drome about four-six weeks after the completion of the treatment. This syndrome is characterized by somnolence, anorexia, and lethargy and is accompanied by EEG abnormalities. The symptoms last one-two weeks and usually subside spontaneously along with normalization of the EEG.

REVIEW OF LITERATURE SUGGESTING ENCEPHALOPATHY DUE TO CENTRAL NERVOUS SYSTEM TREATMENT

Two forms of central nervous system treatment for the control of acute lymphocytic leukemia have been proven to be highly effective in reducing the number of relapses among patients in remission from this illness. These treatments are the intrathecal injection of methotrexate (mtx.) and the administration of a series of cranial irradiations, usually over a ten to fourteen day period and cumulative to about 2400 rads. Some treatment programs use either intrathecal methotrexate or central nervous system (CNS) irradiation, but the most common procedure appears to be the administration of these two forms of treatment conjointly. Evidence is accumulating from a series of studies that both of these treatments are associated with morphological changes in the central nervous systems. Some of these studies deal with the effects of intrathecal methotrexate, others with the effects of CNS irradiation, and still others with the effects of the combined use of these two treatments. In addition, there is some evidence that CNS irradiation facilitates parenterally administered mtx. in infiltrating the central nervous system.

The purpose of this review is to organize the evidence of encephalopathy associated with these treatments in order to determine how convincing a picture of encephalopathy they create, and to see whether reported findings suggest any patterns in how the effects of these treatments might influence the intellectual and cognitive functioning of children. The evidence on the effects of these CNS treatments (in producing changes in the brain) will be used to develop guidelines for the planning of research on expected behavioral changes associated with these treatment effects.

INTRATHECAL METHOTREXATE (I.T. MTX.)

Studies about the neurological effects of i.t. mtx. are few but are persuasive in showing central nervous system impairment as a function of the use of this medication. Such studies tend to be based on clinical and autopsy evidence. Most of the studies which emphasize the effects of mtx. include cases which also received cranial irridation. Despite the use of both forms of treatment, when analyzing their results, many investigators emphasize the effects of mtx. and selectively sort out information that implicates the role of this chemotherapeutic agent in contributing to neurological damage. Kay et al. (1972) describe encephalopathy and severe behavioral symptoms, usually associated with brain injury, among seven patients (six of these patients were between two and eight years of age) who were receiving prolonged methotrexate therapy, in part by intrathecal injections, for meningeal leukemia. The major symptoms consisted of confusion, tremors, ataxia, irritability, and somnolence. Two of the cases exhibited grand mal seizures. These authors felt that the marked EEG abnormalities found among these patients were in keeping with a picture of diffuse encephalopathy. They interpreted the lesions found on autopsy from the one fatal case in their sample as being in keeping with vascular damage.

Smith (1975) did autopsy comparisons on the brains of ten leukemia patients who had received i.t. mtx. and CNS irradiation and on the brains of ten leukemia patients who had not received any CNS treatment. She found evidence of histological changes in the brains of those who had received the CNS treatment. These changes consisted of destruction of cells in the white matter of the cerebrum and cerebellum. She interpreted her results as indicating that it was primarily the i.t. mtx. which was implicated in the brain damage which was observed. Meadows and Evans (1976) studied twenty-three children with leukemia and other forms of cancer who survived for more than five years. They compared these children in terms of the amount of methotrexate (both intravenous and intrathecal) and cranial irradiation they received and found considerably more neurological impairment among those who received the greatest amounts of methotrexate and irradiation. Different diagnoses and confounding factors, such as the presence of meningeal leukemia among several of the patients, make it difficult to apply systematic and quantitative analyses to these data, yet the clinical evidence relating neurological impairment to extent and type of treatment seems quite convincing. The researchers make the point that all those patients who manifested neurological disturbances were administered intravenous methotrexate in high doses over a prolonged period of time. The types of neurological evidence that they cite consisted of seizures, irritability, perceptual-motor deficits, inattentiveness, hyperactivity, and abnormal EEG patterns. Hendin et al. (1974) report autopsy evidence of degeneration of central nervous system tissue among twenty-three children who died of leukemia and who had received CNS treatment. They further note that the case which showed the most severe changes at autopsy had received the most extensive CNS treatment. They interpret their findings as evidence that the neurologic deterioration observed may be the consequence of anti-leukemic CNS treatment. Although many of the patients they report on received both i.t. mtx. and cranial irradiation, they stress the methotrexate as being the implicated treatment in the development of neurological disturbances.

CRANIAL IRRADIATION

Generally, there are two divergent views concerning the vulnerability of the brain to irradiation. The position held by one group of investigators, that the brain is not particularly radiosensitive, is based on some empirical evidence which shows little or no apparent decrement in functioning after exposure to radiation. Support for this point of view also comes from evidence that developing and dividing cells are most sensitive to the effects of irradiation. Because the brain is largely formed with permanent cells at an early age, it is therefore considered to be less vulnerable to radiation. Furchgott (1963), in a review article on the effects of radiation on the central nervous system states, "In general histological studies tend to support the long-held view that adult neural tissues are relatively insensitive to ionizing radiation. It is apparent that doses up to several thousand rads do not interfere with learning of relatively difficult problems whenever radiation malaise or maturational changes do not inhibit performance. Actually the evidence points in the opposite direction. The simplest explanation of the superior learning in the irradiated S's takes into account their decreased distractibility and narrow focus of attention." Contrary to Furchgott's summary statement, there are some scientific reports which present evidence that patients who received cranial irradiation do show brain necrosis and other indications of encephalopathy.

In the treatment of childhood leukemia, cranial irradiation tends to be used in conjunction with i.t. mtx. Therefore, there is greater opportunity to study the independent effects of CNS irradiation by considering investigations where it alone has been used in the treatment of an illness or condition other than leukemia. Hicks and D'Amato (1966) in a review chapter on the "Effects of Ionizing Radiations on Mammalian Development" state that there is consistent evidence of harmful effects of irradiation on young organisms. They point out that the recent widespread practice of using radiation to treat fungus infections of the scalp (ringworm) in children obviously led to radiation penetrating the brain and resulted in serious neurological problems. In a few reported instances where exposures from 50 to 400 rads were made daily for several days, neurologic symptoms began soon after irradiation and progressed over a period of months with convulsions, paralysis, then death. In other children, apathy, sleepiness, irritability, and other symptoms developed some weeks after exposure, but these cleared in a couple of weeks. Electroencephalographic records were made for several weeks or months after the treatment in some series of children so treated; in some they were not changed, in others they were abnormal. Albert et al. (1968) also studied the neurological effects of irradiation which was used for the treatment of ringworm of the scalp. They did a follow-up study where they compared a group who received radiation treatment with a group that did not receive this treatment and found a higher incidence of mental illness in the irradiated group. Some of the findings reported by Hicks and D'Amato (1966) correspond with a post-irradiation syndrome which has been described by other investigators. Freeman et al. (1973) found that children who had received cranial irradiation exhibited abnormal EEG patterns six weeks after the completion of the treatment. These abnormal patterns, which persisted for a short time, were consistent with a diffuse cerebral disturbance, affecting both hemispheres, but without evidence of any focal lesion. Garwicz (1975) studied twelve children who received prophylactic CNS treatment (irradiation and i.t. mtx.) following hematological remission from acute lymphocytic leukemia. Eight of the twelve cases developed a transient postirradiation syndrome consisting of fever, lassitude, anorexia, and somnolence five to seven weeks after the completion of the irradiation therapy. These symptoms lasted one or two weeks and subsided spontaneously. All of these patients showed normal EEG's on follow-up after completion of the CNS irradiation, although there were EEG irregularities during the period of the postirradiation syndrome.

Kramer (1968) summarizes the hazards of therapeutic irradiation of the central nervous system and concludes that although the brain was formerly thought to be highly radio-resistant, recent work has shown it to be much more sensitive. He interprets this recent research as showing that the shorter the time in which a total dose is given, the greater the risk of damage; the higher the dosage, the greater the effect; and, the larger the volume irradiated, the more likely that radiation damage will occur. One line of investigation has been to study the effects of CNS irradiation on the vascular system of the brain. Kramer (1968) cites evidence that radiation seems to have a differential effect on certain blood vessels in the brain and that vascular damage can have a delayed or secondary effect on brain cells which are subsequently deprived of their blood supply. These findings suggest that delayed radiation injury to the central nervous system usually occurs between four months and twelve years after the completion of radiotherapy, with a peak at one to three years. Painter et al. (1975) present evidence supporting this view. They found evidence of symptomatic intercranial occlusive vascular disease in three children following CNS irradiation treatment for CNS tumors. Pennybacker and Russell (1948) also obtained research results, consistent with the conclusion by Kramer (1968), that radiation to the brain results in vascular damage, which in turn contributes to delayed brain damage. They, however, suggest a longer latency period than the one to three year peak period indicated by Kramer. Pennybacker and Russell (1948) studied the effects of radiation therapy on the brains of nine adults and conclude that there is clear evidence of the harmful effects of this treatment on the brain. They feel that this evidence favors the view that the primary effect is on the smaller blood vessels of the brain. In each case there was a long latent period between the radiation treatment and the onset of clinical signs of necrosis. The shortest interval was nine months, the longest five years. They feel that it is unlikely that a progressive effect on nerve cells would so long delay clinical manifestation. They interpret their data to show that the pathology of the brain necrosis appears to be related to damage in the small blood vessels of the brain which eventually leads to damage to brain cells. Thus, there is consistent evidence across studies that radiation may indirectly harm brain tissue through the destruction of blood vessels in the central nervous system. This finding indicates that cranial irradiation is harmful regardless of the radiosensitivity of the brain. Although there appears to be substantial variability in the latency period between radiation treatment and encephalopathy, there is consistent evidence that there is a delay, which may be substantial, before clinical manifestations of the treatment may occur. This finding has important implications for assessing psychological deficits which may be associated with cranial irradiation. That is, one might not expect these deficits to be manifest before one to two years after the treatment.

A few studies have focused on the combined deleterious effects of cranial irradiation and methotrexate when used in the treatment of acute lymphocytic leukemia (ALL). Price and Jamieson (1975) found degenerative changes in telencephalic white matter in thirteen of 231 children who were treated for ALL. All of those children who exhibited leukoencephalopathy showed that methotrexate administered intravenously after a cumulative dose of CNS irradiation of 2000 rads or more can result in degeneration of CNS white matter in patients with ALL. They conclude that their results suggest that chemotherapeutic agents may diffuse through the blood-brain barrier following CNS irradiation of 2000 rads or more. In support of this conclusion they found that the incidence of leukoencephalopathy increased as the total dose of methotrexate increased; patients who received less than 2000 rads did not develop leukoencephalopathy. The authors of this article observed that twelve of the thirteen patients with degenerative changes in the brain showed neurological signs such as seizures and mental changes.

McIntosh et al. (1976) studied prospectively twenty-three children between two and fifteen years of age, who were treated for ALL, in order to determine the effects of central nervous system prophylaxis (cranial irradiation and i.t. mtx.). The CNS treatment consisted of 2400 rads of cranial irradiation distributed over a series of treatments and i.t. mtx. and intermittent maintenance therapy which included the administration of methotrexate intravenously. Neurological symptoms were observed in twelve of the twenty-three patients, all of whom had intermittent limping and mild incoordination between the tenth and eighteenth months of maintenance therapy. Five children had seizures; four had abnormalities in motor, perceptual, behavioral, and language development; and three had learning disability and perceptual motor defects. The eleven children without evidence of motor abnormalities, seizures, or learning disabilities were slightly older (mean age 5$\frac{7}{12}$) than the affected patients (mean age 3½). The mean age of children with seizures was three years at the time of the CNS prophylaxis.

Peylan-Ramu et al. (1978) studied thirty-two children in remission from ALL who had received prophylactic cranial irradiation (2400 rads) and intrathecal methotrexate or cytosine arabinoside. They studied this group by means of CT scans in order to determine whether brain abnormalities were associated with the prophylactic CNS treatment. CT scans also were done on a control group of eleven asymptomatic ALL patients who had never received any CNS therapy. The time interval from the initiation of prophylaxis to the time of the CT brain scan averaged about forty months for the treated group and seventy months for the control group. They found that seventeen of thirty-two ALL patients who had received the CNS treatment showed one or more CT scan abnormalities, whereas the findings for the control patients were normal except for one case in which there was minimal evidence of change. Of the four types of CT abnormalities that were studied, two were found to be equally distributed among patients in both the methotrexate and cytosine arabinoside groups while the other two signs of pathology were observed only for those patients who had received methotrexate.

In summary, there appears to be consistent and convincing evidence that treating the central nervous system in order to control for and reverse disease processes, such as acute lymphocytic leukemia, results in neurological damage. The severity of the damage appears to be associated with the duration and amount of the treatment and the age of the individual at the time of the treatment. There are evidently unknown factors that contribute to the degree of damage which occurs since different studies indicate a range in individual differences in vulnerability to adverse effects from the CNS treatment. Most of the studies that have been done include combinations of factors which have a high likelihood of producing encephalopathy. For instance, programs for treating ALL tend to use both cranial irradiation and i.t. mtx; many of the reported studies include patients with meningeal leukemia; possible changes in the blood-brain barrier because of extensive cranial irradiation facilitate the diffusion into the central nervous system of intravenously administered chemotherapeutic agents; and the various samples studied are heterogeneous as to age, time interval since the initiation of treatment, and the amount and type of treatment. This confounding of factors contributing to encephalopathy makes it difficult to isolate and identify the specific effects of any individual factor. Nonetheless, careful consideration of the various findings provides evidence of suggestive patterns of damage associated with particular treatment procedures. Thus both mtx. and cranial irradiation seem implicated in producing changes in the brain, with the mtx. leading to more immediate and direct changes and the irradiation being associated with more indirect and delayed effects through causing damage to the vascular system supplying blood to the brain. There is both direct and indirect evidence of treatment-related central nervous system damage. The direct evidence consists of histological findings of brain changes from autopsy studies, abnormal EEG records, and abnormal CT scan findings among patients who had received CNS treatment. The indirect evidence of deleterious effects from CNS treatment consists of frequently reported behavioral symptoms such as confusion, tremors, ataxia, irritability, somnolence, depression, apathy, seizures, and an increased incidence of mental disorders.

The physiological and behavioral evidence of neurological damage associated with CNS treatment strongly suggests that the CNS effects of this treatment also would interfere with or impair optimal intellectual and cognitive functioning. On the other hand, recent empirical studies and theoretical views of brain functions would argue that the brain is a highly resilient organ and that when damage occurs other portions of the brain or the nondamaged hemisphere are capable of compensatory activity by taking over functions of the damaged area (Lenneberg, 1967). This theoretical position further suggests that the younger the child (before specialization has occurred) the greater is this compensatory (or redundant) capacity of the brain. The compensatory potential of the brain, however, could be abrogated by the *complete brain treatment* used as a prophylaxis for the care of patients with acute lympocytic leukemia. That is, damage resulting from this generalized type of CNS treatment is probably not localized, but affects the total brain so that areas which might otherwise be available to take over impaired functions also are likely to be affected.

This interpretation of the existing findings leads to an expectation that intellectual abilities will be impaired in ALL patients who have received total CNS treatment. Since the complete brain is affected by this treatment, thereby minimizing the compensatory mechanisms, it seems likely that younger children would be subject to greater intellectual impairment by early CNS damage. In this case younger children would be more vulnerable since the damage might occur before maturation and growth of the brain is completed. Since pervasive brain damage is more likely to impair the ability to learn new or not already acquired skills and is less likely to nullify existing abilities and knowledge, earlier damage seems likely to have a more profound effect on future intellectual functioning. A corollary to this assumption is that the intellectual deficits might be expected to become greater as the time interval since treatment increases. That is, if the ability to acquire new skills and information is more impaired than are existing abilities, as the time interval since the damage occurred increases, the greater will be the developmental lag between the treated patient and the age mates on whom intelligence test norms are based. The data which suggest a delay in brain damage from cranial irradiation (because of damage to blood vessels) also would lead to a prediction that evidence of intellectual deficit might not be expected to occur until a substantial time after the treatment. Thus, the timing of an assessment to evaluate whether or not CNS treatment contributed to any intellectual loss is very important. It seems likely that intellectual difficulties resulting from CNS treatment will be most discernible one to three years after the treatment, with these effects being more apparent with younger children. They will be more apparent with younger children not only because of their greater vulnerability, but because the time interval since treatment will represent a greater proportion of their total life experience. These are a few of the predictions that can be made concerning the effects of CNS treatment on intellectual functioning. There also are important empirical questions concerning these effects. One important question that needs to be studied is whether the CNS treatment results in damage that affects all intellectual functions or whether there is impairment of only selected abilities. The existing data dealing with these types of analyses tend to involve older subjects and be based on more localized brain damage than is the case with the CNS treatment used on ALL patients. Thus, the relation between CNS treatment and the vulnerability of different intellectual abilities remains an empirical question. Another important issue which requires empirical data is whether any observed intellectual loss is progressive or tends to stabilize after a particular interval of time. Also of interest are individual differences and the basis for these differences in deficits associated with the CNS treatment.

Only a few studies present data on the intelligence test performance of children with ALL who have received CNS treatment, and these are in apparent disagreement as to whether or not there is a deleterious effect from this treatment. In addition, generalizing from these studies is difficult because of a series of methodological shortcomings including very small sample sizes, inadequate controls, and apparently inappropriate analyses. At best the findings can be considered tentative and preliminary.

Soni et al. (1975) did a prospective study on a sample of thirty-four children with ALL. They administered intelligence tests to this sample just prior to cranial irradiation and then retested them several times up to eighteen months after CNS treatment. For the prospective study the control group consisted of cancer patients who had received radiation to parts of the body other than the cranium. This group also was tested before and after radiation. In addition, they did a retrospective study in which they administered intelligence tests to eleven ALL patients from an average of two to four years after they received prophylactic CNS treatment. The controls for the retrospective study were ALL patients who had not received CNS irradiation. Examples of the methodological problems associated with this research are: (1) for the prospective study there was a very broad age range in the sample (two and one-half to sixteen years of age); (2) The controls were not well matched for age with the treated patients (median age of five years for the patients and ten years for the controls); (3) The wide age span of the subjects necessitated giving different tests to different subjects. Thus, there was a lack of comparability of measurement across the age span of the sample. (4) There was substantial attrition of subjects so that only fourteen of thirty-four patients from the prospective study, and five of eleven from the retrospective study were still available for the follow-up assessment. With this high rate of attrition it would have been useful to know the initial IQ scores of those cases which dropped out of the study in order to determine whether there were any selective psychological factors associated with those subjects who continued participation in the study. (5) For statistical analyses the samples were attenuated further, since age differences among subjects required the use of different age appropriate tests which were analyzed separately. (Some subjects were administered the Wechsler Intelligence Scale for Children and others the Stanford-Binet.) (6) There was no control or measure of practice effect from repeated administrations of the same instrument.

Because of the extensive methodological shortcoming inherent in this research, it is not surprising that these investigators did not find any significant differences in the level of intellectual functioning between those patients who received cranial irradiation and those who did not receive this treatment. The very small samples reported in this research make it particularly unlikely to be able to demonstrate statistically significant differences between groups. Although their retrospective sample size was too small to do statistical analyses, they assert, based on a qualitative evaluation, that for this group there were "no apparent differences over time." This is an untenable conclusion in terms of their insufficient data base. Moreover, these investigators did not consider important issues (as suggested by other research) in organizing and analyzing their data, such as the age of the child and the interval of time since prophylactic CNS treatment. Since all children were pooled in the analyses, despite their vastly different ages and the difference in time intervals since treatment, results which might have otherwise emerged could have been masked by these confounding factors.

Eiser and Lansdown (1977) studied the effects of cranial irradiation on the intellectual level of nine younger (mean age six years, three months) and six older (mean age nine years) children with ALL. Intelligence test scores were used for comparing these children with healthy control subjects selected from the school classrooms which the patients attended. No information is provided to show that these classmates are indeed of equivalent social class background to the patients. The older group was administered the Wechsler Intelligence Scale for Children (WISC) and the younger subjects were given the McCarthy scale. They report no significant differences between the older ALL patients and their matched controls on any of the measures used, but they did find that the younger subjects performed significantly lower than their controls on a general measure of intelligence as well as on certain select abilities. They did not find any significant correlations between test scores and age of diagnosis, months undergoing treatment, and months since treatment was completed. This is not surprising, however, since it would be necessary to obtain extremely high correlations with samples of only nine and six cases to achieve statistical significance. In addition, correlations are an unreliable and inappropriate statistic for such small sample sizes. In general, all of their findings are of tenuous meaning and at best can be considered only as suggestive because of the extremely small samples which were used. For instance, only six older ALL patients were compared with healthy control cases. In this instance the patients scored six points lower than the controls on the Full Scale IQ. Thus, although there is a trend for the older patients to score lower than their healthy controls, a considerably greater difference in IQ scores than these six points would be needed with this small sample size in order to be statistically significant. Even significant differences would be questionable with samples this small since the IQ level of one or two cases could greatly affect the mean IQ levels of these groups.

In another study Eiser (1978) compared intelligence test scores on three groups of children receiving different treatments for ALL. One group of seven children received no CNS treatment, a second group of nine children had prophylactic CNS irradiation at least six months after diagnosis (delayed irradiation group), and a third group of ten children had CNS irradiation within two months of diagnosis (early irradiation group). It is not made explicit in the article why there should be differences in intelligence test performance between children receiving early or delayed CNS irradiation. Eiser reports negligible differences between the groups having no CNS irradiation and delayed CNS irradiation. Both of these groups obtained significantly higher IQ scores than the group undergoing early CNS irradiation. It is unfortunate that no information is provided concerning the interval of time between CNS irradiation and testing (which presumably differed for the early and late radiation groups), since we assume that variations in this time interval could account for the lower scores of the early irradiated group. This assumption is based on the findings of the previously discussed studies of vascular changes in the brain in which it was found that CNS irradiation caused delayed damage to the brain. Thus, the possibility of vascular damage would predict greater intellectual deficit where there is a longer interval between treatment and testing. Eiser does present correlations between IQ scores, age at irradiation, and time since irradiation. These correlations showed that younger ALL patients who received CNS treatment performed at a significantly lower level than older patients. There was also a nonsignificant trend for IQ's to be lower with increased time since irradiation. As was discussed earlier, however, correlational analysis is an inappropriate and unreliable statistic for the small samples involved in this study. Another factor which makes the findings from this research difficult to evaluate is that no information is given concerning the procedure for assigning patients to the three treatment conditions. Thus, there is no basis for determining whether these three groups were comparable in the initial abilities before treatment or whether there were selective factors involved which might have led to brighter patients being assigned to particular treatment conditions.

The methodological shortcomings inherent in these psychometric studies severely limits the significance and scientific value of the findings reported from these studies. Nonetheless, these studies provide some preliminary evidence of intellectual deficits associated with CNS treatment that are consistent with the neurological and behavioral findings that have been related to this treatment. Other studies are in progress (Kellerman, Moss, and Siegel at Childrens Hospital in Los Angeles and Moss, Nannis, and Poplack at the National Institutes of Health) concerning the effects of CNS treatment on intelligence test behavior. The additional information from these forthcoming studies should provide a clearer and more conclusive picture of the nature and extent to which CNS treatment alters intellectual functioning. In order to obtain findings that can be interpreted with greater confidence, some of the fundamental methodological problems which need to be addressed in future studies, are the need for larger samples and more appropriate control groups. Additionally, research in this area should be designed to evaluate differential vulnerability of different age groups, progressive changes in functioning since the time of treatment, whether changes which occur are continuous, level off, or indicate a potential for recovery, and whether there is a selective nature to the abilities which are affected.

The prophylactic treatment of the CNS has resulted in greatly increased remission rates among children with ALL. This has substantially improved the prospects of these children for a full and complete life. Even if it is learned that some detrimental effects accrue from this treatment, these effects seemingly would be minimal when compared to the vastly improved prognosis of these children. If it indeed becomes established that CNS treatment results in intellectual deficits, it would be important to determine the extent of these deficits, whether or not they lead to specific learning disabilities, and how the overall quality of life and ability to function effectively are affected. Answers to these questions could provide an impetus toward developing training and rehabilitation programs to help compensate for any lost or blunted skills. Knowledge of the effects of CNS treatment also could be put to good use in helping families deal with special difficulties children may be encountering and could provide a basis for understanding and supporting children who are experiencing frustration stemming from a loss in the capacity to master intellectual tasks. Beyond these practical responses to the deleterious side effects of CNS treatment, solid scientific evidence that these effects occur should spur medical researchers to develop new and equally effective treatment procedures with reduced risk of damage.

References
Albert, R. E., & Omran, A. R. : Follow-up study of patients treated by x-ray epilation for tinea capitis. I. Population characteristics, post-treatment illnesses, and mortality experience. *Arch Environ Health*, 1968, *17*, 899-918.

Eiser, C.: Intellectual abilities among survivors of childhood leukaemia as a function of CNS irradiation. *Arch Dis Child*, 1978, *53*(5), 391-395.

Eiser, C., & Lansdown, R.: Retrospective study of intellectual development in children treated for acute lymphoblastic leukaemia. *Arch Dis Child*, 1977, *52*, 525-529.

Freeman, J. E., Johnston, P. G. B., & Voke, J. M.: Somnolence after prophylactic cranial irradiation in children with acute lymphoblastic leukaemia. *Br Med J*, 1973, *4*, 523-525.

Furchtgott, E.: Behavioral effects of ionizing radiations: 1955-61. *Psychol Bull*, 1963, *60*(2), 157-199.

Garwicz, S., Aronson, A. S., Elmqvist, D., & Landberg, T.: Postirradiation syndrome and EEG findings in children with acute lymphoblastic leukaemia. *Acta Paediatr Scand*, 1975, *64*, 399-403.

Hendin, B., DeVivo, D. C., Torack, R., Lell, M. E., Ragab, A. H., & Vietti, T. J.: Parenchymatous degeneration of the central nervous system in childhood leukemia. *Cancer*, 1974, *33*, 468-482.

Hicks, S. P., & D'Amato, C. J.: Effects of ionizing radiations on mammalian development. In D. H. M. Woollam (Eds.) *Advances in Teratology*, Vol. *1*. Cambridge, Academic Press, 1966.

Kay, H. E. M., Knapton, P. J., O'Sullivan, J. P., Wells, D. G., Harris, R. F., Innes, E. M., Stuart, J., Schwartz, F. C. M., & Thompson, E. N.: Encephalopathy in acute leukaemia associated with methotrexate therapy. *Arch Dis Child*, 1972, *47*, 344-354.

Kramer, S.: The hazards of therapeutic irradiation of the central nervous system. *Clin Neurosurg*, 1968, *15*, 301-318.

Lenneberg, E. H.: *Biological Foundations of Language*. New York: Wiley, 1967.

McIntosh, S., Klatskin, E. H., O'Brien, R. T., Aspnes, G. T., Kammerer, B. L., Snead, C., Kalavsky, S. M., & Pearson, H. A.: Chronic neurologic disturbance in childhood leukemia. *Cancer*, 1976, *37*, 853-857.

Meadows, A. T., & Evans, A. E.: Effects of chemotherapy on the central nervous system. A study of parenteral methotrexate in long-term survivors of leukemia and lymphoma in childhood. *Cancer*, 1976, *37*(1), 1079-1085.

Painter, M. J., Chutorian, A. M., & Hilal, S. K.: Cerebrovasculopathy following irradiation in childhood. *Neurology*, 1975, *25*, 189-194.

Pennybacker, J., & Russell, D. S.: Necrosis of the brain due to radiation therapy. Clinical and pathological observations. *J Neurol Neurosurg Psychiatry*, 1948, *11*, 183-198.

Peylan-Ramu, N., Poplack, D. G., Pizzo, P. A., Adornato, B. T., and DiChiro, G.: Abnormal CT scans of the brain in asymptomatic children with acute lymphocytic leukemia after prophylactic treatment of the central nervous system with radiation and intrathecal chemotherapy. *N Engl J Med*, 1978, *298*, No. 15, 815-818.

Price, R. A., & Jamieson, P. A.: The central nervous system in childhood leukemia II. Subacute leukoencephalopathy. *Cancer*, 1975, *35*, 306-318.

Smith, B.: Brain damage after intrathecal methotrexate. *J Neurol, Neurosurg Psychiatry*, 1975, *38*, 810-815.

Soni, S. S., Marten, G. W., Pitner, S. E., Duenas, D. A., & Powazek, M.: Effects of central-nervous-system irradiation on neuropsychologic functioning of children with acute lymphocytic leukemia. *N Engl J Med*, 1975, *293*(3), 113-118.

Chapter Nine

I MAY BE BALD
BUT I STILL HAVE RIGHTS*

JAMES ARONSON

SUPPOSE YOU have just learned you have cancer. And suppose you have never known anyone who had cancer, so your understanding of the word and the disease is limited, at best. Suddenly you find yourself subjected to all sorts of tests, biopsies, and examinations, and people all around you are exhibiting a great deal of concern and interest in you, but you still do not know quite why. Mom and Dad are acting strange, hugging you and crying at the slightest provocation; while family, friends, and strangers alike, are treating you in strange new ways, ranging from obnoxious solicitude to unaccountable anger, and even, occasionally, unbearable ostracism.

What are you to make of it? What are your responsibilities in the new flight, the new problem that has entered your life? And above all, what are your rights, your reasonable expectations of medical aid and emotional support now that your life is suddenly threatened?

My own feelings, as a former cancer patient, is that rights fall into two classes: (1) Inalienable Rights, including the *right to know*, and the *right to the best available treatment*, impeccably administered by well-trained medical personnel; and (2) *secondary or personal rights*, including those which are now ignored or unobtainable in our society. These rights are controlled by no one and cannot be legislated as easily. They are nonetheless important. In this article I will address both categories of patients' rights and consider the problems and complications inherent in both.

Patients' inalienable rights should be considered and respected immediately at the time of diagnosis. The first and foremost right of a cancer patient is the *right to know*. Whether young or old, he has the right never to be lied to, either by doctors, nurses, or family. If a patient is prepared to hear the facts of his case, grim though they might be, then he should be informed, clearly and without jargon or "medicalese," about his situation and his prospects for survival.

The patient's right to know continues throughout the course of treatment and beyond. The physicians and family should be prepared to answer all the patient's questions to the best of their ability whenever

---

* From I May Be Bald But I Have Rights. *The Journal of Clinical Child Psychology*, Vol. 7 No. 3, Fall 1978. Reprinted by permission.

those questions arise. Of course a busy doctor must try to give roughly equal time to all his or her patients, but efficiency and time-saving must never take precedence over communication with the patient. Even a relatively simple procedure, such as a blood test or spinal tap, can be transformed in a young patient's mind, into a horrid, frightening torture. Great care should be taken to make, as much as possible, each procedure intelligible and predictable to the young cancer patient who demonstrates a desire to know.

However, it does not always happen that way. One smokescreen that doctors frequently hide behind when they do not want to answer questions is what they call "therapeutic privilege." But in the current era of malpractice suits, if a doctor keeps vital information from a patient, he/she does so at his/her own risk. Unfortunately, an even more common cause for failure to fulfill the patient's right to know is what appears to be "sheer laziness" on the part of doctors who will not make the effort to talk with their patients beyond the bare necessity. However, despite appearances, I suspect that the real limiting factor in this regard is the extent to which the physician or nurse is defended against the reality of their business with young cancer patients. To take time out to answer questions and respond to the patient's fears and anxieties might trigger more depression and despondency than the doctor or nurse can allow him/herself to have while on the job. Above all, the doctors, nurses, and technicians have the responsibility to relate to their patients as human beings and not as medical punching bags, pincushions, or guinea pigs.

Now, it may sometimes be the case (more often, I suspect, with adults than children) that the patient does not want to know the truth or the rationale of his treatments. In that case, he or she has the inalienable right not to have the truth forced on him against his will. If the patient finds it easier to make the leap of faith by screening out troublesome awareness of the drama of his predicament, to say, in short, to his doctor: "I don't want to know what it is or why, just make me well again!" That too is his right. No one should be forced to confront a reality or an eventuality that he is not prepared to absorb. In many cases, I suspect, this is less a problem than it first might appear, because the mind is amazingly clever at defending itself against the truth.

For example, when I was first diagnosed with cancer, it took me nearly a week to absorb the information. In the meantime, I was in an odd state of euphoria while those around me were counting the months I had left to live. My body/mind simply could not absorb the shock and assimilate the bad news, and thus my blinders went up and stayed up for the better part of a week. Extrapolating from this experience, I imagine that no one will listen to anything before he is prepared to do so.

The second inalienable right is the *right to the most up-to-date treatment.* If the family lives in a town or small city, they should be referred by their doctor to a specialist in the nearest large city. If they are already living in a big city, they have the right to be sure their doctors are informed of all forms and combinations of therapies currently in use and under study for that disease at every major medical center in the country. They should be fully informed of the relative merits and drawbacks of each protocol before being asked to choose between them. When the choice is made, with the advice of their doctor, the patient and his family have the right to be fully informed of all possible side effects, both short- and long-term, that the treatment might entail, as well as the doctor's opinion, based on all available information, of the patient's chances for survival both with and without the treatments.

Of course, if the prognosis is not good, or if the side effects are overwhelming, the patient should have the right to refuse treatment and allow the cancer to run its course. This is particularly relevant in the case of the elderly patient who might not have the stamina or the will to live necessary to make radiation and chemotherapy effective — given the balance between illness from side effects and quality of time remaining.

In the case of the small child with cancer, the problem is far more complex. Invariably, a child under sixteen will have his medical decisions made for him by his parents and physician. But what if his parents, acting out of fear and ignorance, should arrive at some rather dubious decisions about the child's illness? Consider the case of a young child with leukemia whose parents have an active distrust of doctors and hospitals. If caught early and handled judiciously, pediatric leukemia is highly susceptible to cure by modern medical techniques. But despite the fact that young children tend to suffer far less from the side effects of treatment than most adults, some parents cannot bear to see their child suffer nausea, discomfort, and loss of hair at the hands of doctors whose methods they understand only poorly, if at all. Such parents might prefer to take their sick child to a Laetrile clinic or a faith healer. It has been successfully argued in a court of law that the child has the right to the best available treatment for his or her disease, despite the prejudices or reluctance of his parents. Thus, if a qualified oncologist feels strongly that the child's chances for survival might be significantly improved by the techniques at his disposal, the courts have ruled that the child's parents do not have the right to deprive their child of those treatments.

If, on the other hand, the family does decide to opt for modern medical treatment, as is usually the case, both the patient and his family are entitled to full consideration of their emotional and psychological needs throughout the ordeal of long oncological treatment.

Particularly, if the patient does not respond well to some part of the treatment or if there is difficulty in administering the drugs (as was true in my own case), then the doctors and nurses are in the position of asking a great deal from the young patient and should be prepared to give in return. The patient is asked to be brave and strong-willed, to be stoic and heroic in the face of pain and unhappiness. He is asked to endure a variety of iatrogenic ailments all for the sake of a mysterious, invasive treatment which he may never have fully understood. In short, he is required to make a leap of faith in support of the doctors and their clumsy methods, a responsibility that can only be undertaken if he feels himself a full and equal partner in the healing process. To be such an equal partner, he needs access to all the information and truth he can possibly handle.

And, of course, it follows that another inalienable right of the cancer patient, is the right to regularity and continuity of his treatments. Complications and conflicts can lead to modifications in treatment and personnel. But where mid-course changes are unavoidable, the patient should be notified well in advance and allowed ample time to make the transition. Uncertainty and insecurity are pretty enormous problems for the cancer patient to begin with, and should not be aggravated by unpredictable medical treatment. Particular care should be taken to avoid unnecessary switching of the persons responsible for the administration of the child's treatments. I referred earlier to the leap of faith required of the cancer patient. Such a leap is greatly facilitated and perhaps impossible without an emotional transference to, or at least, a friendly relationship with, the nurse or doctor administering treatment. Whenever possible, the person giving treatment, whether of radiation or chemotherapy, should remain the same throughout.

Since the doctor in charge of my case was usually busy with research and administrative responsibilities, my file was farmed out successively to a number of residents and training doctors from Europe, Asia, and South America. I found it rather amusing to meet with the foreign doctors, but then I was considerably older than most of the patients coming into the clinic, and therefore was treated somewhat differently. Also, I was deeply committed to healing myself and believed sufficiently in the doctors' procedures that after a while, I did not much care who gave me the shots. But if I had not had the support of a close-knit, warm family throughout the long ordeal, the frequent turnover of personnel and the concurrent necessity to create rapport with each new person might have been considerably harder to bear.

I also experienced an enormous need, almost a greed, for love, caring, and compassionate attention throughout the two years I was in treatment. And this brings me to the second class of patients' rights which I call "rights" tentatively, since they might be more aptly called blessings. I am enormously fortunate to have my secondary rights and needs met generously, but many cancer patients have not been, and will not be, so fortunate.

These secondary rights, important as they are, can not be controlled in the hospital. In fact it is difficult to say who should be responsible for them. As a result they are often ignored and neglected. But I am convinced that if they are met, the patient will be more likely to survive his disease. Not only will he have greater tolerance and forebearance and thus be able to survive his treatments, but also he will be better able to maintain a positive attitude which I assume to be critical for any patient with a serious illness or disease.

No matter what kind of treatment the patient receives — be it voodoo, Laetrile, or the most sophisticated scientific therapy, half the battle for survival revolves around the issue of whether or not he gives up hope. By providing secondary services and back-up support to the patient, hospital staff and family members can become extremely important links in a whole-life support system for the cancer patient.

For example, the cancer patient has at least a theoretical right to have someone who will listen. Someone with patience, empathy, and compassion, who will give audience to his problems and fears. He needs someone to help him gain insight and understanding of his changing self-image, his new relationships with the world, and his turbulently evolving attitudes about life and death.

Moreover, he needs outlets to express the rage and tension he feels in response to the aggravated stress being placed upon him. This, of course, is impossible to prescribe at the local drugstore or serve up with dinner. There is no guarantee that someone to listen will always be available. Nor is there any way to legislate or orchestrate the expression of feelings. Although a sense of helplessness is probably inevitable, all I ask is for sensitivity and awareness on the part of all concerned that the young cancer patients' emotional needs might be heightened, attenuated, and fluctuating. He will hopefully seek and find satisfaction for his heightened oral and sexual needs and discover constructive ways to vent his anger and frustration. On the other hand, problems should not be exacerbated by overzealous parental protectiveness. The child should be allowed both freedom to regress and freedom to experience periodic explosions of existential rage. In addition, he must be aided in the more subtle task of maintaining a healthy narcissism despite the silent stigma of cancer.

Another problem rests on the fact that, historically, cancer patients always died. Therefore, no one paid much attention to long-term issues. Now that a third to a half of all patients treated for cancer can be cured, it is time to give serious thoughts to some of these other problems. The long-term danger of engraved trauma can be minimized, if, throughout the treatment period and beyond, the young patient is provided with services aimed at insuring ongoing physical and mental well-being of the whole person. These would include:

PROSTHETIC DEVICES. Every effort must be made to minimize the cancer patient's feelings of isolation and alienation from society. His self-image must be maintained at as high a level as possible. If surgical amputation is performed (which fortunately is happening less and less), the patient should have access to plastic surgery and every available kind of prosthetic device. The patient should be provided with advanced devices as soon as possible following surgery and instructed in their proper use. If there are financial problems, these devices should be paid for by the insurance company or, ideally, by the government.

ALOPECIA. In the case of the common side effect of alopecia or loss of hair, the patient and his family should be counseled on the alternatives to baldness. An intelligent counselor should be available to discuss, among other things, whether the child wants to acquire a wig or stick to hats, scarves, or helmets. (Although I hardly endorse this latter choice of headgear, I have in fact seen many young cancer patients wearing football helmets to cover their baldness and perhaps symbolically to defend themselves.) Again, if money is a problem, the cost of a good quality wig should be considered not as a frill but rather as an essential part of the health care of the patient.

NUTRITION. Nutrition is a critical issue, since the loss of appetite and depression can cause severe weight loss and/or malnutrition and anemia in some patients. Chemotherapeutic drugs place a severe strain on the metabolic system of the body, using up proteins and carbohydrates at a prodigious rate. Those proteins, in particular, are essential to the body's immune system. Therefore, a qualified nutritionist should routinely work with all cancer patients to insure that an adequate diet is maintained throughout the period of treatments.

PHYSICAL THERAPY. Very probably, many patients will be in need of reparative or correctional physical therapy following surgery or radiation therapy. This should be considered a fundamental right of any patient who undergoes physical changes as a result of medical treatment. Certain changes, such as fibrosis or the destruction of tissue may be irreversible. But secondary complications due to prolonged misuse or lack of use of parts of the body, as well as psychological overlay in the area of treatment, should be monitored carefully and corrected wherever possible.

At the beginning of my treatment, I received 6000 Rads of radiation in the region of the left scapula and shoulder. Compounded by the effects of radiosensitizing drugs, this dosage reduced the functional mobility of my shoulder and arm. Since no physical therapy was offered, I devised my own series of daily exercises to counteract the progressive shortening and tightening of the muscles in my shoulder. Although I counted the burden of a "bum wing," a small price to pay for the miracle of having had my life saved from cancer, still I resented the constant reminder and handicap of the injured shoulder.

About a year after the completion of my chemotherapy, I contacted a practitioner of Rolfing, which is a new form of psychophysical therapy which concentrates on restructuring the connective planes of organ and muscle encircling sheathes of fasciae within the body. In the course of ten sessions with my Rolfer, I discovered that for over two years I had been "carrying" my arm needlessly, as if it were a useless and lifeless thing. The therapist worked long hours on the fasciae and muscles adjoining the entire shoulder and scapula region, and ultimately, I experienced a tremendous relief of pain while recovering much fuller use of the arm. Needless to say, the psychological benefits from this improvement probably outweigh the physical ones. In a similar fashion, I would think that many cancer patients could benefit from physical therapy — whether conventional, chiropractic, or Rolfing, in the alleviation or elimination of secondary and tertiary trauma and pain.

THC. Finally, it is necessary to mention that THC, the active ingredient in marijuana, has been reported to be anecdotally effective for some cancer patients in counteracting some of the side effects of chemotherapeutic drugs. Mental health professionals are well advised to familiarize themselves with the literature about the use of THC in cancer treatment and glaucoma, now that state legislatures are making its use legal in medical treatment. Preadolescent, adolescent, and adult patients may seek you out to discuss their thoughts about taking this drug and requesting information about its sequelae.

CONCLUSION

Talk is cheap. At this point, the reader will want to ask the following questions: "First of all, where is the money going to come from? And secondly, assuming you get the money, how will you implement these proposals?"

Indeed, the cost of health care for cancer patients is already astronomical. Among the "catastrophic diseases," cancer is considered one of the worst in terms of financial strain on the family of the patient. And to implement the kinds of changes I have outlined for medical institutions would certainly increase the costs still further. So who is to pay?

For many years now, enormous sums have been spent by Congress to fund basic and applied research on cancer and the "cure" of cancer. Great strides have been made and many lives have been saved. But despite thirty years of intensive research (far more than was required to solve the riddles of polio and TB) most investigators feel we are still far from finding a "cure" for cancer. Our understanding of the proliferation of malignant cells is still sketchy and inadequate. And immunotherapy, which holds great promise of someday superseding chemotherapy and radiation therapy, is still in the rudimentary phases of research and development. Consequently, we are liable to remain at our current state of sophistication in the medical fight against cancer for some time to come. I propose, therefore, that a certain amount of the current federal expenditures on cancer be directed for the development and inauguration of experimental programs in selected hospitals designed to meet the primary needs, and, at the very least, the inalienable rights of all cancer patients. In the best units, it would be hoped the secondary rights would be met as well. If every oncological treatment unit contained a physical therapist, a nutritionist, a psychotherapist, and possibly even a family counselor on the staff, I will wager that fewer cancer patients would give up mid-way through their treatments, that more cancer victims could be treated as outpatients, and consequently, that more patients could be restored to full health using the same medical techniques and in the same amount of time as is now customary.

At present, there are few hospitals in the United States where organized support teams such as I have described are working with children and adult patients with cancer. Elsewhere, the cancer patient and his family are left to their own devices to identify their needs and obtain the services they require. If the patient is strong and the family well-united, all will be well and the available resources in the city will be tapped. But if the stability and emotional health of the family are not good to begin with, the blow of cancer in one member of the family might be a fatal blow for all.

Even if not automatically provided as part of a total package of health care for cancer patients, I believe these secondary support services should be readily available in the offices where the patient receives treatment for all those who wish to avail themselves of these services.

As for the inalienable and personal rights that I have described, I would ask that those families and medical personnel already working with young cancer patients ask themselves what they could do to insure that all their patient's rights are honored and respected to the fullest possible extent. Of course, there still can be no guarantee that the patient will be cured, but I firmly believe the fulfillment of patients' rights can help.

There is an old adage that: "Nature cures the disease; the healer merely entertains the patient." In the case of cancer, we have learned to help Nature a little in curing the disease, but the healers must remember not only to entertain the patient but to nurture good health in his whole person as well.

SECTION II
CLINICAL APPROACHES

Chapter Ten

COMPREHENSIVE PSYCHOSOCIAL CARE OF THE CHILD WITH CANCER: DESCRIPTION OF A PROGRAM

JONATHAN KELLERMAN

T HE USEFULNESS of looking at pediatric cancer from the conceptual standpoint of chronic disease has been recognized by authors of several recent papers (Koch et al., 1974; Lansky et al., 1974a, 1974b, 1975, 1977; Holmes and Holmes, 1975; Kagen-Goodheart, 1977; Katz et al., 1977). In this context, investigative emphasis is placed upon identifying adaptive and maladaptive patterns of reactive behavior in the child and family — the latter most often described as "problems of living . . . " (Koch et al., 1974, p. 81) — and clinical efforts are aimed at maximizing optimal postdiagnostic rehabilitation and reintegration.

Despite this, there is a relative dearth of empirical information regarding both the incidence and prevalence of psychological problems among pediatric cancer patients and of detailed, reproducible accounts of comprehensive clinical care.

Lansky (1974a) has noted that, just as a multidisciplinary medical approach, combining chemotherapy, radiotherapy, and surgery has proved most potent in combating the physical ravages of childhood cancer, so might a psychosocial team approach be the preferred modality when addressing the emotional problems associated with malignant disease.

Nevertheless, previous clinical accounts have not emphasized comprehensive, multidisciplinary care and have tended to focus upon the following areas:

Descriptions of the Clinical Activities of A Particular Health Professional

These include the social worker (Nolfi, 1967; Lang and Oppenheimer, 1968; Kagen-Goodheart, 1977), the psychologist (Humphrey and Vore, 1974; Drotar, 1975; Katz et al., 1977), and the psychiatrist (Lansky, 1974a).

Clinical Approaches to Death and Dying

These articles comprise the bulk of the clinical psychosocial literature on pediatric cancer. The large number of papers makes individual citation impractical. (Major references include: Nagy, 1948; Kastenbaum, 1959; Natterson and Knudson, 1960; Nauer, 1964; Easson,

1974; Futterman, et al., 1974; Martinson, 1976; Koocher, 1973, 1977; Spinetta and associates, 1973, 1974a, 1974b, 1975, 1977.)

Descriptions of a Specific Clinical Approach

Modalities described include group therapy (Heffron et al., 1973) and hypnosis (Crasilneck and Hall, 1973; LaBaw, et al., 1975; Gardner, 1976). Individual and family counseling approaches are most often presented within the framework of papers illustrating theoretical or descriptive issues, such as illness impact studies. In general, these deal in very broad terms with clinical techniques. (Included in this group are: Moore et al., 1969; Ablin et al., 1971; Hoffman and Futterman, 1971; Kellerman et al., 1976; Katz et al., 1977; Parodi, 1977.)

It is suggested here that the emotional needs of the child with cancer and his family are best met by the implementation of comprehensive multidisciplinary psychosocial intervention that transcends the expertise of any single type of health professional. Furthermore, the assertion is made that intervention needs to be described in terms that are maximally specific and objectified. Such description is the focus of the remainder of this chapter.

THE PSYCHOSOCIAL PROGRAM

Since November 1, 1976, psychosocial care has been incorporated as part of routine treatment for children with cancer treated in the Division of Hematology-Oncology at Childrens Hospital of Los Angeles. Childrens Hospital of Los Angeles is a three-hundred bed pediatric facility serving the greater Los Angeles metropolitan area and outlying regions. It is a teaching institution, affiliated with the Department of Pediatrics, University of Southern California School of Medicine.

The hospital's Hematology-Oncology division treats approximately 150 newly diagnosed pediatric cancer patients each year and has a total roster of 574 children diagnosed with a variety of malignant diseases (Table 10-I).

These statistics describe a major pediatric oncology center and note must be taken of the possibility that only such a large center can economically afford routine, comprehensive psychosocial care.

Financing of psychosocial services is similar to that of medical treatment, in that patients are billed for both. A large proportion of cost is covered by third party payments from governmental agencies and private insurance programs. Supplemental income accrues to the program in the form of research contracts and grants.

Divisional Affiliation

The Psychosocial Program is part of the division of Hematology-Oncology and the psychosocial staff are members of the division. Because of this, integration of psychosocial care into the oncology treatment program has been facilitated. Shared divisional affiliation has helped to forge a close, amiable working relationship between

TABLE 10-I
CHILDRENS HOSPITAL OF LOS ANGELES
ACTIVE ONCOLOGY PATIENTS

Leukemia	
ALL, AUL	193
AML, AEL, AMMOL, AErythl, APL	20
Chronic myelog.	3
Lymphoma	
Hodgkin's	53
Non-Hodgkin's	20
Central Nervous Tumor	53
Neuroblastoma	31
Retinoblastoma	10
Kidney Tumors	
Wilm's	57
Others	1
Liver Tumors	
Hepatoblastoma	5
Hepatocelluar carcinoma	1
Liver tumor, NOS	0
Bone Tumors	
Osteosarcoma	9
Ewing's tumor	13
Bone tumor, NOS	0
Gonadal and Germ Cell	
Ovary	7
Testis	11
Nongonadal – Malignant Teratoma	3
Soft Tissue	47
Melanoma	0
Reticuloendotheliosis	
Benign histiocytosis	9
Malignant histiocytosis	15
Reticuloendotheliosis	1
	570
Miscellaneous	
Rhabdomyosarcoma 40	
Fibrosarcoma 3	
Synovial sarcoma 2	
Undifferent sarcoma 1	
Benign fibroma 1	

medical and psychosocial staff. Obviously such a relationship needs to grow out of mutually beneficial work experiences. Too often, however, the "outside specialist" never gets the opportunity to build up a level of trust necessary for such cooperation. The consultant may be perceived as being only tangentially involved in pediatric cancer, or as engaging in professional dilettantism. Furthermore, his very participation may imply failure to the referring physician. Placement within the division has aided in preventing such professional xenophobia and has reduced some of the problems noted by Lewis (1978) and Peebles and O'Malley (1978).

Staff

The oncological part of the Psychosocial Program consists of three Ph.D. clinical psychologists, including the director, an M.A. school psychologist, a social worker, a social work assistant, an oncology nurse coordinator, and two patient activity specialists, all of whom work exclusively and specifically with cancer patients. An additional Ph.D. clinical psychologist and social worker work with children with non-malignant hematologic disorders.

TREATMENT PHILOSOPHY

All health care is influenced by the various attitudes and philosophies held by the practitioner toward treatment. This is so even in the more "hard" or "scientific" subspecialities where issues such as radical versus modified surgery or inpatient versus outpatient treatment may surface, but is particularly true when confronting psychosocial issues. In the interests of guiding the reader, it is useful to specify some of the underlying assumptions and attitudes behind the Psychosocial Program, along with their empirical and/or theoretical bases.

Routine Care

The value of incorporating psychosocial care into the routine treatment regimen cannot be overemphasized. The alternative to routine care is that of crisis-reaction. It is felt that "calling in the shrinks" when all else has failed is not advisable for several reasons:

1. Last resort treatment can restrict clinical efficacy by allowing problems to reach a point of severity or chronicity that makes them difficult to treat. This may set a pattern of psychosocial intervention that has a high rate of failure, create a perception, on the part of the referring physician, of the uselessness of such treatment, and may discourage future referral.
2. Last resort treatment depends upon singling out a given patient and family as having behavioral-emotional problems. It may, thus, foster stigmatization. More will be said regarding this in a later section.
3. Relying upon a crisis-oriented treatment approach makes the mental health professional dependent upon the ability of others to recognize, define, and refer problems. Thus, a bias toward disorders that are highly visible and dramatic may be created and a significant proportion of problems may escape attention.

Nonpathologic Emphasis

It is important for the mental health professional to be acutely aware that the child with cancer and his family have not entered into the medical treatment setting due to the existence of a psychiatric disorder.

The appearance of a psychologist, psychiatrist, or social worker may trigger anxiety on the part of the family in terms of how others perceive its mental health. This serves to exacerbate an already heightened sense of anxiety and distress in a population of individuals who have already been dealt more than their share of trauma, and can retard the development of rapport, trust, and a therapeutic relationship.

As has been mentioned, a program that incorporates routine contact between patients and psychosocial personnel goes a long way toward assuring the child and family that no singling-out process has occurred. Psychosocial staff members discuss this during their initial contact with the patient and emphasize the routine nature of the intervention.

The basic model of the program is that of preventing and ameliorating psychological problems in a population of *normal individuals under stress*. Furthermore, a basic posture of confidence in the ability of human beings to successfully cope is assumed. This is in sharp contrast to an approach that predicts inevitable psychopathology. As Tavormina et al. (1976) have noted, there is empirical support for the assumption of normalcy rather than deviance of chronically ill children. Lewis (1978) also stresses the importance of understanding normal childhood behavior when working with pediatric cancer patients. It is felt, by the author, that the tendency to overpathologize — to interpret maladaptive process from routine responses — is countertherapeutic. Consider the following example:

> A seven-year-old boy with non-Hodgkins lymphoma had been treated for several weeks as an inpatient. Though he continued to respond well to the hospital staff, he developed an aversion to the medical intern who administered venipunctures and other painful procedures. Subsequently, he began to withdraw from, and refused to speak to, this house officer. The intern recorded in the medical chart that the child was suffering from psychotic depression related to terminal illness.

As Koocher has noted in another section of this volume, initial observations of the child with cancer are unlikely to be based upon typical behavior. It is important for the clinician to base judgments not only upon empirical information as opposed to value-laden, preconditioned assumptions, but also to make use of a broad range of repeated observations; the child lying inert and silent in a hospital bed may be quite different twenty minutes later when he or she is interacting with peers in a hospital playroom. The youngster who, having just finished undergoing a lumbar puncture and a bone marrow aspiration and who is subsequently restless and fidgety cannot be said to be displaying deviant behavior if one is familiar with normal patterns of reaction to such stress. The thoughtful clinician would be reluctant to diagnose hyperkinesis in such a case.

Similarly, the individual who exhibits conditioned anxiety related to a stimulus that has no inherent noxious properties, such as an elevator or a horse, may be said to be manifesting phobic behavior. That is, there is an element of unrealistic fear to the response. In contrast, the child with cancer who displays conditioned anxiety related to the administration of painful or uncomfortable medical procedures is not behaving unrealistically. This does not mean that the child in the second case cannot be helped through the use of psychological techniques, but such therapy is not enhanced by inferences of neuroticism that are implied by psychiatric labeling and may, on the contrary, be impeded.

In general, the wealth of data presented by Endler and Magnusson (1976) lends support to the efficacy of an interactional approach, one that examines behavior as part of an interplay between personological and situational variables, as opposed to a purely intrapsychic plumbing of hypothesized mental mechanisms.

Children and families have been very receptive to the notion that stress, such as that brought about by a diagnosis of cancer, raises psychological vulnerability; and families have been accepting and appreciative of psychosocial care when it is presented in this context. Of particular value has been the opportunity to familiarize families with the *normal, disease-related patterns of stress reaction.* Parents are grateful to learn, for example, that transitory reactive depression during the initial postdiagnostic period is normal. Providing of such information during early psychosocial intervention helps prevent needless worry and provides a frame of reference. It reassures the parents and children that what they are feeling is normal, and by extension, acceptable. Thus, rather than increasing feelings of stigmatization, psychosocial care can serve an opposite role, that of normalization.

In the event that a child is referred due to the existence of a behavioral problem at some later point, it continues to be important to discuss this with the patient and the family as something that occurs in many children who are under stress, and to avoid psychopathological labeling.

Structured Professional Communication

For a psychosocial program to succeed in a medical setting, it must have the support of the medical staff. Even if such support exists at the outset, it may quickly erode if good communication is not maintained between referring physicians and psychosocial professionals. In the conventional medical setting, the physician bears primary responsibility for the treatment of the child. It is the obligation of the mental health professional to provide information in such a way that aids in this treatment. Some measures that have been useful in accomplishing this have been:

1. Psychosocial consultation is initiated at the request of the attending physician. This does not preclude routine contact between psychosocial staff and patients, nor does it mean that individuals, other than the physician, cannot facilitate referrals. In such instances, however, written physician approval for consultation is obtained. This

places the psychosocial intervention within a reified, structured context, as part of the child's oncological care.

2. All psychosocial contacts are recorded in the medical chart. Copies are sent, routinely, to the referring physician.

3. Psychosocial notes are brief, avoid jargon, and maximize objective behavioral description of clinical impressions and treatment plan. Notations such as "Patient seen, very depressed. Thank you for this fascinating referral." are less useful than are concise summaries of relevant background information, presenting problems, and future plans. It is the omission of the last ingredient that too often characterizes many mental health consultations. Obviously, there are instances when the consultant is at a loss to come up with a viable treatment plan and a note to this effect is important. If further contact is planned with the patient, however, it is necessary to explain the rationale behind treatment and to objectify the intervention to the maximum degree. Consider the example of a child referred due to what is believed to be psychosomatic nausea and vomiting. After psychological evaluation is completed, a useful clinical note might contain the following:

> This six-year-old male, diagnosed with ALL approximately six months ago was referred due to nausea and vomiting occuring on the day preceding administration of intravenous chemotherapy. This pattern began approximately one and a half months after diagnosis and has continued to increase in severity until the present time when emesis occurs up to a dozen times prior to treatment. Possible contributing factors include birth of a new brother around the time the anticipatory vomiting began. Patient is doing well in school and presents no other problems at this time.
>
> Impression: Conditioned anxiety reaction related to treatment for acute leukemia.
>
> Plan: Three to six sessions of brief psychotherapy aimed at clarifying his understanding of and feelings about his disease, its treatment, and possible sibling hostility, as well as examination of changes in family patterns of child rearing. Self-hypnosis for relaxation, and possible use of operant reinforcement of nonvomiting behavior.

4. Written notes are augmented by personal communication with the physician, particularly when information arises that does not lend itself to placement in the medical chart.

Short-Term Rehabilitation

The program's view of psychosocial treatment emphasizes return of the child and family to premorbid patterns of functioning. Obviously, the diagnosis of cancer in a child is a traumatic event and it is unrealistic to expect that the child or family will ever be the same after it occurs. It is therapeutic, however, to encourage a resumption of the set of behaviors that constituted normalcy for a given patient and to use medical feasibility as the major criterion when making decisions about reintegration. Returning children to school is an example of this that has received considerable attention (Cyphert, 1973; Kaplan et al., 1974; Oswin, 1974; Lansky, 1974a, 1974b; Greene, 1975; Travis, 1976; Katz et al., 1977). Other issues are resumption of peer and extracurricular activities, including athletics, and of jobs, in the case of adolescents.

Successful rehabilitation can be maximized by helping the child and family to muster their own strength. An emphasis upon long-term psychotherapy is usually seen as contraindicated for two reasons:

1. The empirical nature of psychological problems related to the disease does not justify extended treatment (Kellerman et al., 1979).

2. Long-term psychotherapy may foster dependency upon the therapist, and, in retarding the development of self-help skills, may be countertherapeutic.

Preparation

An underlying principle of our program is that individuals are better able to deal with stressful events when they are in possession of relevant information about these events than when they are ignorant. This notion has received substantial empirical validation (Janis, 1958; Cassell, 1965; Bandura and Menlove, 1968; Johnson and Leventhal, 1974; Vernon and Bailey, 1974; Melamed and Seigel, 1975; Shipley et al., 1978).

Parent handbooks, open age-appropriate discussions of disease and treatment, laboratory tours, behavioral preparation for medical procedures, and the general avoidance of hidden agenda are all important. It is also essential for psychosocial treatment itself to be open to discussion with the therapist, child, and family sharing an understanding of therapeutic goals and methods.

The Family Adaptive Unit

Comprehensive psychosocial care addresses itself not only to the effects of the disease and its treatment upon individual family members but also attends to the interactions between them. If the entire family is viewed as an adaptive unit, then the usefulness of including family members as observers and, when feasible, participants in treatment, becomes apparent. This reduces the likelihood of distorted perceptions that can lead to increased family friction.

For example, the father who shares in bringing his child to the outpatient oncology clinic will have little difficulty in understanding his wife's long absences from the home when she does the same. Similarly, siblings who watch the ill child leave home, receive an excuse to miss school, go to the hospital for an ill-defined "treatment," and return home with a toy, may be less likely to feel jealous after having observed the host of medical procedures undergone during what was previously seen as a vacation day.

Considering the family as a unit aids in avoiding isolation of the patient and helps preserve the integrity of premorbid adaptive patterns. Needless to say, there are long-standing, prediagnostic relational difficulties that exist in some families that may hinder rehabilitation; when this occurs, treatment is in order. Otherwise, the emphasis is upon helping the family help itself.

Definition of Professional Roles

Overlapping of professional functions can be expected within almost any medical setting. This is, perhaps, most true of psychosocial treatment, for most health professionals believe themselves to possess the basic attributes that are seen as major components of good psychosocial care: empathy, warmth, compassion. In addition within the mental health area a number of different specialties provide care: Psychologists, psychiatrists, social workers, social work assistants, counselors, and paraprofessionals. Though some overlap may thus be unavoidable and, perhaps, even desirable, it is felt that too much blurring of professional roles can lead to confusion on the parts of patients and clinicians, can cause duplication of services, and even worse, bring about inadequate patient care by creating a feast-or-famine situation.

An examination of training and experience will reveal skills that are unique to each of the helping professions. These have been emphasized in order to maximize treatment efficiency and efficacy.

CLINICAL ACTIVITIES OF PSYCHOSOCIAL TEAM MEMBERS

Nurse Coordinator

The Nurse Coordinator has specific masters degree level training in Psychiatry and Oncology and her role can best be described as that of a liaison between the family and the treatment system. She is the first member of the psychosocial team to meet the child and family — as soon as the child is admitted to the hospital with a suspected malignancy — and she participates in the initial diagnostic conference. Her subsequent functions include:

1. *Providing backup information about the disease and its treatment.* During the initial diagnostic conference during which the disease and its treatment are described and informed consents are signed, the parents are most often in shock. Focusing, understandably, upon the fact that their child has cancer, they may go through the motions of attending to the plethora of medical information presented to them and actually retain very little in the way of specifics. The nurse coordinator is available as a supplementary source of facts about the disease, its treatment, and adjusting to the mechanics of the hospital system. This includes helping develop optimal strategies for coping with the treatment regimen and providing a written handbook. This book contains information about the various diseases, treatments, medications and side effects, a glossary of commonly used medical terms and abbreviations, maps of various hospital locations, visitation regulations, and psychosocial issues.

2. *Participating in oncology rounds and serving as a two-way conduit for information between medical and psychosocial staff.* Often the first person to be aware of specific psychosocial issues, the nurse coordinator facilitates referrals from the physicians to the psychosocial team.

3. *Conducting a basic psychosocial intake and family history for each newly diagnosed child and presenting this data at weekly psychosocial case conferences.*

4. *Providing supportive counseling to the child and parent and maintaining ongoing communication with them throughout the child's treatment.* The nurse coordinator does not engage in prolonged or intensive psychotherapy, but, rather initiates the involvement of psychologists and social workers when the need for such treatment arises.

Patient Activity Specialist (Play Therapist)

These therapists hold master's degrees in human development, early childhood education, psychology, or related disciplines and receive specific training in working with physically ill children in a pediatric hospital setting. They are part of a hospital-based program aimed at helping children prepare for and adjust to the hospital experience, and much of the services they offer are carried out within the several playrooms attached to various inpatient wards.

Two play therapists are members of the psychosocial team and work, exclusively, with pediatric cancer patients. One serves as the psychosocial support person for children treated in laminar airflow units and the other supervises an out-patient playroom that operates during Hematology-Oncology Clinic.

Pediatric cancer patients come into contact with the patient activity specialists soon after admission, when the therapist, after being notified by physicians of impending procedures (bone marrow aspirations, transfusions, surgery, etc.) helps prepare the child for these. In addition these specialists are sensitive to the emotional concerns of the child, and they offer psychological support as well as communication of these issues to members of the psychosocial team. Functions of the patient activity specialists include:

1. *Guiding the child in behavioral preparation for medical procedures during hospitalization.* The details of such preparation are discussed in Chapter 8 of this volume.

2. *Designing and running the outpatient playroom.* Situated in the clinic, this room serves as a place of refuge for children who are waiting to be seen for medical appointments or are scheduled for outpatient procedures. The children know that they will not be exposed to pain or discomfort within its boundaries and that they are free to express their feelings about what is happening to them. Drawing paper, easels, paints, crayons, and selected toys are provided. The children engage both in unstructured individual and group activities such as body tracings aimed at eliciting feelings about self-concept, writing of hospital diaries and procedure books, murals, and family drawings.

In addition, a "Doctor Play" table upon which are arranged syringes, swabs, stethoscopes, and other medical paraphernalia, and dolls that serve as surrogate patients, is set up along one wall of the playroom. Here the children are free to engage in procedural preparation.

The pleasant atmosphere of the playroom helps relieve some of the anxiety and tedium associated with clinic visits. An ongoing parent group is scheduled during clinic, and parents find it easier to separate from the ill child when the latter is in the playroom and they then are freer to attend to some of their own needs.

3. *Working with medical and nursing staff in setting up recreational and activity programs for the hospitalized child.* Efforts are made to integrate inpatients into the hospital playroom program. For some children, however, such as those in isolation, or those who are too ill to leave their beds, this is not feasible. The patient activity specialists work with the child, family, and staff in developing an individual activity program in such cases.

Psychologists

After a diagnosis has been reached and a treatment plan has been determined, the psychologists receive a routine consultation request from the attending oncologist to conduct a psychological evaluation. The emphasis of this process is upon gaining rapport with the child and family, getting a picture of the child's premorbid functioning, assessing the existence of psychological problems or potential problems, and providing appropriate treatment. Psychometric tests are used infrequently, and the more common mode of evaluation is a structured interview presented in an unstructured manner. Components of the interview are:

1. *An initial statement that defines and explains the routine nature of the evaluation.* Parents and children are reassured that mental illness is not suspected and that normal individuals under stress may find the providing of information and support helpful.

2. *Subsequent questions regarding the child's school experience, outside interests, hobbies, and social and family relationships.*

3. *Inquiry into the child and family's previous stress history, especially prior experience with major illness or injury.* The family's specific experience with cancer is something that is evaluated along with their perception of the disease; do they regard a diagnosis of cancer as meaning imminent death, or do they harbor hopes for the future? Furthermore the congruence of these attitudes with the medical realities of each individual circumstance is important. Prior experience is particularly relevant here. The family, whose sole encounter with malignant disease was watching the slow, painful deterioration of a relative or friend whose cancer was resistant to treatment, may understandably enter the treatment setting with significant skepticism, if not outright hostility.

Communication to the family of the multiplicity of different types of cancers and treatments is important.

4. *Evaluation of communication styles within the family, those that influence the amount and quality of information the child is provided about his disease and its treatment, as well as those that have implications for the development of future relational problems.* Attempts are made to correct any early misconceptions and to provide the child with age-appropriate information. When a unified approach that encourages honesty is taken by medical and psychosocial staff, parents have been quite open to letting their children know the relevant facts about their illness. As opposed to being adamant about withholding information, most parents are either willing and eager to be open, or confused and uncertain about what and how to tell the child. When parental insistence upon withholding information (rarely) occurs, it is often reversed as treatment progresses, anxiety diminishes, and the unrealistic nature of this attitude becomes apparent. Psychological support and advice is essential throughout this process.

5. *Assessment of the child's response to hospitalization.* The normalcy of transitory reactive depression and anxiety during the immediate post-diagnostic period is explained to parents. Scrutiny is made of patterns of behavior that appear to approach chronicity. Responses of siblings, parents, and members of the extended family are also evaluated. Parents are advised to share in treatment-related behaviors and to encourage siblings to observe the treatment process in order to minimize feelings of isolation.

6. *Inquiry is made into the nature and quality of support systems available to the child.* Does an extended family exist? Are its members perceived as helpful or are there premorbid family conflicts that interfere with the supportive process? What role has religion played for the family? In cases where outside supports are few, there may be greater need for extended psychological support.

7. *Toward the latter part of the initial evaluation, the family's future expectations are explored.* Parents are advised to help the child return as fully as possible to premorbid behavior patterns when medically feasible. School reintegration is often begun at this point. Resumption of prior modes of child-rearing is encouraged. No attempt is made to dictate to parents how to raise their children but rather there is recognition that a multiplicity of satisfactory child-rearing styles exist and that efforts should be made to maintain these despite the child's illness.

8. Finally, *psychological treatment*, particularly hypnosis and relaxation training, is often given during the initial evaluative period. Procedural anxiety is a major problem for children with cancer, particularly those with leukemia, who undergo a large number of repeated bone marrow aspirations, and begins almost immediately after hospitalization (Kellerman et al., 1979). The above self-help modalities have proven useful for this.

The majority of children are not seen for extended treatment after initial evaluation. Structured follow-up is conducted for three weeks. Past this point informal contact is maintained during outpatient clinic visits. A significant minority of newly diagnosed children are seen for treatment, usually short term, for a variety of problems (Kellerman et al., 1979).

In addition to conducting routine evaluations, the psychologists receive problem consultations on previously diagnosed children and engage in an on-going program of clinical research.

Social Worker

The social worker provides services primarily to parents. Despite the program's emphasis upon a family-systems approach, there is a need for individual counseling of parents, particularly with regard to marital issues. While it has not been our experience that the diagnosis of pediatric cancer, per se, causes separation or divorce (Indeed, an examination of several hundred cases failed to reveal one instance of a happy marriage ending due to the child's illness.) in families where premorbid marital stress is high, the illness may serve as the proverbial back-breaking straw. In line with this, the social worker's activities include:

1. *Providing short-term marital counseling and individual supportive counseling for parents, particularly regarding stresses that arise out of the child's illness.* Long-term treatment is sometimes conducted but, more often, is referred to outside agencies or mental health professionals.

2. *Organizing and facilitating group therapy sessions for parents.* Mother's groups exist both within and outside of the hospital's boundaries. In addition, more recent efforts have concentrated upon organizing a father's group that takes place after working hours.

3. *Serving as the professional consultant to an ongoing Hematology-Oncology Parent Association.* This organization raises funds, furnishes toys and wigs for the children, publishes a monthly newsletter containing a disease-related information and runs a reference library of pamphlets, brochures, reprints, and books about childhood cancer.

4. *Acts as a liaison between parents and community service organizations.* Many groups, both governmental and private, offer financial aid, loan medical equipment, and provide help with transportation and child care. The social worker guides parents through what is often a morass of regulations and helps determine eligibility criteria for specific services. She also administers a private fund, raised by parents, that is used to help families experiencing sudden financial crisis.

5. *Provides postmortem counseling.* Those professionals working directly and primarily with the child stand a greater chance of losing contact with the family after the child's death than does the social worker, who works most intensively with the parents. Postmortem counseling is conducted contingent upon the parent's needs and may extend for several months after the death.

Social Work Assistant

The social work assistant's activities include, but are not limited to, those implied by her job title. She does assist the social worker, and maintains active involvement with parent groups and community service organizations. In addition, however, she is the primary psychosocial support for those families who speak only Spanish. This group, primarily Mexican-American, comprises approximately one fifth of our patient roster. The social work assistant is able to establish rapport with Spanish-speaking patients and families by virtue of sharing a common cultural and linguistic background. Her activities include:

1. *Serving as a translator for the medical staff, in the absence of hospital translators.*

2. Through experience in dealing with culture specific issues, she is able to provide unique, effective support. Families from rural Mexican backgrounds may enter the treatment setting with strong beliefs in a variety of faith-healing, spiritualistic, or folk-remedy approaches to medicine. No attempt is made to challenge or denigrate these attitudes and, on the contrary, respect is maintained for the wide range of opinions and beliefs that all families bring with them. The social work assistant does, however, seek to insure that such issues do not prevent the child from receiving optimal conventional medical care. The fact that her input is that of a professional who speaks from a familiar and trusted context lends it potency.

3. *When an exclusively Spanish-speaking child is seen for psychological treatment, the social work assistant often serves as a translator and cotherapist.* In cases where this is not practical, the child is referred to a Spanish-speaking psychologist or psychiatrist.

4. *Helps parents with disease-related communication.* Parents from Mexican-American backgrounds are often reluctant to tell the child anything about his illness. In lieu of receiving information in their language, their own grasp of pertinent details about the disease and its treatment may be deficient. Interestingly, communication abhors a vacuum, and it has been observed that when not offered psychosocial support, some Spanish-speaking parents have formed personal relationships with nonclinical hospital employees, most often custodial staff, and have relied upon the often distorted and inaccurate information they receive from well-meaning but uninformed new acquaintances.

One striking example is the case of an adolescent girl, about to be admitted to a laminar airflow room for chemotherapy, whose Spanish-speaking grandmother appeared on the ward extremely agitated. After talking with her, it was found that she had been discussing her granddaughter's treatment with a hospital housekeeper she had met on another floor. This woman had told her that, though she herself was not familiar with the laminar airflow unit, she had heard that children who entered it rarely left alive. Subsequent counseling, in

Spanish, allayed the grandmother's fears; the girl entered the unit, was treated for several weeks, and released in remission from her disease.

It is impossible to establish rules restricting parental contact with nonclinical staff. Furthermore, after leaving the hospital, both child and family are likely to come into contact with other individuals who offer them misinformation. Thus, the problem of distorted communication is not limited to the hospital setting and needs to be dealt with soon after diagnosis. Providing accurate information in a manner that maximizes its reception and explicitly encouraging questions at any point during treatment are especially useful in this regard. Needless to say, communication issues are not unique to Spanish-speaking patients and families. They run the risk, however, of being intensified due to the additional language barrier. Children and families who speak a foreign language other than Spanish pose special problems in that there is no assigned staff person who can communicate with them. In these cases, attempts are made to obtain competent translators, and religious institutions have been helpful in providing such individuals.

Psychosocial Case Conferences

The members of the Psychosocial Team meet twice weekly. The emphasis of one conference is upon clinical issues and that of the other is administrative. There is usually overlap, however, in the content of these meetings, depending upon the ever-changing clinical realities of any given time period. The order of priorities at the clinical conference is as follows:

1. *Discussion of newly diagnosed patients.* The nurse coordinator presents the psychosocial intake. Psychosocial consultations are often given to the psychologists at this point. A decision as to whether the parents are in need of social work support is made. Unique characteristics of the child and family that may either hamper or aid adjustment to the disease are discussed, as are special needs for supportive services and financial aid. A treatment plan is coordinated and recorded.

2. *Discussion of formerly diagnosed patients who are in crisis.* Typically, this group is made up of children whose disease status has recently taken a downward change. Thus, the special needs of the child who has entered a terminal stage are discussed, as are those of the child in relapse, or who is experiencing increased discomfort. In addition, patients whose family situation has been markedly altered, such as those whose parents are experiencing exacerbated marital problems or other elevated life stress, may be perceived as particularly psychosocially vulnerable and are also discussed.

3. *Presentation of illustrative case material.* Once newly diagnosed patients and those in crisis have been discussed, clinical case material with perceived educational value is presented. Thus, the psychologist who has recently treated a number of patients with similar problems — enuresis, nightmares, anxiety reaction — may describe treatment

modalities, problems, outcome, etc. Similarly, the social worker who has helped a parent resolve a personal conflict may describe the aspects of intervention that are seen as having been particularly effective. Group discussion is encouraged, with the aim of keeping the team abreast of the various clinical activities of its members and of stimulating prospective continuing education.

The administrative meeting is a forum for scheduling the various educational programs and lectures that the team participates in. These include seminars for house staff physicians, school teachers, and the clergy; and both individual and group presentations at scientific and professional conferences.

In addition, high priority is given to providing time for discussion of personal feelings that may arise both out of the inevitable interpersonal conflicts that are part of multidisciplinary care, and the emotional stress of working with children who are seriously ill. There are two approaches that the group uses in an effort to combat some of this inherent tension.

First, a system of peer support is offered so that the staff member who is feeling stressed can discuss this with other members of the team and receive empathy, sympathy, and suggestions. During periods when several children have died, or are dying, at close intervals this becomes particularly important, and there may be several team members who are feeling depressed, fatigued, and otherwise stressed.

Second, the group makes a concerned effort to engage in self-reward. There is a certain irony to the tendency among many health professionals to devote their careers to helping others while quite systematically ignoring their own needs. It has been our finding that martyrs do not make stable, effective clinicians, and that, quite the opposite, the professional who is happy with himself is best able to offer optimal clinical care. Along these lines, the team attempts, periodically, to leave the hospital setting for group lunches, and to get together for after-hours parties. This removes interpersonal relations within the team from a purely clinical context and rescues individual humanity from within the exclusive confines of the helping role.

THE NATURE OF PROBLEMS AND THEIR IMPLICATION FOR PROGRAM DEVELOPMENT

A recent empirical examination of over 100 children with cancer (Kellerman et al., 1979) revealed that the majority of problems for which psychological referral was sought fell into two categories:

1. Conditioned anxiety related to painful or frightful procedures: Chronic pain due to disease is not a major problem for children with cancer. This is in marked contrast with adult cancer patients and is related to the different diseases in these two groups. Acute pain and discomfort, however, usually induced by bone marrow aspirations, lumbar punctures, venipunctures, biopsies, and intramuscular and intrathecal injections of powerful chemotherapeutic agents, is quite

common; and over a third of patients studied were seen for anxiety reactions to this.

Such a reaction commonly takes the form of anticipatory distress prior to the procedure — restless sleep the night before an appointment for outpatient chemotherapy, anorexia, anticipatory nausea and vomiting; and of agitated, often uncooperative behavior during the procedure; followed by a period of emotional depression and listlessness.

2. Behavior problems: These include difficulties at school such as learning disabilities and school behavior problems, oppositional behavior at home, and increased friction between siblings.

Less common, but significant, was prolonged depression, most often related to initial diagnosis or to a downward change in the disease state. Other low-frequency problems included anorexia, enuresis, nightmares, tension headache, and aggressive tantrums. Psychosis was virtually nonexistent in this sample.

Initially, diagnosed children were more likely to present with procedure-related anxiety, and behavorial problems were more common in formerly diagnosed patients. There is some indication from further examination of the data that the period of one to three years postdiagnosis is when behavioral problems are most likely to emerge.

Such empirical examination of the types of problems encountered by children with cancer is important when planning support services. For example, major debilitating psychiatric disorders were not prevalent in this sample, and this casts doubts upon the efficacy of an intensive psychotherapy model in a pediatric oncology setting. On the other hand, the high incidence of conditioned anxiety and behavioral problems can direct those intending to set up psychosocial support programs to seek out professionals who have the requisite skills in methods effective for dealing with these problems. Such modalities include hypnosis and relaxation training, short-term family and individual psychotherapy, behavior therapy, hospital-specific play therapy, and school intervention.

Further research is needed to pinpoint periods of high risk for specific problems along the treatment continuum. Additionally, scientific evaluation of treatment outcome is essential in maximizing clinical effectiveness.

SUMMARY

To the extent that oncological treatment continues to advance and further increase the life expectancy of children with cancer, a concomitant increase in the complexity of disease-related psychosocial problems can be expected. As medical treatment modalities assume an increasingly aggressive and technologically sophisticated stance, treatment-related problems may simultaneously intensify.

The challenge to the health sciences is, and will continue to be, to keep pace with this dynamic system, to conduct systematic, objective research that casts light upon the nature of psychosocial problems and to develop and implement appropriate treatment that helps the child live better, as well as longer. It is the author's feeling that such a joint system of investigation and service can best be carried out within the context of a multidisciplinary, comprehensive psychosocial program functioning as a routine component of oncologic care.

REFERENCES

Ablin, A; Binger, C., Stein, R., Kushner, J., Zoger, S., and Mikkelson, C.: A conference with the family of a leukemic child. *Am J Dis Child, 122:*362, 1971.

Bandura, A., and Menlove, F. L.: Factors determining vicarious extinction of avoidance behavior through symbolic modeling. *J Pers Soc Psychol, 8:*99, 1968.

Cassell, S.: Effects of brief puppet therapy upon the emotional responses of children undergoing cardiac catheterization. *J Consult Psychol, 29:*1, 1965.

Crasilneck, H. B., and Hall, J. A.: Clinical hypnosis in problems of pain. *Am J Clin Hypn, 15:*161, 1973.

Cyphert, F. R.: Back to school for the child with cancer. *J Sch Health, 18:*215, 1973.

Drotar, D.: Death in the pediatric hospital: psychological consultation with medical and nursing staff. *J Clin Child Psychol, 4:*33, 1975.

Easson, W. M.: *The Dying Child: The Management of the Child or Adolescent Who Is Dying.* Springfield, Thomas, 1970.

Endler, N. S., and Magnusson, D. (Eds.): *Interactional Psychology and Personality.* New York, John Wiley & Sons, 1976.

Futterman, E., and Hoffman, I.: Shielding from awareness: an aspect of family adaptation to fatal illness in children. In: S. S. Cook (Ed.), *Children and Dying: An Exploration and Selective Bibliographies.* New York, Health Sciences Publishing, 1974.

Gardner, G. G.: Childhood, death and human dignity: Hypnosis for David. *Int J Clin Exp Hypn, 24:*122, 1976.

Greene, P.: The child with leukemia in the classroom. *Am J Nurs, 75:*86, 1975.

Heffron, W.; Bommelaere, K., and Masters, R.: Group discussions with parents of leukemic children. *Pediatrics, 52:*831, 1973.

Hoffman, I., and Futterman, E. H.: Coping with waiting: psychiatric intervention and study in the waiting room of a pediatric oncology clinic. *Comp Psychiatry, 12:*67, 1971.

Holmes, H. A., and Holmes, F. F.: After ten years, what are the handicaps and lifestyles of children treated for cancer. An examination of the present status of 124 survivors. *Clin Pediatr, 14:*819, 1975.

Humphrey, G. B., and Vore, D. A.: Psychology and the oncology team. *J Clin Child Psychol, 3:*27, 1974.

Janis, I.: *Psychological Stress.* New York, John Wiley & Sons, 1958.

Johnson, J. E., and Leventhal, H.: Effects of accurate expectations and behavioral instructions on reactions during a noxious medical examination. *J Person Soc Psychol, 29:*710, 1974.

Kagen-Goodheart, L.: Re-entry: Living with childhood cancer. *Am J Orthopsychiatry, 47:*651, 1977.

Kaplan, D. M.; Smith, A., and Grobstein, R.: School management of the seriously ill child. *J Sch Health, 19:*250, 1974.

Kastenbaum, R.: Death and development through the lifespan. In H. Feifel (Ed.), *New Meanings of Death.* New York, McGraw-Hill, 1977.

Katz, E. R.; Kellerman, J., Rigler, D., Williams, K. O., and Siegel, S. E.: School intervention with pediatric cancer patients. *J Pediatr Psychol, 2:*72, 1977.

Kellerman, J.; Katz, E. R., and Siegel, S. E.: Psychological problems of children with cancer. Unpublished manuscript, 1979.

Kellerman, J.; Rigler, D., Siegel, S. E., McCue, K., Pospisil, J., and Uno, R.: Psychological evaluation and management of pediatric oncology patients in protected environments. *Med Pediatr Oncol, 2:*353, 1976.

Koch, C. R.; Hermann, J., and Donaldson, M. H.: Supportive care of the child with cancer and his family. *Semin Oncol, 1:*81, 1974.

Koocher, G. P.: Childhood death and cognitive development. *Dev Psychol, 9:*369, 1973.

Koocher, G. P. (Ed.): Special issue on death and the child. *J Pediatr Psychol, 2,* 1977.

La Baw, W.; Holton, C., Tewell, K. L., and Eccles, D.: The use of self-hypnosis by children with cancer. *Am J Clin Hypn, 17:*233, 1975.

Lang, P. A., and Oppenheimer, J. R.: The influence of social work when parents are faced with the fatal illness of a child. *Soc Case, 49:*161, 1968.

Lansky, S. B., and Lowman, J. T.: Childhood malignancy: a comprehensive approach. *J Kans Med Soc,* 1947a.

Lansky, S. B.: Childhood leukemia. The child psychiatrist as a member of the oncology team. *J Am Acad Child Psychiatry, 13:*499, 1974b.

Lansky, S. B.; Lowman, J. T., Vats, S. T., and Gyulay, J.: School phobia in children with malignancies. *Am J Dis Child, 129:*42, 1975.

Lewis, S.: Considerations in setting up psychological consultation to a pediatric hematology-oncology team. *J Clin Child Psychol, 7:*21, 1978.

Martinson, I. M.: *Home care for the dying child: professional and family perspectives.* New York, Appleton-Century-Crofts, 1976.

Mauer, A.: Maturation of concepts of death. *Br J Med Psychol, 39:*35, 1966.

Melamed, B. G., and Siegel, L. J.: Reduction of anxiety in children facing hospitalization and surgery by use of filmed modeling. *J Consult Clin Psychol, 43:*511, 1975.

Moore, D. C.; Halton, C. P., and Marten, G. W.: Psychological problems in the management of adolescents with malignancy. *Clin Pediatr, 8:*464, 1969.

Nagy, M.: The child's theories concerning death. *J Gen Psychol, 73:*3, 1948.

Natterson, J. M., and Knudson, A. G.: Observations concerning fear of death in fatally ill children and their mothers. *Psychosom Med, 22:*456, 1960.

Nolfi, M.: Families in grief: the question of casework intervention. *Soc Wk, 12:*40, 1967.

Oswin, M.: The role of education in helping the child with a potentially fatal disease. In L. Burton (Ed.): *Care of the Child Facing Death.* London, Routledge & Kegan Paul, 1974.

Parodi, A. B.: Psychological aspects in care of the leukemic child. *Hematol, 62:*75, 1977.

Peebles, J. J., and O'Malley, F.: Problems in mental health consultation facing the professional in training. *J Clin Child Psychol, 7:*68, 1978.

Shipley, R. H.; Butt, J. H., Horwitz, B., and Farbry, J. E.: Preparation for a stressful medical procedure: effect of amount of stimulus preexposure and coping style. *J Consult Clin Psychol, 46:*499, 1978.

Spinetta, J. J.; Rigler, D., and Karon, M.: Anxiety in the dying child. *Pediatrics, 52:*841, 1973.

Spinetta, J. J.: The dying child's awareness of death: A review. *Psychol Bull, 81:*256, 1974a.

Spinetta, J. J.; Rigler, D., and Karon, M.: Personal space as a measure of the dying child's sense of isolation. *J Consult Clin Psychol, 42:*751, 1974b.

Spinetta, J. J., and Maloney, L.: Death anxiety in the outpatient leukemic child. *Pediatrics, 56:*1035, 1975.

Spinetta, J. J.: Adjustment in children with cancer. *J Pediatr Psychol, 2:*49, 1977.

Tavormina, J. B.; Kastner, L. S., Slater, P. M., and Watt, S. L.: Chronically ill children: A psychologically and emotionally deviant population? *J Abnorm Child Psychol, 4:*99, 1976.
Travis, G.: *Chronic Illness in Children.* Stanford, California, Stanford University, 1976.
Vernon, D. T. A., and Bailey, W. C.: The use of motion pictures in the psychological preparation of children for induction of anesthesia. *Anesthesiol, 40:*68, 1974.

Chapter Eleven

HYPNOSIS FOR SYMPTOM AMELIORATION

JERRY DASH

INTRODUCTION

Hypnosis was first used with children in 1777, when Anton Mesmer, friend of Haydn and Mozart, and a doctor of medicine, cured a case of hysterical blindness in a young pianist. Since that time, the acceptance of hypnosis has been cyclical in nature, falling in and out of favor with health professionals. (Freud's abandonment of hypnosis contributed to the decline in its use, and hypnosis did not enjoy widespread application again until World War II, when rapid treatment of battle neuroses became necessary.) The recrudescence of hypnosis in the treatment of children may be credited to the British psychiatrist Gordon Ambrose (1961) who used the technique successfully in problems of delinquency, tics, nailbiting, stammering, and other symptoms of anxiety.

Since Ambrose, hypnosis has been used for a variety of psychological and medical problems in children, including severe burns (Bernstein, 1962; LaBaw, 1973), asthma (La Scola, 1968), drug abuse (Bauman, 1970), enuresis (Olness, 1975), psychogenic pain and hysterical blindness (Sarles, 1975), warts (Clawson, 1975), and school phobia (Lawler, 1976). Hypnosis is also used as an adjunct to psychotherapy with children (Ambrose, 1968; Gardner, 1974; Kroger, 1977), and is being used as a pain control measure in children and adolescents with sickle cell anemia (Zeltzer, Dash and Holland, 1979).

Children undoubtedly make the best hypnotic subjects because of their trust, vivid imaginations, and the ease with which they intertwine fantasy and reality. Erickson (1958) has pointed out other factors that make children good hypnotic subjects, including their hunger for new experiences, openness to new learning, willingness to receive ideas, and enjoyment in responding to them. The limited experiential background of children is not cluttered with myths and misconceptions about hypnosis, so that "preinduction talks" are usually brief or unnecessary with children.

Gardner (1974) has developed a theory that helps explain the ready hypnotizability of children. Cognitively, the concrete thinking and limited reality-testing of children facilitate their acceptance of appropriately worded suggestions. On the emotional level, the child's willingness to experience regressive states and his ability to move

215

quickly from one intense feeling state to another, contribute to his increased hypnotizability. On the interpersonal level, children are usually more ready than adults to enter into a relationship of trust and closeness, and more often perceive the offer of help as assisting rather than interfering with their quest for mastery and autonomy. Of equal importance, Gardner notes, is that the child who moves from the waking state into hypnosis does not have so far to go as the adult, whose waking behavior is easily contrasted with hypnotic behavior. (Actually, children enter hypnotic states several times each day through activities such as daydreaming, watching television, and fantasy play.)

The studies of London (1965), London and Cooper (1969) and Morgan and Hilgard (1973) are frequently cited to show that children between the ages of five and fourteen make the best hypnotic subjects. These studies used the Children's Hypnotic Susceptibility Scale (London, 1963), which has twenty-two items that employ verbal inductions and standardized instructions and challenges and is therefore probably inappropriate with younger children. In fact, hypnotic approaches have been successfully used with preschool children and even infants (Crasilneck and Hall, 1973; Cullen, 1958; Jacobs, 1962; La Scola, note 1); and the present author has found older adolescents to be excellent hypnotic subjects. There appears to be no sex difference in hypnotic susceptibility in children (Cooper, 1966).

In spite of the apparent ease and utility of hypnosis with children, Gardner (1976a), in a survey of 229 children's health professionals, found that her sample had positive attitudes towards hypnosis, but little knowledge of its specific advantages and applications. Such a situation merely contributes to hypnosis being used as a technique of "last resort." This chapter will review the use of hypnosis with adult and pediatric cancer patients, discuss theoretical and practical considerations in the uses of hypnosis, and report on representative cases from among the fifty cancer patients with whom the author has worked over the past three years. In so doing, it is the author's hope that more pediatric cancer centers will implement hypnosis as adjunctive treatment and that hypnosis will come to be used as a first resort in reducing the distresses of childhood malignancy.

BACKGROUND

Hypnosis with Adult Cancer Patients

At the present time, any review of the existing literature on the uses of hypnosis with cancer patients is by necessity brief. This is somewhat surprising considering the excellent results when employed. The myths and misconceptions concerning hypnosis that have prevented its wider acceptance will be discussed later in this chapter.

Probably the earliest reference to be found concerns the case of a patient with stomach cancer treated by Taplin and cited in a book by Miller (1912). The patient responded with improved sleep, increased appetite, and diminished pain. Two other isolated cases are those of

Hollander (1932) who helped a female patient achieve relief of pain from uterine cancer, and Rosen (1951) who used hypnosis for pain control in a patient with bone metastases from breast cancer. The best known of the early studies is the one by Butler published in 1954. He reported favorable results on the use of hypnosis in conjunction with pain medication in twelve cases of gynecologic cancer. Butler made a plea for more extensive efforts to understand hypnosis and its physiological effects.

Erickson (1959) presented three case reports in which he used a variety of hypnotic techniques, teaching his subjects the use of analgesia, anesthesia, positive and negative hallucinations, body disorientation and dissociation, amnesia for previous pain experiences, and time distortion. These techniques were taught in one prolonged hypnotic session. He cited the main advantage of hypnosis over pain-relieving medications: "In terminal painful illness, sedatives, analgesics and narcotics are employed that may deprive the patient of the privilege of knowing that he is alive and of enjoying what pleasures yet remain; also, they deprive his relatives of adequate contact with the patient."

In an addendum to Erickson's article, Schon (1960) relates his experiences using hypnosis with another terminal case. Other favorable reports have come from Lea, Ware, and Monroe (1960) and from Cangello (1961), who found decreased use of narcotics in 59 percent of his patients (N = 22).

More has been written on the uses of hypnosis with adult cancer patients by Paul Saccerdote than by any other author. In numerous papers (Saccerdote, 1965, 1966a, 1966b, 1968a, 1970) he has developed a theory and practice of pain control from twenty-five years experience with patients suffering many forms of protracted painful illness. In addition to the techniques used by Erickson, Saccerdote has pioneered the use of induced dreams and sensory hypnoplasty (the latter of which consists of the patient molding an hallucinated piece of clay, representing the afflicted body area, into a pleasant and pain-free work of art.) The reader is referred to the above papers and others in the present reference list (Saccerdote, 1962, 1967, 1968b) for a detailed description of Saccerdote's work. The present author has incorporated many of Saccerdote's ideas into his work with children and finds them equally applicable and effective. These will be described in later sections.

Hypnosis with Pediatric Cancer Patients

Reports on the uses of hypnosis with pediatric cancer patients appear to be limited to three published articles. Crasilneck and Hall (1973) describe the case of a four-year-old child with inoperable brain cancer who was in continual pain, refused to eat, cried constantly, and demanded that his mother remain with him most of the time. It was necessary that he be given narcotics several times daily for his pain. To the authors' knowledge, the child had no idea of the concept of hypnosis. They produced a state of somnambulism in the patient by having him stare at a cigarette lighter flame for fifteen minutes. Suggestions were given that he would have less pain, eat better, sleep well, and enjoy television and magazines. All of the suggestions were realized, and it was possible to reduce narcotic injections from five or six daily to a minimal amount of Demerol®.

La Baw, Holton, Tewell, and Eccles (1975) have reported on the results of hypnosis and self-hypnosis with twenty-seven children ranging in age from four to twenty years old. Over a period of two years their patients were trained in group self-hypnosis sessions. A registered nurse and a clinical social worker performed a large part of the training. The induction technique employed was a progressive body relaxation method followed by guided imagery of restful scenes common to children's experiences, such as a tranquil mountain view. Obtained with the trance state were more rest, easier and longer sleep, more adequate food or fluid intake and retention, and greater tolerance for and manageability during diagnostic and therapeutic procedures. Anxiety, depression, and anticipatory vomiting prior to treatment were also diminished.

Gardner (1976a) has published a detailed clinical report on hypnotherapy used with other treatment modalities to help a terminally ill child and his family cope effectively with problems encountered as a result of the illness. She points out that the induction and treatment were selected to enhance the child's sense of control and mastery at a time when the disease itself was out of control. Her approach was geared to the child's need to feel that hypnosis was not something done to him by another powerful person, but a state he could achieve for himself after proper training.

HYPNOSIS FOR PAIN CONTROL:
THEORETICAL CONSIDERATIONS

The effectiveness of hypnosis for pain control is easily demonstrated at the bedside. The reality of hypnotic analgesia and anesthesia has been well established, from the more than three hundred major surgeries performed by Esdaile in India in the nineteenth century, in which the only anesthetic used was hypnosis, to the temporal lobectomies performed under hypnosis reported by Crasilneck and Hall (1973).

At the experimental level, as Saccerdote (1970) has noted, the elimination of uncontrollable variables often produces an artificial pain and artificial hypnosis. Hilgard (1969) states that "Clinicians are at the present time far ahead of our laboratories in the hypnotic reduction of pain." Much of the difficulty with the laboratory studies stems from incomplete agreement over how to define, measure, and interpret pain, and how to correlate it with social, personality, and cultural variables. For an excellent and thorough review of the pain literature, the reader is referred to the recent article by Weisenberg (1977).

Defining Hypnosis

Although ambiguities in the definition and measurement of pain do exist, it is nonetheless important to clarify what hypnosis is, and attempt to explain its contribution to pain reduction. Erickson (1959) has defined hypnosis and the rationale for its use with cancer patients:

> Essentially, hypnosis is a state of intensified attention and receptiveness and an increased responsiveness to an idea or set of ideas. There is nothing magical or mystical about it . . . In medicine, as well as in denistry, this normal everyday capacity for intensely directed attention can be employed to concentrate a patient's attentiveness and responsiveness in an altered fashion so that he benefits through a new and learned responsiveness to selected stimuli. This constitutes the use of hypnosis in painful terminal illness.

Hilgard (1973) has also approached hypnosis on the basis of different systems of cognitive functioning and levels of consciousness. Hypnosis produces an altered state of consciousness. The pain stimulus is able to reach one level of consciousness but is blocked from the more immediate level of awareness. That is, the person does perceive the pain stimulus at some lower level. However, he is capable of keeping it from coming to the level of awareness that makes it distressing.

NEUROCHEMICAL ASPECTS. In the author's experience, the hypnotized individual who is taught to control pain often reports in the same manner as the patient medicated with Demerol® or morphine, i.e. "I know the pain is there, but it doesn't bother me so much." In this regard, Beecher (1957) has noted that morphine (and all related narcotics, synthetic or not), although assumed to act mostly by changing the central perception of pain, actually, to a great extent, modifies the psychic reaction to pain. Beecher's opinion is especially interesting in light of the recent identification of morphine receptor sites and the existence in the body of two endogenous pentapeptides with opiate agonist action (Hughes, Smith, Kosterlitz, Fothergill, Morgan and Morris, 1975; Simon, Hiller and Edelman, 1975). Saccerdote (note 2) currently instructs hypnotized pain patients to increase the "brewing" of these endorphins and enkaphalins in their own brain for self-produced, nonaddictive pain control.

NEUROPHYSIOLOGICAL ASPECTS. It is also possible to approach the modifications obtainable by hypnosis from a neurophysiological standpoint. Saccerdote (1970) has noted that the presence or absence of pain is an expression of the balance between sensory (peripheral) and central (centrifugal) inputs occurring at the synaptic stations. Centrifugal inputs are activated not only by what occurs at the periphery, but also by psychological activities: memories of past experiences, attention, emotions, etc. These psychological activities are, of course, directly modifiable by hypnotic suggestions for amnesia, time distortion, and dissociation.

BEHAVIORAL ASPECTS. Behavioral principles afford another frame of reference for understanding the effects of hypnosis. In one of Pavlov's (1928) classical experiments, dogs exposed to electric shocks or other painful stimuli, consistently followed by presentation of food, developed conditioned responses indicating expectation of food, without any evidence of pain, when subjected to the noxious stimuli alone. It is possible to conclude that the dogs had either learned to prevent the transmission or the perception of pain or that the noxious stimuli, through conditioned learning, had been modified into a pleasant experience. Saccerdote (1970), in commenting on these studies, notes that Pavlov's experiments were conducted with dogs in a state of almost complete sensory isolation. In his opinion, they were in a psychophysiological state similar, if not identical, to hypnosis. It is therefore acceptable that humans, too, can be trained, during one or more hypnotic sessions, either to alter conduction, or to utilize different pathways (associations) so that noxious stimuli either are not perceived, or else are experienced as a different, preferably pleasant, subjective sensation. This is especially plausible in light of the general agreement that in hypnosis, the subject's critical faculties are reduced and his susceptibility to suggestion is heightened. Thus, as Kroger (1977) states, this situation causes "unreality to be interpreted as reality." It should be apparent that this line of reasoning coincides with Erickson's definition of hypnosis cited above.

Wolpe (1969) has suggested that relaxation is antagonistic to the elicitation of anxiety. Most clinicians can attest to the role of anxiety in hyperesthesia to medical procedures. It would follow, therefore, that relaxation should increase pain tolerance. Thompson (1977) saw great benefits in reducing pain reactions by relaxing her patients, and produced a film showing the use of hypnosis in dermabrasion surgery. Case reports presented below will help illustrate that relaxation, being incompatible with anxiety, significantly reduces not only pain reaction, but also nausea, anticipatory vomiting and gagging in cancer patients.

PLACEBO AND RAPPORT. Finally, the role of rapport and placebo effects in hypnosis should not be overlooked. In many ways, hypnosis may be the most powerful of placebos. The author is in no way discouraged by this, and in fact, makes a point of capitalizing on this factor. Frequently, the hypnotherapist is the only staff person who causes the patient no pain. Simple procedures such as removing an adhesive bandage can elicit pain and fear reactions in the sensitive or anxious patient. The patient soon realizes that the hypnotherapist's sole purpose is to minimize discomfort. Rapport, without which hypnosis probably cannot occur, is frequently established as a result of this factor alone.

As Cullen (1958), an anesthesiologist, has observed, "If the child has confidence in the hypnotherapist and the latter, in turn, has confidence in his ability to hypnotize or relax the patient, the rest will follow." Whatever the neurophysiological, neurochemical, psychodynamic, or behavioral reasons for the effectiveness of hypnosis, its efficacy is rooted in the motivation and expectation of the patient, and in the confidence and intuitiveness of the hypnotist. In pediatric hypnotherapy in particular, the hypnotherapist must be able to meet the child on his own level, without talking down to the young patient. He must also be willing to tolerate regressive and playful states in himself. The imaginative processes of hypnotist and subject are major catalysts in producing the perceptual state of hypnosis.

PRACTICAL CONSIDERATIONS

Not only is patient rapport and cooperation an essential component of successful hypnotherapy, but staff and parental cooperation must be obtained as well. In addition, it is important to remove the myths and misconceptions that will inevitably be held by patients, parents, and staff members. Some of the more commonly held *misconceptions about hypnosis* are the following:

1. *Loss of control* (including fear of not being dehypnotized, and fear of revealing secrets about oneself). This mistaken notion stems from the Svengali-like mystique that frequently is attributed to hypnosis even by enlightened individuals. Supposedly, the subject is under the control of the hypnotist, who shapes and molds his thoughts and behaviors. It should be explained that all hypnosis is self-hypnosis, that is, a person goes into hypnosis because he wants to and can come out of hypnosis when he wants to. The hypnotist is only a guide who teaches the subject how to enter the hypnotic state. Also, the person in hypnosis is not asleep or unconscious (numerous physiochemical, brain wave and blood pressure studies show that hypnosis more closely resembles the waking state than sleep). The subject hears everything that goes on, and will not say or do anything he does not wish to. The person in hypnosis is actually hyperalert and concentrated in his attentiveness. A useful analogy is to the music-lover at a concert who listens to the music with his eyes closed. He looks like he is asleep, but is probably paying closer attention to the music than one whose eyes are open and finds his attention wandering to the interior design of the auditorium or to the clothes and hairdo of the person in front of him. The author does not use the word "sleep" in his inductions or deepening techniques. The word may have anxiety-arousing properties for some children; furthermore, we do not wish the subject to fall asleep.

2. *Weakmindedness.* Susceptibility to hypnosis is held by many people to indicate some defect in character or intelligence. In fact, intelligent individuals with good imaginations make the best hypnotic subjects. This remark, by inference, also tends to increase motivation, as most people like to regard themselves as being of at least average intelligence.

3. *Hypnosis is dangerous.* Anything that has a prosocial use can be

put to antisocial uses: syringes, drugs, etc. The fact that something can be misused is no argument for its disuse. It is conceivable that an unscrupulous hypnotist, by producing a total amnesia and establishing a valid motive, could get an individual, already predisposed, to commit an antisocial act. Naturally, such circumstances do not exist in a doctor-patient relationship.

Patient Preparation

As mentioned earlier, preinduction talks with children are usually brief or unnecessary, because children, as a rule, have not built up mistaken (or any, for that matter) notions about hypnosis. It is usually sufficient to ask the child what he knows or has heard about hypnosis. In most instances, children will have seen a television or movie dramatization of hypnosis. They need to be told that, "Lots of times things are exaggerated on TV. You know, police shows and doctor shows are not always very true to life. In the hospital, we only use hypnosis for important things like helping children feel better. I'm not going to make you do anything silly like quack like a duck." (Occasionally, of course, a particular child may want to be made to quack like a duck, in which case, you go along with the playfulness for a time before getting down to serious business.)

Parent Preparation

It is the author's opinion that hypnosis should not be attempted if parents object to its use — the possibilities for undermining treatment are too great in such cases. This is the rare exception, however, as most parents are only too eager to support efforts at relieving their child's discomfort. What's more, parents can and should be actively used to extend and reinforce the hypnosis by having them periodically encourage the child to practice his new skills. This should be done in a careful and nonintrusive manner and is probably unnecessary and perhaps inadvisable with adolescents. If acceptable to the child, it is often a good idea to have the parents observe one or more hypnotic sessions.

Staff Preparation and Participation

In general, it is helpful to give as many presentations as possible (at ward rounds, in-service training seminars, etc.) on the uses of hypnosis with children. The more commonly held misconceptions may be gone over, followed by case examples and perhaps demonstrations with one or more patients.

On the wards, medical personnel involved with the child need to be informed and kept advised of the patient's use of self-hypnosis. The first hypnotic session should be detailed in the patient's chart, with instructions to the staff, for example: "Prior to procedures, please allow patient two to three minutes to go into self-hypnosis. You may assist in deepening the hypnosis by placing your hand gently on the patient's right shoulder after he has relaxed himself, and reminding him to drift even deeper into the hypnosis." The patient is also instructed to ask the doctor or nurse or blood drawing team to give him a couple of minutes to go into self-hypnosis before they start their procedures. This assures that the hypnotherapist need not be present for all procedures.

In sum, prior to conducting any hypnosis, it is imperative to remove any misconceptions that may be held by patients, parents, or staff. Most of these will stem from demonstrations of stage hypnosis or dramatizations seen on television or in movies. Because the hypnotherapy can be undermined by opponents of its use, it is essential to secure the cooperation of all those concerned in the child's care and treatment.

SPECIFIC TECHNIQUES

A frequent objection to the use of hypnosis is that it is time consuming. This is simply untrue. The following verbalization, which is sufficient to produce a medium to deep trance state in most children, takes but a few minutes:

Now, I am going to teach you a very easy and interesting way to control your discomfort. I'd like you to look at my watch, and keep looking at it as I move it slowly up above your eyes. As I move it away, just take a nice deep breath, and hold it. Now as the watch moves down, keep looking at it, and let your breath out slowly. When you can't see my watch any more, just close your eyes, and keep them closed until I ask you to open them again. Now, take three more nice deep breaths, and let yourself get more relaxed with each breath. In a moment, I'm going to touch you on the shoulder, and when you feel my hand touch your shoulder, just let all of your muscles go real loose and floppy, just like cooked spaghetti. That's very good. Now I'm going to ask you to use your imagination, and to see yourself in your imagination standing at the top of a flight of stairs, the kind you'd find in an old hotel. Very wide and sturdy steps, with a sturdy handrail going down along the side that you can hold on to as you walk down these steps. And you can see deep, thick carpeting covering the steps all the way down. There are fifteen steps here, and I'm going to be counting backwards from fifteen down to one. With each number that you hear, take another step down, and with each step down, get more and more relaxed. Alright, fifteen . . . fourteen . . . etc.

Now at the bottom of these stairs is a very comfortable easy chair. Just see yourself walking over to the chair, and getting real nice and comfortable as you relax completely into the chair. Now in front of you you can see the television set that you watch at home. Is it color or black and white? (child answers). Does it come on right away, or do you have to wait for it to warm up? (child answers). I'm going to count to three, and on three, the set will light up, and you'll see your favorite television show, and you'll see the whole show from start to finish. Alright, one . . . two . . . three. Now the set's on, the screen lights up, there's a commercial, and now, your favorite show. (Allow about thirty seconds). Alright, another commercial now, and maybe you'd like to tell me what show you just saw?

This verbalization does not make use of any of the so-called "susceptibility tests" or challenges, which are really unnecessary with children. It begins with the notion that the child is going to be taught something, and this notion of a "teacher-student" relationship ought to be employed throughout the hypnotherapy. It fits in nicely to the child's need for mastery. Also, the word "pain" is avoided, and substitutes such as "discomfort" are used instead. For the sensitive or anxious patient, the word "pain" can elicit a pain reaction. Once a suitable level of relaxation is achieved, any of the following techniques may be employed for specific problems.

"Favorite Place" Technique

The child is instructed to see himself getting up out of the chair in which he sat to view his favorite show. In front of him he can see a very large and beautiful wooden door. When he pushes through this door, he'll find himself in a very favorite place of his, a place he has visited on a vacation or with friends, in which he feels very relaxed and happy. Preferably, a place he was at before he ever got sick, and before he ever was worried about doctors, shots, spinal taps, bone marrows, etc. This is a very simple and effective way of achieving age regression with children. In the author's experience, even children who have had to be amputated because of osteogenic sarcoma will readily and without anxiety recall a time and place when they were very active and happy prior to their amputation. After the child has clearly visualized this favorite place, he is instructed that he can return to this time and place whenever he wants to, merely by closing his eyes, taking three deep breaths, seeing himself push through the door, and he will once again be extremely relaxed and comfortable. It is possible to condition the child to do this at the first sign of nausea, or prior to any procedure, so that these unpleasant experiences become the cue for relaxation.

Anesthesia and Analgesia

When the child is in hypnosis, it is a simple matter to teach him to achieve numbness in his hand which he can then transfer to any part of his body. Numbness can be achieved by having the child imagine he has had his hand in a bucket of ice water; or that he had been sitting on it for a long time; or that he has pulled a thick leather glove over his hand, making his hand feel numb, heavy, and woodenlike. He can then achieve the same numbness in his arm or back by simply placing his numb hand elsewhere on his body and "rubbing it all into the spot where you're going to get your shot."

Using the simile of electric wiring, the child is presented with a simplified version of his nervous system, and told that he can switch on and off circuits in different parts of his body. For example, if an intravenous injection is to be started in the wrist area, the child is asked to visualize the nerve in his arm, and to see a switch that controls the electricity in this arm located just above the area where the needle will be inserted. He can see a wall switch, or a dimmer switch, and when the switch is on, he can see the nerve "lit up" with electricity. Most children will describe the nerve as a "piece of silver wire" or as a "red tube" (similar to a vein). The child is then told to turn the switch to "off," to see the nerve (or "wire" or "tube") grow dim, and then to notice that the area beneath the switch is numb.

Another excellent method for scientifically-minded children is the "light bulb" technique described by La Scola (1968). In this method, the brain is described as a control panel with rows of switches above which are different colored light bulbs, each of which controls feelings in different parts of the body. By turning off the switch beneath a certain bulb, and seeing that bulb grow dim, the feelings in that part of the body disappear.

Posthypnotic Suggestions

A posthypnotic suggestion is simply an idea suggested to the subject that is to be carried out after the hypnosis is terminated. In this regard, each patient is given a suggestion to practice self-hypnosis, and to be sure to ask the nurse or doctor for a couple of minutes to go into self-hypnosis before starting the procedure. The child is to go into hypnosis by the method taught in his session with the hypnotherapist. In the author's experience, most children go on to develop their own methods of entering, deepening, and terminating hypnosis. The simplest method of terminating hypnosis is to count from A to E, and on "E" the eyes open, and the child comes all the way out of the hypnosis, feeling awake, alert, clear-headed, refreshed, and relaxed. Many children profit from their skills in self-hypnosis by using it not just for medical procedures but for improvement in other areas such as study habits, athletics, self-confidence, etc.

Dissociation

Certain chemotherapeutic agents can cause burning sensations during intravenous administration severe enough to go unameliorated by techniques of hypnotic anesthesia. In such cases, it is possible to suggest the development of dissociative phenoma in various body parts. A hand or an entire upper extremity can be induced into catalepsy, and from then into a totally dissociated state by suggesting that the limb has a mind of its own and a life of its own, and that it will respond to suggestions from the hypnotist without any need for the patient to consciously attend to what the hypnotist is saying. Erickson (note 3) frequently employs a technique of *total dissociation,* in which the hypnotized person is instructed to come out of hypnosis from the neck up, leaving his body in a trance state. The author has used this method successfully for pain reduction in patients recuperating from exploratory laparotomies.

CASE REPORTS

The case reports that follow will illustrate some practical applications of the aforementioned techniques. Seldom will one induction or treatment method be used exclusively with a child. Typically, a patient will be taught a variety of inductions and deepening techniques and will be encouraged to change his "favorite place" visualization from time to time.

Case One

E. W. was a seven-year-old child diagnosed with acute undifferentiated leukemia who was first seen after being admitted for terminal care. In spite of twenty-five mg dosages of Thorazine® every four hours, he was vomiting up to thirty-five times each day. This was much greater than to be expected as a side effect from the chemotherapy. His mother was unwittingly maintaining and reinforcing the vomiting by leaping to his side with a basin each time he complained of nausea, and stroking him tenderly at each emesis. In hypnosis, the patient was told that he could control his nausea by closing his eyes, taking three deep breaths, placing his hand on his tummy, and the nausea would disappear. The mother was asked to respond to her son's nausea in a more restrained manner, to avoid tactile reinforcement, and instead to reinforce him verbally only after the nausea had subsided.

After the first hypnotic session, the vomiting recurred only three times in eighteen hours. At this point, it was agreed that Thorazine would be administered only at the mother's request. Three more hypnotic sessions were conducted over the next seven days. For the remainder of the child's care, antiemetics were used no more than twice a day, and vomiting occurred from zero to three times on any given day.

Case Two

M. G. is a very active and athletic eleven-year-old lymphoma patient whose intern requested hypnosis after this patient punched him in the jaw when told he was scheduled for yet another spinal tap. Prior to the introduction of hypnosis, the patient was medicated with a combination of Demerol, Phenergan®, and Thorazine to sedate him for procedures. The DPT had only a paradoxical effect, however, as the patient felt a great deal of discomfort during the procedure and only after the needle was removed would he fall into a narcotized sleep for six to eight hours.

This child was an excellent hypnotic subject who entered a somnambulistic trance state very quickly. He was hypnotized in his room during two daily sessions and became convinced that he could use hypnosis for helping him with procedures. Hypnosis was induced a third time in the treatment room. The patient produced anesthesia in his hand, which he then assiduously rubbed into the lumbar region of his spine. Only a local anesthetic was used. It was suggested to the patient that he would sleep deeply for ten minutes and wake up feeling fine all over. Ten minutes after the spinal tap he was on his feet enjoying unrestricted freedom of movement.

Case Three

M. H. is a thirteen-year-old female patient with Stage II Hodgkin's disease. She was eager to be "put to sleep" to help her overcome a longstanding problem of gagging on pills. This is a fairly common problem in pediatric patients. It is usually aggravated by well-intentioned parents who, out of understandable frustration, use heavy-handed methods to get their children to swallow needed medications. In hypnosis, after watching her favorite television show, this patient was told that she would "see a special documentary show on the screen. This would be about a young girl who learns a very easy way to take medicine." The documentary used close-up cameras and zoom lenses to "show everyone how this girl is able to relax all her throat muscles so that the pills tumble past her tongue and on down into her tummy."

She awoke smiling and a little hesitant about sharing the source of her pleasure. Finally, she said that she really didn't like watching news programs. Instead, she watched a musical variety show in which she was the star. She saw herself dancing around the stage, laughing, and letting her mouth and throat open wide each time she would sing. Naturally, the girl was commended for her creativity and resourcefulness. She went on to use this visualization successfully for subsequent ingestions of medication.

Case Four

Another example of creativity and imaginativeness comes from a thirteen-year-old girl with Ewing's sarcoma. A. H. was seen originally because she had become very withdrawn and depressed and suffered a great deal of nausea and vomiting during chemotherapy. She grudgingly conceded to try hypnosis and surprised herself and others with her trance capabilities. Her favorite place was a farm in Iowa where, prior to being diagnosed, she had enjoyed a large family picnic. She returned to this scene at least a dozen times in hypnotic sessions. Each time she recalled more and more details of what took place there. She remembered the colors of the frisbees she played with, counted the fruits that were eaten, and described the surrounding countryside in the minutest detail. In later sessions, she revealed various forms of mischief she had entered into with her cousins. She delighted in describing the time she and her playmates set up ears of corn on the highway and then hid in the cornfields to watch passing cars smash the corn into the pavement.

This patient was taught to anesthetize her arm by imagining it submerged in a bucket of ice water. She wanted to learn another technique, so she was taught to visualize a long leather glove being pulled up over her arm. She used self-hypnosis for several administrations of intravenous medication during which she was unaware that the needle had even been inserted. She said that to produce this state she combined the image of the glove with that of the ice water. When asked if dunking the glove in the ice water did not ruin the leather, she replied, "Of course not!" This child's mood improved greatly. She returned to school for a while and resumed activities such as cheerleading and bicycle riding.

SUMMARY

Hypnosis is a state of relaxation and concentrated attention in which critical faculties are reduced so that susceptibility and receptiveness to ideas is greatly enhanced. Children make the best hypnotic subjects because of their trust, vivid imaginations, and hunger for new experiences. Establishing the hypnotherapy as a teacher-student relationship coincides nicely with the child's need for mastery. Hypnosis thus becomes demystified, and takes on the character of a new skill which, like other skills, becomes easier with practice.

Commonly held myths and misconceptions about hypnosis need to be removed prior to conducting any hypnosis. Most of these stem from stage hypnosis or television and movie dramatizations and are more common among staff and parents than among children. Staff and parent cooperation must be obtained if treatment is to be successful. Parents should be allowed to observe one or more hypnotic sessions. Staff members need to be informed of its potential uses at ward rounds, in-service training seminars, etc.

In this regard, the work of Karen Olness (1977) at Minneapolis Children's Health Center is extremely noteworthy. During eighteen months of in-service training, the following groups were taught the uses of hypnosis and self-hypnosis: registered nurses; residents; medical students; administrative, secretarial, and housekeeping staff; full time and voluntary physician staff. The increased awareness of the usefulness of hypnosis led to an increase both in the personal use of self-hypnosis by hospital staff and in the use of hypnosis among community physicians. Olness found that phraseology used with patients was favorably altered. For example, there was less use of the phrase, "this is going to hurt." Substituted was the phrase, "would it be all right with you if the hurt doesn't bother you?" Familiarity with hypnosis tends to increase one's sensitivity to the role of suggestion in the communication of words and ideas.

Efforts such as those at the Children's Hospital and Health Center of San Diego, the University of Kansas Medical Center, and Childrens Hospital National Medical Center in Washington, D.C., are to be commended to other pediatric centers as well. There, the author provided training to the hematologist-oncologists themselves, as well as to the psychologists, nurses, and social workers, in the uses of hypnosis. It is a great advantage to have those who actually perform the bone marrow aspirations, spinal taps, and other procedures to be trained in hypnotic techniques and sensitized to their communications to their patients.

At Childrens Hospital of Los Angeles, the success of hypnosis with cancer patients has encouraged other physicians and psychologists to develop skills in hypnotherapy. Hypnosis is thus being increasingly used with patients in other divisions. Additionally, a major research grant, funded by the American Cancer Society, is currently in progress for teaching the uses of self-hypnosis and biofeedback to adolescent cancer patients. In the near future, we hope to teach self-hypnosis routinely to all newly diagnosed cancer patients, and to do so in group as well as individual training sessions.

More and more children's hospitals in the United States are moving towards comprehensive psychosocial care for patients with chronic and life-threatening illnesses. It is hoped that the uses of hypnosis will become thoroughly recognized and incorporated into such programs, not only for reduction of distress but for the sense of mastery it imparts to those who use it.

REFERENCE NOTES

La Scola, R. L.: Personal Communication.
Sacerdote, P.: Self-Hypnosis and the Control of Pain. Workshop presented at the Society for Clinical and Experimental Hypnosis, 29th Annual Meeting; Los Angeles; October, 1977.
Erickson, M. H.: Personal Communication.

REFERENCES

Ambrose, G.: Hypnosis in the Treatment of Children. *Am J Clin Hypno 11:*1, 1968.

Ambrose, G.: *Hypnotherapy with Children.* London, Staples Press, 1961.

Bauman, F.: Hypnosis and the Adolescent Drug Abuser. *Am J Clin Hypn, 13:*17, 1970.

Beecher, H. K.: The Measurement of Pain. *Pharmocol Rev, 9:*59, 1957.

Bernstein, N. R.: Management of Burned Children with the Aid of Hypnosis. *J Child Psychol, 4:*93, 1963.

Butler, B.: The Use of Hypnosis in the Care of the Cancer Patient. *Cancer, 1:*1, 1954.

Cangello, D. W.: The Use of Hypnotic Suggestion for Pain Relief in Malignant Disease. *Int J Clin Exp Hypn, 9:*17, 1961.

Clawson, T. H.: The Hypnotic Control of Blood Flow and Pain and the Potential Use of Hypnosis in the Treatment of Cancer. *Am J Clin Hypn, 17:*160, 1975.

Cooper, L. M.: Sex and Hypnotic Susceptibility in Children. *Int J Clin Exp Hypn, 14:*55, 1966.

Crasilneck, H. B. and Hall, J. A.: Clinical Hypnosis in Problems of Pain. *Am J Clin Hypno, 15:*153, 1973.

Cullen, S. C.: Hypno-Induction Techniques in Pediatric Anesthesia. *Anesthesiology, 19:*279, 1958.

Erickson, M. H.: Hypnosis in Painful Terminal Illness. *Am J Clin Hypn, 1:*117, 1959.

Erickson, M. H.: Pediatric Hypnotherapy. *Am J Clin Hypn, 1:*25, 1958.

Gardner, G. G.: Attitudes of Child Health Professionals Towards Hypnosis: Implications for Training. *Int J Clin Exp Hypn, 24:*63, 1976a.

Gardner, G. G.: Childhood, Death and Human Dignity: Hypnosis for David. *Int J Clin Exp Hypn, 24:*122, 1976b.

Gardner, G. G.: Hypnosis with Children. *Int J Clin Exp Hypn, 22:*20, 1974.

Hilgard, E. R.: A Neodissociation Interpretation of Pain Reduction in Hypnosis. *Psychol Rev, 80:*396, 1973.

Hilgard, E. R.: Pain as a Puzzle for Psychology and Physiology. *Am Psychol, 24:*103, 1969.

Hollander, B.: Hypnosis and Anesthesia. *Proc Roy Soc Med, 25:*597, 1932.

Hughes, J.; Smith, T. W.; Kosterlitz, H. W.; Fothergill, L. A.; Morgan, B. A., and Morris, H. R.: Identification of Two Related Pentapeptides from the Brain with Potent Opiate Agonist Activity. *Nature, 258:*577, 1975.

Jacobs, L.: Hypnosis in Clinical Pediatrics. *NY State J Med, 62:*3781, 1962.

Kroger, W.: *Clinical and Experimental Hypnosis,* (Second Edition). Philadelphia, Lippincott, 1977.

La Baw, W.: Adjunctive Trance Therapy with Severely Burned Children. *Int J Child Psychother, 2:*80, 1973.

La Baw, W.; Holton, C.; Tewell, K., and Eccles, D.: The Use of Self-Hypnosis by Children with Cancer. *Am J Clin Hypn, 17:*233, 1975.

La Scola, R. L.: Hypnosis with Children. In Cheek, D. B., and Le Cron, L. M. (Editors), *Clinical Hypnotherapy.* New York, Grune and Stratton, 1968.

Lawlor, E. D.: Hypnotic Intervention with "School Phobic" Children. *Int J Clin Exp Hypn, 24:*74, 1976.

Lea, P.; Ware, P., and Monroe, R.: The Hypnotic Control of Intractable Pain. *Am J Clin Hypn, 3:*3, 1960.

London, P.: *Childrens Hypnotic Susceptibility Scale.* Palo Alto, Consulting Psychologists Press, 1963.

London, P.: Developmental Experiments in Hypnosis. *J Proj Tech Pers Assess, 29:*189, 1965.

London, P., and Cooper, L. M.: Norms of Hypnotic Susceptibility in Children. *Dev Psychol, 1:*113, 1969.

Miller, H. C.: *Hypnotism and Disease: A Plea for Rational Psychotherapy.* Boston, Gorham Press, 1912.

Morgan, A. H. and Hilgard, E. R.: Age Differences in Susceptibility to Hypnosis. *Int J Clin Exp Hypn, 21:*78, 1973.

Olness, K.: In-Service Hypnosis Education in a Childrens Hospital. *Am J Clin Hypn, 20:*80, 1977.

Olness, K.: The Use of Self-Hypnosis in the Treatment of Childhood Nocturnal Enuresis. *Clin Pediatr, 14:*273, 1975.

Pavlov, I. P.: (Collected Writings). In Gnatt, W. H. (Editor and Translator). *Lectures on Conditioned Reflexes.* New York, International Publishers, 1928. Three Volumes.

Rosen, H.: The Hypnotic and Hypnotherapeutic Control of Severe Pain. *Am J Psychiatry 107:*917, 1951.

Sacerdote, P.: Additional Contributions to the Hypnotherapy of the Advanced Cancer Patient. *Am J Clin Hypn, 7:*308, 1965.

Sacerdote, P.: Involvement and Communication with the Terminally Ill Patient. *Am J Clin Hypn, 10:*244, 1968a.

Sacerdote, P.: On the Psycho-Biological Effects of Hypnosis. *Am J Clin Hypn, 10:*10, 1967.

Sacerdote, P.: Psychophysiology of Hypnosis as it Relates to Pain and Pain Problems. *Am J Clin Hypn, 10:*236, 1968b.

Sacerdote, P.: Theory and Practice of Pain Control in Malignancy and Other Protracted or Recurring Painful Illnesses. *Int J Clin Exp Hypn, 3:*160, 1970.

Sacerdote, P.: The Place of Hypnosis in Severe Protracted Pain. *Am J Clin Hypn, 4:*150, 1962.

Sacerdote, P.: The Uses of Hypnosis in Cancer Patients. *Ann NY Acad Sci, 125:*1011, 1966b.

Schon, R. C.: Addendum to Hypnosis in Painful Terminal Illness. *Am J Clin Hypn, 1:*61, 1960.

Simon, E. J., Hiller, J. M., and Edelman, I.: Solubilization of a Stereospecific Opiate-Macromolecular Complex from Rat Brain. *Science, 190:*389, 1975.

Thompson, K. F.: Hypnosis in Dental Practice: Clinical Views. In Weisenberg, M. (Editor), *The Control of Pain.* New York, Psychological Dimension, 1977.

Weisenberg, M.: Pain and Pain Control. *Psychol Bull, 84:*1008, 1977.

Wolpe, J.: *The Practice of Behavior Therapy.* New York, Pergamon Press, 1969.

Zeltzer, L. K., Dash, J. and Holland, J. P.: Hypnotically Induced Pain Control in Sickle Cell Anemia. *Pediatrics, 64:*533, 1979.

Chapter Twelve

INITIAL CONSULTATIONS WITH THE PEDIATRIC CANCER PATIENT

GERALD P. KOOCHER

THE PSYCHOLOGICAL management of the pediatric cancer patient is complicated by many factors. The variability of developmental differences, the variety of different disease entities which are called "cancer," and the individualized medical treatments and complications each patient faces, make each one's concerns quite different. The pages which follow are intended as a basic outline for the clinician who is about to meet with a pediatric cancer patient for the first time. I shall attempt to focus on key clinical issues common to many cases and to illustrate these points with relevant case materials.

EVALUATING THE CHILD'S EXPERIENCES

It is important for the mental health professional who will be working with pediatric cancer patients to become familiar with the nature of the illnesses, treatments, and complications that are a part of each child's experience at the treatment center (Koocher and Sallan, 1978). This information will help put both the child's and the family's emotional frame of reference in perspective. Such information will also help the clinician to anticipate potential concerns and take steps to prevent as much psychological distress as possible.

It is unlikely that a clinician's first encounter with the child who has cancer will be in a relaxed setting or otherwise be typical of the youngster's "normal" behavior. The usual interaction cannot be predicated on the model of a professional helping emotionally troubled people to overcome long-standing maladaptive behavior patterns. Instead, one can expect to encounter basically sound families confronting inordinate amounts of stress which they are powerless to control. In the face of such events even the best adjusted families will be unable to escape reactive emotional difficulties linked to powerful reality events. When a family has pre-existing emotional problems, the onset of cancer certainly adds considerable stress.

The mental health professional's usual focus in the course of psychotherapeutic intervention is the uncovering of unrecognized or unconscious material and its interpretation to clients in constructive fashion. With pediatric cancer patients this focus becomes secondary to more direct supportive measures, including facilitating communication among family members, encouraging the expression of significant

231

emotional concerns, assisting in the management of reactive behavior problems, and sensitizing clients to the emotional subtleties which are easily overlooked. These tasks are not limited solely to pediatric patients and their families but also apply to the mental health professional's work with other members of the treatment team (Geist, 1977; O'Malley and Koocher, 1977).

Key Issues

During the initial contacts with a pediatric cancer patient there are a series of basic concerns which the clinician will need to consider. These are probably best framed as questions to be answered.

WHAT DOES THE PATIENT KNOW? Knowing exactly what has been communicated to the patient and family is very important, but it is also important to recognize that what has been comprehended may differ substantially from what information was allegedly offered. It is important to ask the child or adolescent, "Why are you here at the hospital? What is the name for your illness? What do you know about it? How will the doctors be treating you?," and other similar questions. Only in this way is it possible to reconcile the patient's understanding of events with the actual state of affairs as reflected in the medical record or treatment protocol. Such questioning also tends to reveal additional concerns or fantasies which the patient may not have had the opportunity to verbalize. This approach also establishes the mental health professional's role as a concerned listener at a time when the patient has had many things done to him or her with relatively little listening.

WHAT SURFACE CONCERNS DOES THE PATIENT HAVE? While the nature of the anxieties a patient may face is quite complex there are some facets which will be more easily verbalized than others. One example of this may be found in a child's varying awareness of his own death (Spinetta, 1974). A child may focus on expressed concerns about separation from parents or about physical symptoms of the disease, while remaining seemingly oblivious to the potential terminal nature of the illness. In such cases it is wisest to address the surface or expressed concerns of the child than to raise the unspoken concern which may be far more salient to parents or adults on the treatment team than to the child at that point in time. By providing educative information and assurances in direct response to the patient's expressed concerns it is possible to provide a maximum amount of support, while not imposing unsolicited and potentially anxiety-provoking data on the child. At the same time, responding openly and honestly to the surface concerns will establish a climate within which the child will be able to raise more threatening fears as they come to mind. The importance of an open and honest communication network in the treatment of pediatric cancer patients cannot be overemphasized (Vernick & Karon, 1965; Binger et al., 1969).

WHAT SOURCES OF SUPPORT ARE AVAILABLE? Sources of support include the patient's own personality and coping abilities as well as the emotional support available from family members. Under the ideal circumstance the family will be able to offer the patient considerable emotional support, but there are times when their own grief, distance from the treatment center, general disorganization, or other such factors will make it difficult for family members to be as available as they should be to the patient. In such circumstances members of the treatment team may deliberately or inadvertently become strong support sources for the pediatric patient. It is important to assess the nature of these supports from time to time, since they are variable within the family, treatment team, and patient as a function of many changing events. The change in a nurse's shift rotation, the illness of a sibling requiring a parent's presence at home, or the emergence of a new side effect may all contribute to a rather dramatic change in patient's coping ability. Some forethought to the meaning of the child's support systems can be helpful in anticipating these factors and providing substitutes for losses.

In assessing the family support mechanisms it is important to be aware of the hierarchical concerns of the family, patient, and treatment staff, especially when these may be heading toward a conflict point. When, for example, the family is most interested in having the patient at home and the treatment staff is of the opinion that hospital management is indicated, it will be critical to prevent the child from feeling a loss of support in the face of a conflict between these two sets of caretakers. As a result, the mental health professional will need to be mindful of both the family's structure and coping needs and the basic history of the child's illness to date. All this is a part of knowing and being sensitive to the complex emotional support systems of the pediatric cancer patient.

WHAT SOURCES OF STRESS ARE ANTICIPATED? While it is not always possible to predict the temporal sequence of stress events commonly associated with the treatment of cancer in childhood, the events themselves are well known to those who work with these patients. The recent diagnosis of a life-threatening illness is, of course, a substantial stress as is the hospitalization which may attend the diagnosis. The need for surgical alterations to one's body, side effects of chemotherapy (e.g. nausea and alopecia), relapses, infections, and even the cessation of treatment when it has proven successful are all predictable psychological stress events.

It is often possible to lessen the psychological stresses associated with such stress events by preparing the child for them in advance. This preparation can take many forms, and alopecia provides a fairly common event to use as an example. If one knows that the child will begin to experience the hair loss four to six weeks following the initial chemotherapy, this can be explained along with the information that the hair usually grows back after the treatments are over. Children can be introduced to others who have already lost their hair and told about the availability of wigs. Some may begin to wear a wig even before the hair loss is fully underway. The point to be made is that one can do a degree of stress prevention by informative and supportive desensitization.

Case Examples

I have selected three brief case examples for presentation, because they represent the range of issues that might reasonably turn up in most pediatric cancer treatment settings. While all of the case material is true, some of the "children" described are composites drawn from several similar patients. The first case will present the experiences of a newly diagnosed young child, the second case will illustrate some concerns of an older child in mid-treatment, and the third case will describe some of the difficulties faced by the patients who are on the way to being "cured." These are not intended as comprehensive therapeutic examples, but rather as illustrations of material which might be elicited in an early or initial patient interview based on the questions noted above.

Case One

Ginny, age six, had not complained about any specific symptoms prior to her initial hospitalization. Her parents noted that she had begun to walk with some unusual posturing, and with some inquiry had learned that she was experiencing some pain on inhaling deeply. A chest x-ray and other tests led to a hospital admission for pneumonia and the subsequent tentative diagnosis of a stationary blood clot in the chest wall. Only after exploratory surgery to "remove the clot" was a malignancy diagnosed. By this time Ginny had undergone two hospitalizations at different facilities, a number of invasive tests, and an operation all because of "pneumonia and a blood clot" which had been moderately well described to her. The adults involved had made admirable efforts to advise Ginny of planned procedures and the rationales for these, but their own uncertainties regarding the actual diagnosis left the six-year-old somewhat anxious and confused.

Ginny's parents sought a consultation. They felt ill at ease with the whole concept of discussing the illness with their daughter but knew that it was important. After I became acquainted with Ginny on the hospital ward, she and her mother accompanied me to my office. I explained that we were going to have a conference about her disease and asked if it would be alright to make a tape recording of our conference so that Ginny's father, who was at work, could hear all about what we said. Ginny very much liked the idea of making a taped message for her father and seemed comfortable with the idea of getting some information.

I began by asking Ginny why she had come to the hospital, and she informed me that she had "pneumonia and a blood clot to take out." I acknowledged this information and noted that the doctors had found a tumor when they went looking for the blood clot and had taken it out so that it would not hurt her. I asked if she knew what a tumor was and after getting a negative reply, I explained that it was like a lump under the skin that grew where it was not supposed to. Together we drew a picture of a human body and using her scar as a reference point added the tumor to the picture. I noted that some people call this kind of tumor "cancer," and helped her to repeat the words so that she could remember them. Next I asked what Ginny thought would happen if the doctors had not found the tumor and taken it out. Rather spontaneously and with firm emphasis she replied, "It would have hurt me a real lot more!"

I agreed with that assessment and began to explain that while we did not know how she happened to get that tumor, the doctors wanted to make sure it did not grow back. This led us into a discussion of chemotherapy and radiation therapy, followed by some initial information about hair loss. Ginny had a number of questions of her own in the days that followed including some wondering about whether the doctors might have taken out any parts of her that she needed. In the atmosphere of open communication that had been established she was able to voice this concern and hear that indeed only the tumor and none of the other parts of her had come out.

Both parents were able to participate fully in discussions with Ginny using the taped interview as a kind of model. Any doubts I may have had about her understanding of our discussion vanished some days later when her three-year-old sibling came in to visit. The youngsters met for a while in the lobby of the hospital, but when the time came for Ginny to return to her room the younger brother began to cry, "I want Ginny to come home." According to her parents, and much to their amazement, Ginny put her arm around the three-year-old and said, "I want to come home too, but I have to stay here and get chemotherapy to help the doctors fight my tumor."

Case Two

Karen, age fifteen, had been diagnosed as having a bone tumor six months before I met her. Her left leg had been amputated above the knee and she routinely commuted about 300 miles to the treatment center for chemotherapy every three weeks. During her three-day hospital stays for chemotherapy she was generally brusque and somewhat hostile to the staff, much to the dismay of her mother who continually apologized for Karen's rudeness. Because of the brief hospital stays and Karen's general aloofness, she had not been seen by anyone from the mental health service team. The event which precipitated the request for a consultation was the departure of her primary physician for vacation. Upon hearing that news Karen greeted the substitute with the news that she was soon " . . . going to croak" and the hope that the plane carrying her vacationing doctor would crash.

When I arrived to talk with Karen she was alone in a single-bed room. I introduced myself as a psychologist whose job it is to talk with patients in the hospital about, "the things that worry them." At that point Karen rolled over and faced the wall without comment. I asked if she would like to talk for a while but got no reply. Next, I asked if she would prefer that I leave, but again I got no reply. I commented that I had talked with a lot of teenagers who had cancer and needed amputations, and noted that many of them had similar worries. I also noted that it is hard to talk to a stranger sometimes but that I would be glad to start by talking about some of the common worries that other teenagers in her situation some-times have. Again, I was met with silence. Finally, I suggested that if she did not tell me to go I would sit for a while and tell her about some of these common concerns. Taking the subsequent silence as a positive cue, I pulled up a chair.

I began by commenting on how angry some teenagers get about having no privacy in the hospital, how hard it is to go back to school after losing a limb and hair, how short-tempered people can be at home, and other frustrations of that sort. Karen turned back toward me with tears in her eyes and began talking about her fear that her illness would lead her parents to divorce. She felt that their quarreling at home, especially around the issue of trips to the treatment center, were her responsibility and she feared that she was unable to stop hurting these two most important people in her life.

Following this session and a few family meetings it became obvious to Karen and her parents that all were attempting to "protect" each other from emotional distress in ways which prevented them from supporting each other in the most crucial areas of need. Communication in the family was facilitated, tensions were released, and Karen (to the amazement of the staff and her parents) became a much friendlier person and was noticeably more relaxed.

Case Three

Bob, age seventeen, had been diagnosed as having Hodgkins Disease six years earlier. He had experienced a three-year remission of disease symptoms, followed by a relapse, more treatment, and another prolonged remission. When I first met him he was again off treatment, having completed his second round of therapy two years earlier. He was a high school senior within a few months of graduation. His school had waived certain elective courses so that Bob could graduate with his class, but he was depressed and was not looking forward to graduation. His parents had encouraged him to come in for an outpatient psychological consultation.

During our initial interview Bob talked mostly about his illness and the time it has "robbed" him of during high school. He spoke of teachers who would not believe that he was too weak from his treatments to do some assignments, and of the loneliness he felt by not being physically able to keep up with his peers. In many ways he was mourning disappointments and social losses he had experienced over the past several years. It was striking that despite the fact that he had been off of all treatments for twenty-four months he continued to be past-oriented and was unable to focus much attention on his future.

When asked directly about his focusing on the past Bob's first association was to relapse three years earlier. He had not wanted to believe it at the time and had delayed reporting the return of his symptoms in the hope that they would go away. Now he felt that the return of the disease was again imminent and sheepishly noted that he often spent considerable time checking himself for the return of disease symptoms.

It is not at all unusual for the "long-term survivor" or the patient who has hopefully been "cured" of cancer to worry about recurrence. It is especially not unusual in the case of those who have had one or more relapses during the course of their treatment. In Bob's case the approaching anniversary of his relapse, some lingering guilt about his delay in reporting it, and his mixed feelings about nearing the end of his high school career all combined to hinder his planning for the future.

Several more interviews with Bob followed in the next few months, but one of the most important interventions was set up at our first session. I suggested that he schedule a check-up physical exam immediately, rather than wait until the next regular appointment two months hence. I also helped him to give himself permission to call for a medical appointment whenever he found himself worrying about his physical status. In this way he was able to get immediate feedback on his condition rather than worry by himself. Bob has remained well and is now attending college.

SUMMARY

In order to work effectively with the pediatric cancer patient a mental health professional must be able to carefully evaluate the child's experience of the illness. This would include consideration of the child's knowledge and understanding about the disease, as well as the conscious fantasies and concerns (s)he may have in relation to causes, prognosis, or treatments. Noting the sources of support available to the child and anticipating potential stresses in the foreseeable future will also enable the mental health professional to plan the most appropriate intervention when needed. Psychological consultations with the pediatric cancer patient require a special set of data about the specific natural histories of the illnesses involved, but the consultant must also be a creative "team player" who can work together with the family, physicians, nursing staff, and other caretakers toward the child's best interests.

REFERENCES

Binger, C. M., Ablin, A. R., Feuerstein, R. C., Kushner, J. H., Zoger, S., and Mikkelsen, C.: Childhood leukemia: Emotional impact on patient and family, *NE J Med, 280:*8, 414-418, 1969.

Geist, R. A.: Consultation on a pediatric surgical ward: Creating an empathic climate, *Am J Orthopsychiatry*, 47, 432-444, 1977.

Koocher, G. P. and Sallan, S. E.: Psychological issues in pediatric oncology. In Magrab, P. R. (Ed.): *Psychological Management of Pediatric Problems*. College Park, Maryland, College Park Press, 1978.

O'Malley, J. E. and Koocher, G. P.: Psychological consultation to a pediatric oncology unit: Obstacles to effective intervention, *J Pediatr Psychol., 2:*2, 54-57, 1977.

Spinetta, J. J.: The dying child's awareness of death: A review, *Psychol Bull, 81:*4, 256-260, 1974.

Vernick, J. and Karon, M.: Who's afraid of death on a leukemia ward?, *Am J Dis Child,* 109, 393-397, 1965.

Chapter Thirteen

PREPARING CHILDREN FOR MEDICAL PROCEDURES

KATHLEEN MCCUE

A S RECENTLY AS TEN YEARS AGO, most of the problematic emotional reactions experienced by a child with a malignant disease and his family were centered around the issues of separation and eminent loss. More currently, with advances in medical treatment, the problems these individuals must deal with reflect the chronic long-term nature of the disease. The focus on death has been deemphasized, while much greater attention is being given to coping with the medical realities and returning to a normal way of life.

Despite this life-oriented focus, however, children with cancer are subjected to many physical and psychological stresses during the course of their illness and treatment. Continuing major causes of psychological trauma to pediatric cancer patients are the number and nature of the medical events they must undergo. Painful and intrusive medical procedures, surgeries, and frequent hospitalizations can all be sources of stress to the child and his family.

There are numerous techniques for helping individuals deal with this stress, among which are included play therapy, puppet therapy, preprocedural teaching, modeling, and medical education. These terms are used to describe the various methods by which medical and mental health professionals communicate with the patient and his family about an upcoming medical event. In the present chapter, techniques will be reviewed as they are discussed in the literature and an analysis of what actually goes into an optimal educational session will be presented. The term "preparation" will be used throughout when referring to any of these many techniques.

PSYCHOLOGICAL EFFECTS OF TREATMENT

The development of techniques for preparation emerged out of a body of literature which demonstrated that hospitalization and medical procedures are potentially traumatic events for children and can lead to varying levels of psychological upset. In the 1940s, exploratory work was done (Jackson, 1942; Senn, 1945; Langford, 1948) which documented some of the psychological consequences of hospitalization on children. Regression, severe withdrawal, aggressive and acting-out behavior were noted as sequelae of hospitalization. These early studies were usually psychoanalytically oriented, and tended to hypothesize about the effects of acute illness and separation without presenting objective data.

Several of these initial reports presented information on the effects of surgery (Deutsch, 1942; Jessner and Kaplan, 1948; Levy, 1945) and in some instances anecdotal data was included. Due to the high frequency of tonsillectomy in children, a substantial number of articles were published which presented information on the psychological effects of this particular surgical procedure (Coleman, 1950; Bellam, 1951; Jackson et al., 1952; Jessner, Bloom and Waldfogel, 1952). Jackson et al. (1952) presented early data comparing tonsillectomy patients in a hospital where psychological factors were considered to those in other hospitals and found that "children treated with consideration for emotional factors gave less evidence of trauma." The highest incidence of trauma was found in children under four years of age. In each of these articles the authors attempted to outline what they considered to be appropriate preparation for the children and were universally critical of the kinds of "pragmatic lies" used by parents to get their children to the hospital with the least resistance. All authors advocated at-home preparation.

Around the same time that these parasurgical articles were appearing, Prugh et al. (1952), completed what is now a classic in the literature on children's reactions to hospitalization, studying 100 families, fifty in a control or unsupported group and fifty in an experimental group. Control patients were subjected to usual hospital procedures including minimum parental visitation, with no effort to include parents in care of patients and no attempt to prepare or especially support the child during medical events. For the experimental group, a new kind of ward management was instigated including " . . . daily visiting for parents, early ambulation for patients, a special play program, psychological preparation for and support during potentially emotionally traumatic procedures, more integration of parents in care of the child. . . . " The two groups were matched for age, sex, diagnosis, and other factors. Data was collected from both groups, including interview material before, during, and after hospitalization, behavioral observations of the patients by the hospital staff, and psychometric evaluations of personality structure and adaptation in the children and their families. Results were discussed in terms that considered patient age, since this proved to a significant variable, and data analysis including follow-up information indicated that "an experimental program . . . appears to have produced a significant lowering of the incidence and severity of reactions at all age levels, most marked among children over four years of age."

During the decade following the Prugh study, references continued to appear which evaluated the effects of hospitalization on children. Most of these (Eckenhoff, 1953; Falstein et al., 1956; Vaughan and Lord, 1957) supported the value of preparation but offered few suggestions for its application. Because several authors had stressed

that children four years of age and younger were particularly susceptible to the trauma of hospitalization, there was an increased attention
paid to this age group. Robertson and Freud (1956) presented a detailed case history of a four-year-old girl undergoing a tonsillectomy,
including information on the child's reactions to her surgery from as
early as six weeks prior to the hospitalization to approximately twenty-
four weeks after discharge, and found long-standing reactions.
Erickson (1958) conducted a series of play interviews with twenty-two
four-year-old children and evaluated their reactions using ten four-
year-old, nonhospitalized nursery school children as comparison subjects. Although no statistical evaluations were done, the results were
interesting and suggestive. Hospitalized boys were more verbal and
more aggressive than were hospitalized girls. Hostility in the hospitalized children, after they returned home, was three times as great as
in the control children. Most of the hospitalized children showed
hostile behavior in their play sessions to the doctor and nurse dolls,
while almost none of the control children exhibited such hostility. In
addition, hospitalized children were less active in their play than control children, averaging about half as many activities in play sessions of
equal duration.

Most studies reported responses of children to hospitalization without attempting to specify likely causes of stress in a medical setting. In
1958, however, Gellert identified factors most likely to result in trauma
for pediatric patients, including separation from parents and home
environment; inadequate support from parents; spatial and psychological isolation; unfamiliar routines; schedules and procedures;
physical constraint; enforced dependency; shame, embarrassment,
and fear; misunderstandings; and ignorance. Gellert offered clinical
suggestions for dealing with potential stress in each category.

A similar method of organizing determinants of psychological distress in hospitalized children was used by Vernon et al. (1965) in their
extensive review of the literature. Throughout their book, Vernon et
al. delineated three major foci for preparation: (1) providing information to the child; (2) encouraging emotional expression; and (3) establishing a trusting relationship between the child and hospital staff. No
mention was made of reduction of anxiety or increased cooperation as
therapeutic goals, and those factors which were included were very
difficult to operationalize. Therefore, it was not particularly meaningful to discuss the "success" of psychological preparation. Vernon et al.
considered this in their discussion of research problems.

It should be noted that the literature does not uniformly support the
notion that hospitalization can produce psychological trauma in children, nor is there agreement that preparation is useful for all pediatric
patients. Sipowica and Vernon (1965) in comparing hospitalized and
nonhospitalized twins obtained ambiguous data. Although results indicated that twins who experienced surgery showed more indications
of distress than their at-home cohorts, no statistical differences were

found when the groups were compared along numerous psychological variables. Jessner et al. (1952) found no differences between prepared and unprepared children when these groups were compared in terms of behavior problems during hospitalization. In this study, preparation was done at home by parents and parental report was used to determine whether it was adequate preparation. In evaluating postoperative play responses of hospitalized children, Vredevoe et al. (1969) found no differences between the play of hospitalized children and that of a control group of nursery school children. There were methodological issues in these reports, just as there are in those which support preparation, which make interpretation of contradictory results difficult.

TECHNIQUES OF PREPARATION

Given a growing amount of data suggesting that hospitalization could be traumatic for children, researchers began turning their attention to method of preparation and education. Early references dealt with the specifics of preparation, included no data, and were by and large theoretical presentations (Plank, 1963; Mellish, 1969; Smith, 1960). The focus of these reports was preparation for surgery and the method recommended was preoperative instruction.

Several articles in nursing journals (Webb, 1966; Scahill, 1969; Abbott, Hansen and Lewis, 1970) discussed guidelines for preparation and presented anecdotal supportive data. Methods recommended were preadmittance/preoperative instruction and parent education, but the goals differed from some of the more psychodynamic studies in that they emphasized improved management of patients and increased compliance. Using manageability as a dependent measure, Sauer (1968) compared two groups of children, an experimental group (N = 50) who received preadmission orientation and a control group (N = 59) who did not, and found significantly increased manageability in the experimental group, as rated by nursing staff using single blind measurement.

Dimock (1960) advocated the use of play therapy techniques for preoperative preparation of children, commenting that "Play is the true language of children and a child's natural medium of self-expression," and recommended that children be encouraged to draw or act out with dolls the events that they were to experience, and through these activities express their fears and master them. Cassall (1965) compared two groups of children, one group who received puppet play therapy before cardiac catheterization and one which received no special preparation. The prepared group was found to be significantly lower in disturbed behavior during catheterization, but there were no significant differences between groups either before or after the procedure, or on standardized measures of psychological distress.

In the last decade, several articles have been published which offer a script to the reader to be followed when preparing a child for medical procedures (Petrillo, 1972; Tesler and Hardgrove, 1973; Lucano, 1974). The goal of such techniques is to help the nurse or patient-care individual optimally manage the child, by maximizing knowledge and cooperation. Prehospitalization educational programs with similar goals are well documented (Johnson, 1974; Parsonage, 1971; Lowery, 1975), resulting in the existence of preadmission tours in most major pediatric facilities. Hunnisett and Knowles (1970) emphasized the preparation of parents rather than patients, indicating that parents contribute to the trauma and anxiety of the child because they are not capable of fully discussing the hospitalization with him.

Although the vast majority of the literature on preparation is either theoretical or anecdotal, several studies have been published in recent years which attempt to experimentally explore specific aspects of preparation. Conducted with adult subjects, the work of Andrew (1970) is nevertheless of interest. In this study three groups of subjects were divided according to personality type along the regressor-sensitizer dimension (sensitizers, who use information as part of an intellectual defense system; neutrals; and avoiders, who seldom use intellectualizing defenses). Prepared and unprepared subjects in each personality group were evaluated to determine who would show most improved recovery from surgery. Dependent measures used were days from surgery to discharge and amount of pain medication. The sensitizers, who were expected to show the most improvement, did not differ depending upon preparation. The neutral group recovered in less time and with less medication when prepared than when unprepared. Prepared avoiders recovered in the same amount of time as their unprepared peers but needed more medications. These results indicate that the effects of preparation may be significantly affected by these and other adaptive styles.

Johnson (1972) reported two studies, one done in the laboratory and the other in a clinical medical setting, which offer further information about optimal preparation techniques. In the first, adult subjects were exposed to ischemic pain using a blood pressure cuff. Factors investigated were subjects expectation and direction of attentional focus. All subjects were given pretest information, with one being told what sensations and feelings they would experience and the other half receiving factual description of procedures. With regard to attentional focus, half of the subjects worked multiplication problems while experiencing pain, while the others were asked to attend to the sensations and report what they felt. Subjects who were given a description of the sensations reported significantly less distress than those who were given procedural descriptions. There was no relationship between distress and the distraction/attention dimension. In the second study, ninety-nine patients scheduled to undergo a gastrointestinal endoscopy were divided into three experimental conditions: one group received no information; one received a description of the procedure; and the third group was given sensory information. Both groups receiving preprocedural information had less anticipatory distress than did nonprepared patients, as measured by quantity and dosage of prescribed tranquilizing medication and the sensation information group significantly demonstrated the least distress. Thus, description of sensory experience appears to be an important variable to consider when preparing medical patients.

Wolfer and Visintainer (1975) studied pediatric surgical patients and their parents. A two-group experimental design was used, with the treatment group receiving special psychological preparation and continued supportive care, and a control group receiving regular hospital care. Dependent variables included blind observer ratings of distress, pulse rates, resistance to induction, pattern of recovery room medications, ease of fluid intake, time to first voiding, mother's self-report of anxiety, maternal satisfaction, and mother's rating of adequacy of information. Patients' preparation included information, sensory expectations, role rehearsal, and support. Parents were provided supportive counseling at stress points (admission, blood tests, and just prior to preoperative medication). Parents were also given factual information and encouraged to express their fears and feelings. The experimental group was significantly less upset and more cooperative than the control children on all measures, including physical indices. Parents reported significantly less anxiety and more satisfaction in the experimental group than in the control group. Visintainer and Wolfer (1975) replicated and expanded this study, using a four-group design. Patients were assigned to receive either stress point preparation, single session preparation, consistent supportive care, or no specific preparation. The results demonstrated that the most useful method of preparation was one that combined support, factual and sensory information, and opportunity for rehearsal. The consistent care group did only minimally better than the control group.

Recent studies of preparation have used modeling films to reduce children's fear and anxiety and promote cooperative behavior. Melamed, Weinstein and Hawes (1974) investigated the use of modeling to prevent fear-related behaviors in a group of children undergoing first-time dental work and demonstrated that observational learning significantly prevented dental management problems, even though the children's subjective estimate of fear did not change. Melamed and Siegel (1975) used a modeling film to prepare children for surgery using dependent measures similar to the physiological indices employed by Wolfer and Visintainer (1974). In addition, a first effort was made to distinguish between "state," or situational anxiety, and "trait," or long-term anxiety. The experimental group who had viewed the peer-modeling film showed less state anxiety than the control group, but preparation did not affect levels of trait anxiety. In their most recent article, Melamed et al. (1976) used a modeling film with children scheduled for surgery. Patients were divided into two groups, one which saw the film six to nine days prior to admission, and the other which viewed it on the day of admission. Unlike an earlier study (Melamed and Siegel, 1975), there was no preoperative education program in existence at the hospital from which the sample was drawn. Results indicate reduction in anxiety in prepared patients on a variety of behavioral, psychological, and self-report measures after viewing the film. There was no main effect for time of viewing, but there was an interaction between this variable and patient age in that younger children did better after being prepared immediately before a procedure, while older children benefited from more advanced preparation. The data also supported the hypothesis that similarity between patients and peer-models in the film, in age, race, and sex was positively correlated with subsequent anxiety reduction.

It can be seen from the literature that there has not been enough controlled, replicated research to state unequivocally what the best method is for preparing children for medical events. Methods of preparation presently being used differ widely depending on the attitude of the institution toward preparation, the theoretical orientation of the therapist, the amount of time available and numerous other factors; however, even given the inconsistencies in the clinical application of preparation, it is still possible to present a model of intervention that is consistent with the available data and can be generally used for medical events experienced by pediatric cancer patients. Such a model grew out of extensive clinical experience and can be applied, with flexibility to any medical event a child must undergo, from hospital admission to blood tests and bone marrow aspirations, and even for complex procedures such as major surgery.

A MODEL FOR PSYCHOLOGICAL PREPARATION FOR MEDICAL EVENTS

Stage I. Introduction and Assessment
    A. Introduce self to patient and parents.
    B. Inform child about upcoming event, and allow child to express his feelings.
    C. Let child and parents know that you will be preparing them, explaining the medical event.
        1. Assure child that you will not be doing anything directly to him.
        2. Do not begin preparation or show the child any equipment at this time.
    D. Assess emotional state of child and parents.
    E. Confirm actual medical information from individual who will perform procedures.
Stage II. Education Session
    A. Explain why procedure is being done.
    B. Explain and demonstrate entire procedure.
        1. Use actual equipment, if acceptable to child.
        2. Use doll and/or diagrams for accuracy.

    3. Identify feelings and sensations.

    4. Allow child to express his feelings and reactions.

  C. Encourage child to handle equipment and demonstrate his knowledge of procedure.

  D. Provide appropriate peer models using films or live demonstrations when available.

  E. Repeat demonstration several times, if indicated.

  F. Show child and parents any other rooms or areas of institution, as is appropriate.

Stage III. The Medical Event

  A. Stay with child as much as possible.

  B. Facilitate separation, if necessary, by supporting parents and reducing parental anxiety.

  C. Verbalize during procedures, identifying equipment and sensations.

  D. Do not attempt to distract child.

  E. Help child and parents take an active role in medical events.

Stage IV. Follow-Up (Postprocedure)

  A. Spend as much time as possible with child and parents after procedure. This is a good time for learning.

    1. Go over procedure again and give child a chance to show what happened.

    2. Validate child's feelings, including anger or disorientation and anxiety.

    3. Make physical contact with child only if he indicates that he wants it.

  B. Encourage the child to work toward future mastery of the repeated medical event. Do not distract.

  C. Determine whether parents need further information.

The initial stage of preparation is one of the most important and most frequently overlooked. The manner in which the preparation therapist introduces himself and explains his purpose to the patient can set the emotional tone for the entire preparation. Several things should happen during this initial meeting. First, an assured, mastery-oriented approach should be taken. Comments like, "I'm going to tell you about your operation so you won't have to be scared," or "Most children feel better when they know exactly what the doctor will be doing," help to create a positive atmosphere. However, it is important not to promise responses which the child may be incapable of, such as "after I talk to you, you will be able to hold still during your test." Comments to the child need to be somewhat indefinite, and the child must be given permission not to be helped if he so chooses. Second, a beginning foundation of trusting communication between staff and child is laid by assuring the child that he will be told about and allowed to see everything that he wishes. Finally, the child must be assured that it is all right to feel whatever he is feeling. At any point in the preparation that the therapist perceives a shifting of rising emotional response, it is useful to comment ("You seem pretty scared right now," or "I think you must be pretty mad about having to have this test") and to give permission for the child to have these feelings. It is then appropriate to let the child know that there are things he can do to make his feelings change, if he wants to. Anger and fear are the two most common emotions a child will exhibit in response to medical events.

At some time during the initial contact, the therapist needs to inform the parents whether they will be allowed to attend the procedure, and what their involvement may be. If the parents have the option of attending, it is better to let them know this out of hearing of the child. Some parents will choose not to attend, either because they believe their child will be more cooperative without them, or because they cannot handle watching their child in pain. Whatever the reason, parents should be supported in their decision and not made to feel guilty by being confronted in front of the child. If parents or child are particularly upset at this stage of preparation, or if the parents are not present but are expected soon, the therapist can sometimes facilitate a postponement of the medical event until an emotionally more appropriate time.

During the Education Session stage of the preparation, the child and his parents will receive as much information as they are willing to accept about the upcoming event. It is very important at this point to remember that children respond differently to stressful events than adults. Children need to absorb, integrate, and master an event in a concrete manner, since they usually cannot succeed in doing this abstractly. A classic example is the way adults usually turn away from a blood test, avoiding visual contact with the equipment, while most children will look at the equipment and intently watch the procedure. Attempts by adults to turn the child's head away or prevent his involvement with the test are usually met with increased anxiety and struggling on the part of the child.

If a doll or diagram is used to illustrate the upcoming event, it is useful to draw in as much detail as possible. Veins, spinal columns, and organs can all be drawn on a doll, and such drawings help the child to understand concretely what will be done. It can be very provocative to use the child's own personal doll or stuffed animal, and this should not be done unless the child specifically requests it. If the child will be undergoing complicated procedures involving multiple dressings, I.V.'s, tubes, or casts, it is very useful to simulate these things on a doll and then leave the doll with the child. When the tube is removed or the dressing changed on the child, the child can help perform the same function on the doll.

Children should always be allowed to choose whether they wish to see the actual medical equipment or not. Most children will ask to see real equipment, including needles. When given the opportunity to handle this equipment, many children will belligerently and forcefully stab the doll with the needles, thereby acting out their feelings of rage and impotence.

It is common for children to demonstrate heightened anxiety during the Education Session and may cry, cling to a parent or act in a hostile manner. This behavior can be very useful for the child and the preparation therapist should not attempt to curtail it. Frequently this is the child's first chance to really express his feelings and with the proper support it can be a cathartic experience. If the child becomes upset at this point, it indicates that he really understands what is about to happen and is attempting to come to grips with the information. This response may offer much more potential for growth than that of a child who floats through the Education Session, blithely playing with the equipment, without ever really understanding or believing that anything is going to happen to him. For the second child, the actual medical event is usually extremely traumatic. If children have the opportunity to act out their feelings during an earlier stage of preparation, they frequently can demonstrate more self-control during the medical event.

Some institutions have films or videotapes of child actors modeling appropriate responses to various medical events. These should be used, when possible. Sometimes other children are available to demonstrate or be role models. For example, in any inpatient pediatric setting, there will be children with I.V.s and these children can be asked to tell the child being prepared how the I.V. feels now, how it felt when being started, and what the acceptable behavior was. Obviously, these real-life models must be chosen very carefully. The peer model must be behaviorally stable and should be quite familiar with the procedure he will discuss. Children who are under stress or at risk themselves should not be asked to act as models for other children. Dolls, puppets, or stuffed animals can be a model for younger children, if the therapist acts as a ventriloquist and makes the surrogate respond realistically to the medical event.

The Education Session does not, in fact, have to be a single session. If there is a great deal of information to impart, if the child has a short attention span, or if the session is interrupted for some reason, it can be continued at another time. It is best not to spread the Education Session out over several days, however, because children may not be able to remember the earlier explanations. If the child is scheduled to go to an ICU, experience his procedure in another room or for any reason will be in some other area of the institution he and his parents should be shown that area during the Education Session.

There are a number of things the preparation therapist can do during the medical event stage to support the child and promote mastery. If possible, the therapist should accompany the child during any specific procedures. If parents are allowed to attend, they will benefit by the positive, nondistractive example which the therapist can set. If the child must separate from his parents, the therapist can facilitate this process and sometimes just his familiar presence will make the child feel more secure.

It is very important to verbalize during any procedure, letting the child know what will happen and how it will feel. Even if the child is screaming or crying, many of the things that are said to him will be heard, and the commitment made by the therapist to tell him what is happening will have been met. A child should never be given fictitious choices, nor should his permission be asked to do things. If there are decisions he can make, such as which leg he wants a shot in, it is good to allow him this control. However, sometimes even simple decisions are too burdensome for an anxious child.

As discussed earlier, most children need to attend closely to the medical procedure in order to be able to integrate and master it. No attempt should be made to distract the child or take his mind off the event. If the child begins to talk about school or some other extraneous matter, it is acceptable to follow his lead and converse about these things. However, as long as the child is concentrating on what is happening to him, the content of the conversation should focus on the immediate situation.

Even those children who do not understand what is happening or who have a difficult time during a medical event can have a positive experience during the follow-up stage of preparation. In essence, this stage repeats much of what happened during the Education Session. The difference is that the child is usually less anxious and more angry.

The most common adult response to a child who has experienced pain, fear, or discomfort is to hold and cuddle him, and try to make him forget what happened. This can make a child feel better temporarily but will not help him in his general mastery of medical situations. Providing immediate comfort, especially by a parent, is best followed by a chance for the child to work out some of his feelings and frustrations. Sometimes offering the doll or equipment will give the child an opportunity to resolve things for himself. Alternatively, children may not want to touch the medical equipment but will draw pictures of what happened, or will even punch a punching bag or engage in some other aggressive play. Since the hospital staff are the most likely targets for the child's anger, they should refrain from engaging in all but the most basic physical contact until the child indicates that he is ready to be touched or held. It is interesting to note that often when preparing a child for a specific medical event, the therapist will observe that the child is using the equipment to perform a different procedure on a doll. Frequently the Education Session stage of one preparation will also provide for Follow-Up from some separate event. This demonstrates the child's ongoing need to work on and resolve these very intense experiences.

FACTORS AFFECTING PREPARATION

Developmental Level of Patient

Although the preparation model is applicable to children of all ages, certain considerations must be made for children outside the preschool/school age range. Very young, preverbal children obviously cannot cognitively incorporate the facts pertaining to an upcoming medical event, nor can they be expected to exhibit much self-control, but it is still important that they receive comprehensive preparation. Infants and toddlers can become familiar with the medical equipment, sometimes demonstrating surprising understanding of how the equipment is used. This familiarity will help to reduce the child's anxiety when confronted with such items.

Case One

Tiffany, a two-and-a-half-year-old girl, was developmentally delayed, functioning at about a one-year-old level. When she was scheduled for a bone marrow aspiration to rule out Histiocytosis, the nurse informed the preparation therapist about the procedure, assuming that the child would not benefit from any education. When preparation was attempted however, Tiffany eagerly seized the equipment and proceeded to perform many shots and blood tests on the doll, probably in response to the things that had happened to her. During the actual procedure, she seemed to listen to what the therapist was telling her, and responded appropriately to painful stimuli.

Later, the lab technician stated that Tiffany was completely changed in her behavior toward blood tests: during previous tests, she had struggled and screamed and seemed terrified, but later that same day she was calmer and more responsive and cried just when it hurt. Tiffany kept the rag doll and syringes, and could be seen engaging in "doctor play" during much of her hospitalization.

It is logical that if any item, such as a syringe, is used as much for play as for pain, a unilaterally negative association can be avoided. It is especially important when preparing a baby, to have the parents observe the preparation. When the parents know in detail what to expect, their own anxiety is lowered, and they can be calm and supportive to their child.

At the other end of the age spectrum, adolescents and preadolescents require a different kind of sensitivity on the part of the preparation therapist. Individuals in this range function sometimes as children and sometimes as adults. Some adolescents will state that they do not want to know or see anything and then will proceed to ask detailed questions about an upcoming medical event. Teens and preteens resent being infantilized and struggle to maintain as much personal control as possible. Therefore, the therapist must not approach these patients in a patronizing or demeaning way. However, it is incorrect to assume that, because of their age, adolescents will not wish to handle equipment, work with dolls and diagrams, or do some of the other things done by younger children. It is also important to avoid the assumption that, because they are older, adolescents do not need specific emotional support during stressful medical events. They may be more reluctant to request a hand to hold during a painful event but are frequently in as much need of this sort of help as are younger children.

Recently, a workshop was begun on a CHLA adolescent inpatient unit to allow the patients to engage in medical "play," and receive medical information. The prediction from the staff was that the patients would reject the workshop, finding it babyish and silly. However, it was extremely well received. Patients learned how to regulate IVs, gave shots to oranges, examined procedure needles carefully, and even set up complicated surgeries. The adolescents requested precise details and sought specific medical and biological facts. Physicians and nurses were brought in to provide information and were impressed at the level of understanding and expertise demonstrated by the teenage patients.

Goals of Preparation

One problematic area within the field of preparation is the inconsistency with which the goals are defined. In much of the early anecdotal literature, the goal was simply stated as helping the child develop a trusting relationship with the institution and the staff. While admirable, such a goal is very difficult to operationalize or evaluate. Later, precise variables such as amount of pain, medication, or discharge time from the hospital were used to assess the success of preparation. This sort of data was much easier to collect, but the personal, emotional component was often neglected. To date, the issue of how to measure therapeutic efficacy of preparation has not been satisfactorily resolved.

Problems can occur when various adults working with a child have different goals for preparation. The physician or nurse may evaluate success in terms of how cooperative the child can be during a procedure; the parent's primary goal may be to reduce the child's expressions of anxiety, while the preparation therapist may be most interested in establishing a consistent positive relationship. It is necessary for there to be communication among those working with the patient, and it is also important to establish goals which are realistic. For example, it is unfair to expect a child to refrain from crying during a painful event. Adults should be united in their willingness for a child to express his emotions, and crying is the most natural way for a pediatric patient to do this.

Parental Involvement in Preparation

The advantages of having parents participate in their child's preparation have already been mentioned with regard to the very young patient, but parental participation can be useful for children of any age. Parents make up the primary support system for most children, and with the proper information and education, they can do more for their child, emotionally, than even the best trained staff. When parents attend the actual preparation, not only do they receive detailed medical information, but they can observe and model the calm, mastery-oriented approach of the preparation therapist.

Many parents initially object to having their child prepared. They often truly believe that the child will do better and be less traumatized if no one tells him anything. This is understandable in light of the fact that parents want to protect the child and postpone any potentially frightening experience for as long as possible. It is especially common in the case of pediatric cancer patients, since these patients are under particularly high levels of stress. Usually, endorsement of preparation by the physician, plus a full explanation of what preparation involves will convince the parent to allow the medical education. It is very important, when dealing with reluctant parents, to explain how the child will probably react to the preparation and to expedite the medical event so the child does not experience undue anticipatory anxiety. Parents need honest feedback after the event, letting them know what they might do to further help the child cope with subsequent procedures.

Procedural Variables

The format for preparation has been presented as if it applies uniformly to any medical event. Although this is generally true, there are certainly variables within the procedures themselves which influence how the child is likely to react and thus must be accounted for during preparation.

Children with cancer undergo certain medical procedures quite routinely, and others on an emergency or one-time basis. The routine, regular events vary in intensity from blood tests to bone marrow aspirations, and sometimes include regular hospital admissions for children treated with certain chemotherapy protocols. Emergency or one-time events include surgeries, emergency admissions, and crisis-oriented procedures such as thoracentesis. For regular or expected events, preparation can follow the outlined model quite specifically. Since the event is planned, there is time to schedule the preparation, gather full information, and make any additional arrangements that will help the child and his parents to cope. However, for special or emergency medical events, time is usually at a premium and frequently staff and parents are rushed and upset, and the emotional needs of the child can be easily overlooked. The preparation therapist can act as an advocate for the child in this sort of situation giving him information and providing a calming influence. Preparation must frequently be on-the-spot, while the medical event is proceeding. As long as the verbal description remains one step ahead of the actual physical event, the child can integrate this experience.

The use of anesthesia is another variable which has an effect on how the preparation session proceeds. There are three levels of anesthesia which are commonly used with pediatric patients: General anesthesia as in the case of surgery; local anesthesia for painful procedures such as bone marrow aspiration; and no anesthesia for such events as blood drawing, IVs and intramuscular injections. In the situation where there is to be no anesthesia, the focus of the preparation is on the procedure itself and how it will feel at different stages. Since these procedures usually involve only one painful component, and sensations are relatively uniform for most children, the preparation therapist can be very specific about the child's probable reaction.

Procedures that include a local anesthetic are less consistent. They involve an injection of some sort of numbing medication which is usually quite painful, and then the procedure itself. Children seem to react very individually to the anesthetic: some children feel little or no pain during the rest of the event, while others are in great discomfort during the entire procedure. Thus, it is important for the preparation therapist to make no definite promises concerning the lack of pain after local anesthesia, but it can be helpful to offer the suggestion that "many children don't feel very much after the numbing medicine has been put in." The level of trust which the therapist has established with the child will determine the potential for the child to believe what he has been told, as will the child's past experiences with medical events. The more honestly the child is dealt with the more susceptible he will be to suggestions of pain control.

When a general anesthetic is to be used, the major focus of the preparation will be on the application of the anesthetic and how the child will look and feel when awakened. It has already been discussed how difficult it is for most children to give up attention to, and control of, a medical event, so it is easy to understand why the thought of breathing something or getting a shot of something which causes sleep can be much more frightening for children than for adults. Much attention should be given to having the child practice breathing into a mask, if that will be the method of induction. A brief explanation of what will happen while the child is asleep is indicated, but these events should be minimized. Children always want to know who will be present when they awaken, and when they will see their parents. Due to advanced techniques in anesthesiology, it is likely that children will be awake enough to recall their experience in the recovery room, and so this period should be covered. It is always important with surgery and other major procedures to confirm the actual medical information beforehand, since types of dressings, sutures, and drainage devices differ from surgeon to surgeon.

The use of sedatives for children undergoing minor medical events has become a very controversial issue. On the one hand, since pediatric cancer patients go through so much pain and invasion of their bodies, it seems logical to use any chemical means available to reduce their discomfort. On the other hand, it has already been demonstrated how frightening the loss of control is to preschool and school-age children, and sedation can produce such a loss of understanding and self-control. Another factor to consider is that children with malignancies must undergo certain procedures regularly, and there is risk involved in the frequent use of sedatives or tranquilizers.

In the final analysis, the decision about whether to use sedating drugs prior to a medical event depends on the child, his age, and his previous history in adapting to procedures. Children under the age of ten or eleven seem to respond poorly to sedation. They frequently become agitated and fight the effects of the drugs more than they might have fought the procedure.

Case Two

A four-year-old boy, Christopher, was sedated with DPT, a combination of Demerol®, Phenegran®, and Thorazine®, prior to a bone marrow aspiration. The child, who was quite anxious before the sedative, became relaxed and sleepy until the procedure began. He then became extremely upset and aroused, and fought the procedure wildly. It finally took five adults to hold this small child still so the procedure could be completed. One intern commented that the sedative seemed to give the child extraordinary strength. After the procedure, the child slept for several hours as he allowed the medication to take effect.

Preadolescent and adolescent patients may respond very well to sedatives, if they choose to not attend to the medical situation. One eleven-year-old leukemia patient could not tolerate lumbar punctures unless he took oral Valium® beforehand. He was given several chances to prepare for the event and cooperate prior to use of sedation but was incapable of doing so. For this child, who was denying most of the medical experience, sedatives made the procedure tolerable.

If sedation is to be used, it is important for the preparation therapist to spend time working with the child before he is sedated. Once a child is sleepy and nonattentive, it is virtually impossible for him to integrate information about the upcoming event. Even though the child may awaken fully during the procedure itself, it is too late at that point to offer much more than simple supportive measures.

The Future of Preparation

The general area of medical preparation is just beginning to emerge as a professional discipline with many needs for change and development. Twenty years ago, most staff members who worked in medical settings operated under the philosophy that children responded best to stressful events when separated from their parents and when knowing as little as possible that might frighten them. Those few individuals who believed that psychological preparation had value, functioned purely by intuition, since there was little literature to assist in developing medical education for children. As studies began to appear which supported preparation, it became more widely accepted and many institutions began various programs to provide some sort of medical education for their young patients. Unfortunately, although the need for preparation is now recognized, there is still no consistent use of specially trained staff to provide these services. Frequently, preparation is done by whoever is available, without regard for their knowledge of child development and child psychotherapy and certainly without attention to interpersonal skills with children.

The first step toward providing medical environments staffed with skilled and highly trained preparation therapists will be to achieve a secure level of financial support for preparation services. Since insurance companies and third party carriers are the primary resources for subsidizing medical expenses, these groups must be convinced of the value of preparation therapy. When it can be clearly demonstrated that the expense of providing quality preparation is more than offset by savings in other hospital costs, the use of preparation will be supported by financial backing. Some of the recent literature indicates that preparation results in less administration of pain medication, reduced nursing care, and less overall time spent in the hospital. More of this type of data must be collected in order to prove the fiscal value of preparation. There is a general move toward preventative health care, and preparation is certainly an important aspect of this trend.

Along with the need for more research on the outcome of preparation therapy, there is a definite need for evaluation of the different techniques of preparation and comparison of outcome. Very few preparation studies have been replicated, because most are too vague about the specific nature of the intervention. As in most fairly new therapies, preparation therapists rely a great deal on their own intuitive and individual methods and techniques, and thus make it very difficult to train others to provide the same service or, to replicate results produced by these people.

Much of the recent literature indicates that modeling is one of the most successful methods of preparation, and yet it is not widely used because of the lack of generalized modeling films or tapes and also because of the lack of proper audiovisual equipment. In order to provide efficient as well as effective preparation, prerecorded modeling films will soon be in great demand. Since the use of mixed media for all kinds of education is on the increase, by the time good modeling materials are available most medical settings may very well enjoy access to necessary equipment. It should be possible within the next ten years to widely distribute pre-packaged preparation materials, including audiovisual aids, to be used by trained professionals, which will provide education and preparation for most pediatric patients.

The general community is now becoming aware of the need for and uses of preparation for children, and this will be an area of very rapid change in the next few years. Several books are available that aim to help parents prepare their children for medical events. A few pilot projects are occurring in schools to help familiarize children with medically related materials and further programs like this are expected to develop. Since people learn best when not under high stress, it is logical to teach children about hospitalization and prepare them for medical experiences before they are in the situation of needing such education. Medical staff, educators, and parents are all much more aware of the value of preparation, and, hopefully, that awareness will continue to grow. As preparation proves itself to be fiscally responsible and important for quality medical care, it will become incorporated into all parts of a child's medical experience. For the child with cancer, this means he will understand more, trust more, and fear less, thus gaining more control over his body and his destiny.

REFERENCES

Andrew, J. M.: Recovery from surgery with and without preparatory instruction for three coping styles. *J Pers Soc Psychol, 15:*223, 1970.

Abbott, N. C., Hansen, R. and Lewis, K.: Dress rehearsal for the hospital. *Am J Nurs 70:*2360, 1970.

Bellam, G.: Tonsillectomy without fear. *Am J Nurs, 51:*244, 1951.

Cassell, S.: Effects of brief puppet therapy upon the emotional responses of children undergoing cardiac catheterization. *J Ans Psychol, 29:*1, 1965.

Coleman, L. L.: The psychologic implications of tonsillectomy. *NY J Med, 50:* 1225, 1950.

Deutsch, H.: Some psychoanalytic observation in surgery. *Psychosom Med, 4:*105, 1942.

Dimock, H. G.: *The Child in Hospital: A Study of His Emotional and Social Well-being.* Philadelphia, Davis, 1960.

Eckenhoff, J. D.: Relationship of anesthesia to postoperative personality. *Am J of Diseases in Children, 86:*587, 1953.

Erickson, F. H.: *Play Interviews for Four-year-old Hospitalized Children.* Monographs of Society for Research in Child Development, 23, 1958.

Falstein, E. I., Judas, I., Mendelsohn, R. S.: Fantasies of children prior to herniorrhaphy. *Am J Orthopsychiatry, 27:*800, 1957.

Gellert, E.: Reducing the emotional stresses of hospitalization for children. *Am J Occupational Therapy, 12:*125, 1958.

Hunnisett, F., Knowles, D.: Orienting prospective patients. *Hospitals J Am Hosp Assoc, 44:*51, 1970.

Jackson, E.: The treatment of the young child in the hospital. *Am J Orthopsychiatry, 12:*56, 1942.

Jackson, K.: Psychological preparation as a method of reducing emotional trauma in children. *Anesthesiology, 12:*293, 1951.

Jackson, K.: Winkley, R., Faust, O. A., Cermak, E. G., Burtt, M. M. Behavior changes indicating emotional trauma in tonsillectomized children. *Pediatrics, 12:*33, 1953.

Jessner, L., Bloom, G. E., Waldfogel, S.: Emotional implications of tonsillectomy and adenoidectomy on children. *Psychoanalytic Study of the Child, 7:*126, 1952.

Jessner, L., Kaplan, S.: Observations on the emotional reactions of children to tonsillectomy and adenoidectomy. *Problems of Infancy and Childhood.* (M. J. E. Senn, Ed.) New York, Macy Ed., 1948.

Johnson, G. H.: Before hospitalization: A preparation program for the child and his family. *Child Today, 3:*18, 1974.

Johnson, J. E.: Effects of structuring patients' expectations on their reactions to threatening events. *Nursing Research, 21:*499, 1972.

Langford, W. F.: Physical illness and convalescence: Their meaning to the child. *J Pediatrics, 33:*242, 1948.

Levy, D.: Psychic trauma of operations in children and a note on combat neurosis. *Am J Dis Child, 69:*7, 1945.

Lowery, C. H.: Preparing children for the hospital. *Am Family Physician, 12:*136, 1975.

Luciano, K.: The who, when, where, what and how of preparing children for surgery. *Nursing '74, 4:*64, 1974.

Melamed, B. G., Meyer, R., Gee, C., Soule, L.: The influence of time and type of preparation on children's adjustment to hospitalization. *J Pediatr Psychol, 1:*31, 1976.

Melamed, B. G., Siegel, L. J.: Reduction of anxiety in children facing surgery by modeling. *J Cens Clin Psychol, 43:*511, 1975.

Melamed, B. G., Weinstein, D. and Jawes, R.: *Preparation of Children for Dental Work by Film Modeling.* Midwestern Psychological Association Convention, Chicago, 1974.

Mellish, R. W.: Preparation of a child for hospitalization and surgery. *Pediatr Clin North Am, 16:*543, 1969.

Parsonage, J.: Preparation of children going into hospital. *Dist Nurs, 14:*30, 1971.

Petrillo, M.: Preparing children and parents for hospital and treatment. *Pediatr Ann, 1:*24, 1972.

Plank, E.: Preparing children for surgery. *Ohio State Med J, 59:*809, 1963.

Prugh, D. G., Staub, E. M., Sands, H. H., Kirschbawm, R. M. and Lenihan, E. A.: A study of the emotional reactions of children and families to hospitalization and illness. *Am J Orthopsychiatry, 23:*70, 1953.

Robertson, J. and Freud A.: A mother's observation on the tonsillectomy of her four-year-old daughter. *Psychoanalytic Study of the Child, 11:*410, 1956.

Sauer, J. E.: Preadmission orientation: Effect on patient manageability. *Hospital Topics, 46:*79, 1968.

Scahill, M.: Preparing children for procedures and operations. *Nurs Outlook, 17:*36, 1969.

Senn, M. J. E.: Emotional aspects of convalescence. *The Child, 10:*24, 1945.

Sipowicz, R. R. and Vernon, D. T. A.: Psychological responses of children to hospitalization. *Am J Dis Child, 109:*228, 1965.

Smith, R. M.: Preparing children for anesthesia and surgery. *Am J Dis Child, 101:*142, 1961.

Tesler, J. and Hardgrove, C.: Cardiac catheterization: Preparing the child. *Am J Nurs, 73:*80, 1973.

Vaughan, G. F. and Lond, M. B.: Children in hospital. *Lancet, 272:*1117, 1957.

Vernon, D. T. A., Foley, J. M., Sipowicz, R. R. and Schulman, J. L.: *The Psychological Responses of Children to Hospitalization and Illness.* Springfield, Thomas, 1965.

Visintainer, M. A. and Wolfer, J. A.: Psychological preparation for surgical pediatric patients: The effect on children's and parent's stress responses and adjustment. *Pediatrics, 56:*187, 1975.

Vredevoe, P. L., Kim, A. C., Dambacher, B. M. and Call, J. D.: Aggressive post-operative play responses of hospitalized pre-school children. *Nurs Res, 4:*3, 1969.

Webb, M.: Tactics to reduce a child's fear of pain. *Am J Nurs, 66:*2699, 1966.

Wolfer, J. A. and Visintainer, M. A.: Pediatric surgical patients' and parents' stress responses and adjustment as a function of psychologic preparation and stress point. *Nursing Care Nursing Research, 24:*245, 1975.

Chapter Fourteen

DISEASE-RELATED COMMUNICATION: HOW TO TELL

JOHN J. SPINETTA

OW DOES ONE TELL a child that he or she has a potentially fatal illness? Both parents and professionals alike find themselves in a dilemma. Parents often try to spare their children the necessity of facing adult-like tasks before their time; they try to keep them in a happy, somewhat protected environment. While it may be possible though not advisable to avoid the topic of death with some young children, the task of avoidance becomes increasingly difficult when the child has been diagnosed with a life-threatening illness. When the changes in the emotional climate surrounding the child become so obvious that the child senses that something very serious is wrong (Spinetta, 1974), it becomes necessary to deal honestly with the child's questions at the child's level of understanding. Over the years medical practices have greatly increased the lifespan of many children. Twenty years ago, leukemia, for example, was an acutely fatal illness. Today, for many, it has become a life-threatening chronic illness. With this changed perspective, one may respond to the child's questions early in the diagnosis with a reality-based hope and optimism, and parents are encouraged to keep their own hopes very much alive (Clapp, 1976; Koocher & Sallan, 1978; Lansky & Lowman, 1974; van Eys, 1977). Yet the potential threat to life remains ever present, and one cannot hide the truth for very long. Whether told or not, the child will learn very quickly that he or she has cancer or leukemia and learn eventually that the disease is potentially fatal (Bluebond-Langner, 1974, 1977; Spinetta, 1974).

The ideal is to have the family communicate with the child in sharing the family heritage regarding the place of death in life, and in listening and responding to the child's expressed concerns. The professional can be highly supportive of the family's attempts at communication. By establishing an atmosphere of open and honest communication and encouraging and supporting the family in its efforts, the professional can be in a position to share openly with the child when the child is ready for that sharing. Communication with the child about death need not take away from that child hope and a reality-based optimism. Addressing the issue of the seriousness of the child's illness from the time of diagnosis will allow energy that would otherwise be wasted in maintaining a deceit to be applied to the very real problem of living with a life-threatening illness. Helping the child live as normal and full a life as possible within the physical limits imposed by the diagnosis and treatment is the goal of that treatment. Discussing death honestly will allow the child the freedom to go on with the task of living.

While hope of cure must be maintained, it would be unrealistic to think that a child over six years of age can be protected indefinitely from awareness of the potential fatality of the illness. Open use of the terms "cancer" and "leukemia" from the start, even with young children, will not necessarily lead to depression (Kellerman, Rigler, Siegel, & Katz, 1977); on the contrary, avoidance of the terms "cancer" and "leukemia" may compound the problem and lead to isolation and distrust when the child eventually discovers that the adults in his environment have been deceiving him (Spinetta, Rigler, & Karon, 1974). It is our own distinct belief and conviction that in this particular area of concern, it is far better to address the issue in advance (Spinetta, 1977). The task of telling a child about his own potentially shortened lifespan is not an easy one and certainly cannot be accomplished bluntly and in a single statement. While the present chapter will stress the need for open and honest communication, the issues remain complex and very much related to the child's level of development. The chapter will address the complexities surrounding the task.

When one writes a "How to . . . " chapter, the chapter becomes inevitably prescriptive and highly subjective. The author makes no apologies for either. What is presented here is an approach to "telling the child," based on a decade of both rigorous research and clinical practice in this area. The topic will be addressed in the following manner:

A. Five Prerequisites to Communication with the Child about Death.
1. The Parental Stance on Death: Philosophical Position.
2. The Parental Stance on Death: Emotional Position.
3. The Child's Age, Experience, and Level of Development.
4. Family Coping Strategies.
5. The Difference between Content (what to tell) and Process (how to tell).
B. Objections to Explaining Death to Children.
C. How to Talk to a Child about Death.

FIVE PREREQUISITES TO COMMUNICATION WITH THE CHILD ABOUT DEATH

The Parental Stance on Death: Philosophical Position

An essential prerequisite to communication with the family is a basic understanding of the family's view of life (Kantor & Lehr, 1975; Lewis, Beavers, Gossett & Phillips, 1976). It is especially important when dealing with an issue so basic to the human condition as death that one understand both the force of the basic parenting demand (Sheposh,

Spinetta, Chadwick and Elliott, 1978), and the critical role of the family as the prime emotional and intellectual environment for the child (Spinetta & Maloney, 1978). A family resides within a larger social and cultural context, both intrafamilial and extrafamilial. A family has a manner of facing death, a manner of placing meaning to the mystery of death that may be long-standing within the traditions of past generations, or of brief standing within the context of new-found cosmology, or even lacking altogether, for want of ever having had the need or courage to face the issue previously (Toynbee, 1976). This social context of the family's private cosmology/theology/philosophy of death is the environment from which the child will draw his or her own meaning and strength. It is necessary that the professionals both understand the parent's philosophy of life and also come to terms with their own view of the purpose of life and death. Should there be a discrepancy between the professional's view and the parent's view, it is not advisable for the professional to attempt to change the parent's beliefs at this time. To attempt to replace the parental cosmology at so critical a time as the crisis point of diagnosis of cancer can lead to ultimate failure in coping and adaptation for the child while he is alive (Spinetta, 1978, Spinetta & Maloney, 1978), and most especially to a failure in ultimate adaptation of the parents and surviving siblings after the death of the child. In a recent study (Spinetta, Swarner, Kard & Sheposh, 1978), it was demonstrated that firm commitment to a family-consistent and time-honored view of the place of death in life was critical to the ultimate adaptive efforts of the surviving family members.

In brief, professionals who talk to the child must keep in mind that families differ in what they bring to the illness in terms of philosophical stance on the place of death in life. The professional must guide the family in its efforts to tap its own basic strengths rather than attempt at this critical time to pursue a course of radical change in the parental views.

The Parental Stance on Death: Emotional Position

As important as the parental cosmology is to the family's ultimate adaptive efforts, even more important is how well the family has incorporated that stance (Glock, 1965). It is not so much what death is that concerns most of us; it is rather how we feel about death (Feifel, 1977; Jackson, 1965; Kastenbaum, 1977). When someone close to us dies, we grieve, we cry, we may feel angry. If that person was an essential part of our daily existence, we may feel that our whole life has fallen apart, that we will never be the same, that we cannot go on living. When the person who dies is someone not as closely tied to our own personal life, we may still feel a grief that is tied to the basic social condition in which we find ourselves. When a United States president is assassinated, the world weeps. When a loved comedian takes his own life, we are sad. When we read in the papers of floods and devastation and automobile accidents and airplane crashes, we feel that a part of us has been taken. "Every man's death diminishes me."

When one is dealing with the parents of a child who has been diagnosed with a life-threatening illness, it is critical to be patient, to allow time to become aware of, and help the parents become aware of, both their general and their specific attitudes and emotional responses toward the concept of death. Has the family experienced death before? Was it a grandparent? An uncle or aunt? A close friend or neighbor? What was the mother's reaction? What was the father's reaction? Did they grieve at the same pace or in different manners? Did they share their feelings of grief with each other and with other family members, or did they suffer in isolation and silence? Did they involve the children? At what age? Knowledge of the general and specific history of the family's emotional approach to the concept of death is the second prerequisite to talking to the child about death.

The Child's Age, Experience, and Level of Development

A third prerequisite to communication with a child about the concept of death is a basic understanding of developmental levels in the growth of the child's thought processes, notably those surrounding the concept of death. There are many references which speak to this issue (for example, Easson, 1970; Grollman, 1967; Hostler, 1978; Jackson, 1965; Spinetta, Spinetta, Kung & Schwartz, 1976). Although it is difficult to do justice to so complex a topic in so brief a space, we will address this issue at this point in an overview fashion, so that we can place the issue in proper perspective. We will address the topic in two phases: (1) The Healthy Child and Death, and (2) The Seriously Ill Child and Death.

THE HEALTHY CHILD AND DEATH. Concepts of death are age-related in children and differ with intellectual ability and development (Spinetta, Spinetta, Kung & Schwartz, 1976). It is generally believed that during the first two years of life, there is no understanding of death as such, but fear of separation from protecting, comforting persons is present in its most terrifying intensity. While death is not yet a fact of life for the child going on three, anxiety about separation remains all pervasive. Sometime between the ages of three and five, most children first comprehend the fact of death as something that happens to others. At this time, the concept of death is still vague. It is associated with sleep and the absence of light or movement and is not yet thought of as permanent. In contrast to toddlers, most children of this age are able to withstand and understand short separation. They often respond more spontaneously and with less anxiety to questions about death than do older children. They are also curious about dead animals and flowers. But children between three and five typically deny death as a final reality. They believe death is accidental and they themselves will not die (Aradine, 1976).

Attitudes and concepts of children do not change abruptly at any given age, but evolve gradually and with wide individual variation. This is true whether one is talking about the concept of time, the concept of space, or the concept of death. From approximately the age of six onward, the child seems gradually to be accommodating herself to the proposition that death is final, inevitable, universal and personal. Many six- and seven-year-olds suspect that their parents will die someday, and that they too may die, but only in the very distant future. Children in these early school years show a strong tendency to personify death. Many children, at their initial awareness and discovery of death, are horrified, confused, and angered. Although some recent authors feel that a child in the present day and age is coming to grips with the concept of death at a younger age than ever before because of exposure (Hansen, 1973), most still agree that the child under ten has not yet attained a well-developed understanding of death. As children approach adolescence, they are equipped with the intellectual tools necessary to understand time, space, life, and death in a logical manner. At about the age of ten or eleven the fact of the universality and the permanence of death becomes understandable.

What we have discussed up to this point is the normal development of the ability to conceptualize in the healthy child. A speeding up of the process occurs when the child is faced with death at an early age, at a level preceding the ability to conceptualize it (Bluebond-Langner, 1974, 1977; Spinetta, 1974).

THE SERIOUSLY ILL CHILD AND DEATH. How does all this apply to the child who has been diagnosed with a potentially life-threatening illness? Recent studies of six- to ten-year-old leukemic children reveal that, despite efforts by parents and medical personnel to keep the child from becoming aware of the prognosis, he somehow picks up a sense that the illness is no ordinary illness. The fear of abandonment and separation, characteristic of the younger child, has added to it a fear of bodily harm and injury and possible awareness of his own impending death, or, at the very least, the awareness at a level preceding his ability to conceptualize it, that something very serious is happening. The awareness of one's own impending death becomes stronger as the child nears death (Bluebond-Langner, 1974, 1977; Spinetta, Rigler & Karon, 1973, 1974).

Despite the great efforts often expended on the part of physicians and parents to protect the young children from awareness of the prognosis, the children can and do become aware of the seriousness of their illness, at an age much younger than such awareness occurs in their healthy counterparts.

It is important, then, in speaking with children with cancer about the concept of death, to understand differences in ability to conceptualize that are due to the child's age and level of development, but at the same time, to keep in mind that a child who is experiencing the cancer and the often drastic changes in the emotional climate around him often becomes aware of his own impending demise at a much younger age than his healthy peers and at a level that often the child himself cannot conceptualize.

Family Coping Strategies

A fourth prerequisite to communication with a child about the potentially fatal nature of the cancer is an understanding of the family's usual manner of dealing with crises. An understanding of the past, present, and possibly changing coping modes of the various family members as individuals, and of the family as a social group is essential if a professional is to tap the family's own resource pool. Individuals have different levels of stress tolerance, different levels of ability to deal with stress, different histories of success and failure in overcoming stresses (Selye, 1974, 1976). What works for the professional may not work at all for the family, especially when the family is in the middle of sustaining the burden of the diagnosis of cancer in their child. The very diagnosis itself can shift the family's central survival skills to a newer mode. At this stage in the family's development, the individual members need a professional who is willing to understand and help them piece together their usual mode of coping with crises, help them grow into facing this crisis, give them the tolerance and patience they will need themselves to make the transition, and remain noncritical in the process. This is not a time for imposition. It is a time for support.

The Child's Affinity for Process over Content

The fifth and final prerequisite for communicating with a child about the potential threat to his own life is a basic understanding of how a child works. Process is process and content is content; a child prefers the former over the latter. In this author's experience, it is more important to know how to talk about death than it is to know what to say. At a level long preceding the ability to verbalize, a young infant can pick up subtle and not-so-subtle cues of tension, anger, or happiness from the mother. As children grow, they remain very much attuned to nonverbal cues in their environment (Mussen, Conger & Kagan, 1974). They are very dependent on the adults around them to help explain to them what they are feeling. In a warm and close family, the parents will try to explain to the child what she is feeling and soothe the child's expressed concerns. However, when the parents reach an area that may be of some emotional distress for them as adults, such as the areas of sex and death, they may fall short of their usual attempts at explanation. If children do not find a real explanation to fit what they sense, they may let their imaginations take over. They may assume that they did something wrong, and that is why mommy and daddy will not explain this to them. They may feel that the medical intrusions are punishments for wrongdoing. Unless the parents explain to the child, at his level, what is happening, the child may have to deal with imagined fears, distresses, and concerns that are much more disturbing and difficult to deal with than the actual facts.

Children are attuned to nonverbal cues in their environment. An understanding of this concept is a prerequisite to meaningful communication with the child.

OBJECTIONS TO EXPLAINING DEATH TO CHILDREN

It is understandable that the experienced professional has had and will continue to have reasonable objections to talking to a child about death. In this section of the chapter, we will raise the most common objections to talking to a child with cancer about his possible impending death. We will then attempt to respond to the objections with data from research studies. Eight objections will be discussed in logical order.

OBJECTION ONE. The child does not know about death, let alone his own possible impending death. We should not add to his burden by telling him things that he may not even imagine.

RESPONSE ONE. The child does know, at an age much younger than we have previously imagined (Bluebond-Langner, 1974, 1977; Spinetta, Rigler & Karon, 1973, 1974). By talking to the child about the possibility of his own early death, one is not telling him anything new; one is merely giving him permission to speak freely of his concerns.

OBJECTION TWO. If it is true that one is confirming the child's suspicions, then it would seem clear that even if the child suspects, he is better off not being told outright.

RESPONSE TWO. The fear of the unknown is worse than the fear of the known, most especially in a child (Kastenbaum, 1977; Mussen, et al. 1974). The child who is not allowed to share becomes isolated, depressed, and filled with malaise (Spinetta, 1974; Spinetta & Maloney, 1975, 1978).

OBJECTION THREE. Communicating with the child will not help him; it will only open up a Pandora's box that had best be left alone. The adults in the child's world have the strength necessary to shoulder the burden and it is not fair to force the child to share such a burden at so young an age.

RESPONSE THREE. Communication reduces feelings of isolation, self-dislike, and despair (Spinetta & Maloney, 1978). Allowing the child a chance to express concerns, both negative and positive, eventually leads that child to a healthier self-concept and to the ability to live as normal a life and as full a life as possible within the context of the illness.

OBJECTION FOUR. Communication will hurt the siblings and parents in the long run because they will have to live with the knowledge that they failed to protect their young child from the burden of awareness.

RESPONSE FOUR. Communication is best for the parents in the long run (Binger, Ablin et al., 1969; Futterman & Hoffman, 1973; Hofer, Wolff, Friedman, & Mason, 1972; Spinetta, Swarner, Kard & Sheposh, 1978; and Stehbens & Lascari, 1974). Those parents interviewed one full year after the death of their child who showed the healthiest and most advanced level of adaptation to life without their child were those parents who reported having spent the years of the diagnosis and illness communicating openly with their child upon request and in a manner appropriate to the child's age and developmental level.

OBJECTION FIVE. Talking about death with your own child may prove harmful to other parents and families and children who may overhear you talking, for example, in a hospital waiting room. You must be sensitive to the needs of others.

RESPONSE FIVE. It helps other parents to talk about it, to get their feelings out in the open, reduces tension and allows the families to be prepared for untoward eventualities (Spinetta, Spinetta, Kung & Schwartz, 1976; Townes, Wold & Holmes, 1974).

OBJECTION SIX. Not all families can endure or sustain such levels of openness. You must be sensitive to the needs and abilities and levels of readiness of specific families.

RESPONSE SIX. This is very true. Our research (Spinetta 1977, 1978) has shown that there are at least three types of family approaches to the issue of communication and support: (1) supportive, (2) quasi-supportive, and (3) noncommunicative.

There are some families who, because of a past history of dealing with crises; because of personality, philosophy, and basic view of life not only talk openly within their family about life's concerns, but allow their children and themselves the freedom to openly express both positive and negative feelings. Such families prove themselves most supportive to the needs of individual members.

Other families, those we term quasi-supportive, may talk openly about the illness, but seem to fall short of allowing the child and other family members, including themselves, to talk openly about feelings, both positive and negative. In such families, there is often a nonmalicious, well-intentioned resistance to open communication that forces the levels of support underground. In some such families, the levels of support may be less than genuine (Spinetta, 1978).

Finally there are those families we term noncommunicative, that openly admit to not being able to even mention the word cancer, and who do not allow conversation either about death or about other crises in the family structure. While such families may appear to need greater levels of communication, it is critical to allow such families the time and room to move forward at their own pace in dealing with their response to the illness.

OBJECTION SEVEN. If I, as a professional in the hospital structure, take the time out of my busy medical day to discuss with a family the psychosocial issues surrounding the prognosis, then I have opened up a new plateau of communication with that family. I will no longer be able to deal solely with the medical. I will be forced to deal with problems at the more time-consuming level of the psychosocial. I cannot deal with all of my other patients in this way. Thus, I won't even begin. I am not trained to handle such problems. It would be unfair to try to do so.

RESPONSE SEVEN. This is a very true point, and very well taken. Alby and Alby (1973) spoke to this issue when they discussed the necessity of having a "psy-person" on each team dealing with childhood cancer. It is not only unfair to the doctors to demand that they take the effort to deal with the family's psychosocial problems, it is unfair to the family to have a physician not trained in the psychosocial or unwilling to do so, attempt to deal in a haphazard manner with the problem. Some physicians in institutional settings may have the time to deal with such problems and may wish to do so with certain families. However, in most institutions and for most physicians, it may be reasonable to assign a "psy-person," when finances and institutional agreements permit, to deal with such issues.

OBJECTION EIGHT. I can't take it. I'll burn out. There is no way that I, as a professional dealing with these areas, can continue to deal at an intense personal and familial level, on a daily basis, and keep giving of myself at this level over time. I cannot continue doing this without burning out.

RESPONSE EIGHT. Very true. There really is no way that any person can continue to respond to the needs of families, parents, children, siblings, fellow staff members, and oneself continually over time, without burning out. There are several solutions to this: (1) Remove oneself from the feeling level. Deal with the children as objects to be studied and cured. Have the "psy-person" deal with the feelings, or (2) Give totally and completely to each family that demands it; burn out early, leave the profession, or (3) Deal with burn-out before it occurs by: (a) talking to one's medical peers about the problems that occur in working with families at this close a level; and (b) learning to "get away." Getting away could mean taking long weekends off, days off, vacations, or learning to reduce levels of stress by a variety of self-relaxation techniques now in vogue (Lecron, 1964; Selye, 1974, 1976; Axelrod, 1978; Schowalter, 1978; Viles, 1978.)

HOW TO TALK TO A CHILD ABOUT DEATH

Now that we have dealt with prerequisites and addressed several objections to communication with the child about the potential fatality of the illness, what are our suggestions about the process of talking to the child about death? The following points are suggested as topics to be raised with a child, in an age-appropriate manner, at the child's own level of readiness. It is important to keep in mind the prerequisites mentioned above, and to place the conversation within the context of the specific and personal environmental history of the child, in the specific familial and institutional environment.

In the author's own experience, the following points have proved beneficial to the child when couched in the child's own language and raised in a tactful process-oriented manner. Some of the points may be raised at the child's initial expression of concern over a possibly impending death. Others are best reserved for the child whose disease course has brought him very close to the actual point of death. In all cases, it is important to remain aware of the child's level of concern. The author has found it helpful to explain to the child that:

(1) Death is a part of the natural order of things.

(2) Death has a social significance. We have special feelings for the other persons we share our lives with, as they do for us.

(3) Death is a separation on both sides. Not only does the person who dies lose the people left behind, but they lose their child as well.

(4) The loss is never complete. The deceased lives on in some way. (Here the specific cosmological stance of the family is critical; some feel that the child will live on in spirit; others that the child will have passed on a legacy of the meaning of life to friends; others that the child will live on in both body and soul for eternity.)

(5) The child will not be alone at death and after. (What the child is looking for is parental presence and support throughout, both during the death process and after death. It is important to reassure these children that they will not be suffering death alone, and that the parents will remain with them even after death. This last point is critical, essential to the child, and of necessity to be phrased within the context of the parent's cosmological stance, as with point 4.)

(6) People at the point of death, whether adults or children, have the need to know that they have done all that they could with life. This is a universal human concern that is shared by children as well as by adults. Even young children can live fulfilled and happy lives before they die. It is not necessary to live to eighty-five to make a lasting contribution to the human condition. Young children can touch the minds and hearts of those they deal with at school, in the hospital, at home, in a manner that will live on in others' memories. If the child's life, manner of facing the illness, and death can help modify a parent's, sibling's, or professional's attitude in a manner that helps move the human condition one step further forward, that child will have contributed to humanity and will have led a highly effective life in a short period of time.

(7) It's all right to cry and to feel sad.

(8) It's all right to feel angry and resentful.

(9) It's all right not to want to talk to anyone anymore about it for a while.

(10) When the child is ready to talk about it, the adult will be there to listen and support. (This had better be true.)

(11) It is not necessary to express how you feel in words. Sometimes it's all right just to sit there and not have to talk. And if what you say when you want to talk sounds confused or silly, that's all right too. Adults don't always know what to say either.

(12) Death will not hurt. The dying process itself may be painful,

and the doctor will do all that can be done to reduce the pain to a minimum, but death itself won't hurt. The pain will never return again. (Children are very concerned with having the pain finally end. It is important to reassure them that it will finally end.)

(13) When someone that you love dies, it is important for you to be able to say goodbye. People have a social custom of saying their last goodbyes together, crying together, talking over what happened. Sometimes people do this in the privacy of their homes; sometimes they do it in church. These goodbye group-happenings are usually called funerals. Don't be scared of them. They are very important for your mother and father and your brothers and sisters.

(14) We grown-ups sometimes don't know very much about death either. If we talk to the doctor a lot, and cry afterwards, or if mother and dad talk about your illness and are teary-eyed, that's because we love you and don't want to lose you, and don't know how we're going to be able to get along without you. If someday you won't be here with us anymore, we will be very unhappy. But we will remember the happy times, and you will live on with us (in body, mind, spirit, memory, see #4 and #5 above). We will be happy knowing that you have been happy. And we will always be with you.

The above points are highly subjective and are listed here because they have proved helpful in the past in the author's conversations with children. They remain suggestions to be applied with caution and judgment, at the child's own bidding, and at a level with which the child is comfortable. The most important of all the suggestions and pre-scriptions listed above, to be kept in mind throughout any conversation with a child, is that a child is more process-oriented than content-oriented. Children pay less attention to what you say, and more atten-tion to your concern, how you say what you are saying, and the body language you use when you are attempting to communicate your concerns and offers of help. Although the content of your communi-cations is not unimportant — what you say is critical — you can say all sorts of things and make all sorts of "mistakes" in what you say, and the child will overlook that, if your manner is in tune with the child. However, no matter how well rehearsed and "correct" your content is, if your manner is lacking or not in tune with the child, you may find that the conversation was in one direction only.

How do you talk to children about their own possible early death from cancer? With great difficulty, with great concern, with care for the child, and with a heavy price on your own emotions and feelings. But the reward for your efforts will be a child who is able to face you in turn as a mature person, at whatever age and developmental level, and feel with you that he or she is not alone in facing the most difficult task any one of us has to face in our lives, the fact of our own death. The failure to make the attempt can only lead to isolation, loneliness, and ultimate despair in the child. Making the attempt, giving the child the social support and understanding most needed at that time, has as its reward the fullest gift we can share with the child with cancer: our own love, understanding, and shared concern for each of our roles in the basic human condition.

REFERENCES

Alby, N., & Alby, J. M.: The doctor and the dying child. In E. J. Anthony & C. Koupernik (Eds.), *The Child in His Family, Vol. 2: The Impact of Disease and Death.* New York, Wiley, 1973.

Aradine, C. R.: Books for children about death. *Pediatrics, 57:*372, 1976.

Axelrod, B. H.: The chronic care specialist: "But who supports us?" In O. J. Z. Sahler (Ed.), *The Child and Death.* St. Louis, C. V. Mosby, 1978.

Bluebond-Langner, M.: I know, do you? Awareness and communication in terminally ill children. In B. Schoenberg, A. Carr, D. Peretz, & A. Kutscher (Eds.), *Anticipatory Grief.* New York, Columbia, 1974.

Bluebond-Langner, M.: Meanings of death to children. In H. Feifel (Ed.), *New Meanings of Death.* New York, McGraw-Hill, 1977.

Clapp, M. J.: Psychosocial reactions of children with cancer. *Nurs Clin North Am, 11:*73, 1976.

Easson, W. M.: The dying child: *The Management of the Child or Adolescent Who Is Dying.* Springfield, Thomas, 1970.

Feifel, H.: Death in contemporary America. In H. Feifel (Ed.), *New Meanings of Death.* New York, McGraw-Hill, 1977.

Glock, C. Y.: *Religion and Society in Tension.* Chicago, Rand McNally, 1965.

Grollman, E. A. (Ed.): *Explaining Death to Children.* Boston, Beacon Press, 1967.

Hansen, Y.: *Development of the Concept of Death: Cognitive Aspects.* (Los Angeles, California School of Professional Psychology, 1972). Ann Arbor, University Microfilms, 1973. (73-19,640).

Hofer, M. A., Wolff, C. T., Friedman, S. B., & Mason, J. W.: A psychoendocrine study of bereavement, Part I: 17-Hydroxycorticosteroid excretion rates of parents following death of their children from leukemia. *Psychosom Med, 34:*481, 1972.

Hostler, S. L.: The development of the child's concept of death. In O. J. Z. Sahler (Ed)., *The Child and Death.* St. Louis, C. V. Mosby, 1978.

Jackson, E. N.: *Telling a Child About Death.* New York, Hawthorn Books, 1965.

Kantor, D. & Lehr, W.: *Inside the Family.* San Francisco, Jossey-Bass, 1975.

Kastenbaum, R.: Death and development through the lifespan. In H. Feifel (Ed.), *New Meanings of Death.* New York, McGraw-Hill, 1977.

Kellerman, J., Rigler, D., Siegel, S. E., & Katz, E. R.: Disease-related communication and depression in pediatric cancer patients. *J Pediatr Psychol,* 1977, *2(2),* 52-53.

Koocher, G. P. & Sallan, S. E.: Psychological issues in pediatric oncology. In P. R. Magrab (Ed.), *Psychological Management of Pediatric Problems.* 2 vols. Baltimore, University Park Press, 1978.

Lansky, S. B. & Lowman, J. T.: Childhood malignancy. *J Kans Med Soc, 75:*91, 1974.

Lecron, L. M.: *Self-hypnotism: The Technique and Its Use in Daily Living.* Englewood Cliffs, N. J., Prentice-Hall, 1964.

Lewis, J., Beavers, W., Gossett, J., & Phillips, V.: *No Single Thread: Psychological Health in Family Systems.* New York, Brunner-Mazel, 1976.

Mussen, P. H., Conger, J. J., & Kagan, J.: *Child Development and Personality.* Fourth Edition. New York, Harper & Row, 1974.

Schowalter, J. E.: The reactions of caregivers dealing with fatally ill children and their families. In O. J. Z. Sahler (Ed.), *The Child and Death.* St. Louis, C. V. Mosby, 1978.

Selye, H.: *Stress Without Distress.* Philadelphia, Lippincott, 1974.

Selye, H. *The Stress of Life.* Rev. Ed. New York, McGraw-Hill 1976.

Sheposh, J. P., Spinetta, J. J., Chadwick, D. L., & Elliott, E. S.: Parental Participation in Decisions Regarding Extraordinary Life-sustaining Measures. Manuscript submitted for publication, 1978.

Spinetta, J. J.: The dying child's awareness of death: A review. *Psychol Bull, 81:*256, 1974.

Spinetta, J. J.: Adjustment in children with cancer. *J Ped Psychol, 2:*49, 1977.

Spinetta, J. J.: Communication patterns in families dealing with life-threatening illness. In O. J. Sahler (Ed.), *The Child and Death.* St. Louis, C. V. Mosby, 1978.

Spinetta, J. J., & Maloney, L. J.: Death anxiety in the out-patient leukemic child. *Pediatrics, 56:*1034, 1975.

Spinetta, J. J., & Maloney, L. J.: The child with cancer: Patterns of communication and denial. *J Consult Clin Psychol, 46:*1540, 1978.

Spinetta, J. J., Rigler, D., & Karon, M.: Anxiety in the dying child. *Pediatrics, 52:*841, 1973.

Spinetta, J. J., Rigler, D., & Karon, M.: Personal space as a measure of the dying child's sense of isolation. *J Consult Clin Psychol, 42:*751, 1974.

Spinetta, J. J., Spinetta, P. D., Kung, F., & Schwartz, D. B.: *Emotional Aspects of Childhood Cancer and Leukemia: A Handbook for Parents.* San Diego, Leukemia Society of America, 1976.

Spinetta, J. J., Swarner, J., Kard, T., & Sheposh, J. P.: *Effective Parental Coping Following the Death of a Child from Cancer.* Manuscript submitted for publication, 1978.

Stehbens, J. A., & Lascari, A. D.: Psychological follow-up of families with childhood leukemia. *J Clin Psychol, 30:*394, 1974.

Townes, B., Wold, D., & Holmes, T.: Parental adjustment to childhood leukemia. *J Psychosom Res, 18 (1):*9, 1974.

Toynbee, A.: Various ways in which human beings have sought to reconcile themselves to the fact of death. In E. S. Shneidman (Ed.), *Death: Current Perspectives.* Palo Alto, Mayfield, 1976.

Van Eys, J.: What do we mean by "the truly cured child"? In J. van Eys (Ed.), *The Truly Cured Child: The New Challenge in Pediatric Cancer Care.* Baltimore, University Park Press, 1977.

Viles, P. H.: Reflections of a physician caregiver. In O. J. Sahler (Ed.), *The Child and Death.* St. Louis, C. V. Mosby, 1978.

Chapter Fifteen

GROUP THERAPY

BETSY SACHS

T HERE ARE AS MANY models for group therapy as there are needs for
groups to fill. Medical settings have found group work useful to
offset the problems that accompany chronic illness and physical handicaps. In a 1976 lecture, Irvin D. Yalom reported the use of group
therapy with terminally ill cancer patients. There are self-styled, lay-led
groups such as Make Today Count, begun by Orville Kelly (1977), a
cancer patient who felt the need to communicate with others. Bozeman
et al. (1955) found that parents of leukemic children often formed
their own unstructured groups in hospital waiting rooms and lounges.
There have been reports of on-going professionally led groups which
are presently taking place on oncology units, but only a few have
discussed this modality as an intrinsic part of the treatment in pediatric
settings.

The purpose of this paper is to review some of the literature regarding the use of group therapy for pediatric cancer patients and their
families and to describe the history, context, techniques, and results of
several years of group therapeutic involvement on the oncology service
of Children's Hospital of Pittsburgh.

REVIEW OF THE LITERATURE

The literature on group work in pediatric oncology is sparse. Heffron, Bommelaere, and Masters (1973) described preclinic group sessions at the University of New Mexico where parents (mostly mothers)
developed a better understanding of leukemia and learned useful
techniques for coping with the psychosocial aspects. Heffron (1975)
again reported on one hospital's means of offering help to parents,
patients, and staff concerned with pediatric cancer management. He
stated that there was no set format for discussion at the meetings but
rather that "each meeting was allowed to go wherever the needs of the
group dictated."

Kartha and Ertal (1976) detailed a seven-session series for mothers
of leukemic patients who were free of psychosis. Initially, this was done
experimentally and the authors did not make clear whether the groups
became an integral part of total treatment. Kartha and Ertel (1976), on
the other hand, took a more structured approach. "The topics for
discussion were selected in advance consultant with the mothers."

David and Donovan (1975) discussed two groups, not directly con-

270

cerned with cancer but nevertheless relevant, one composed entirely of mothers of multihandicapped children which met during clinic hours like the previously mentioned groups, and one which met in the evening so that both parents could attend. Ablin, Binger et al. (1971) write of a family conference with the entire family of a leukemic child, including parents, siblings, attending physicians, psychiatrist, and social worker, which was scheduled sufficiently after the diagnosis to maximize trust and confidence.

Hamovitch (1964), in his study of parent participation in a hospital pediatrics department, says that mothers of leukemic children expressed three needs: the need for tangible services, the need for temporary escape from the oppression, and the need for emotional support. "Parents of other children with leukemia are regarded as the most valuable source of emotional support." Like several others, Hamovitch highlights the need for parental support but limits the involvement to mothers. These findings will be discussed in another section.

McCollum (1975) devoted one section of her book to parent groups. She separated self-help groups into two kinds: educational-information and experiential-therapeutic, and urged that the therapeutic groups be led by a professional. My own experience corroborates the following quote from her book:

> The formation of a new group requires time and energy, especially if its nature is determined entirely by those parents who expect to participate. The very process of developing into a working group invariably involves a struggle for leadership, an effort to evolve goals, agree on procedures, resolve disagreements and personality conflicts, and develop a sense of unity and trust. Parents whose time and energy are already drained by their child's illness may prefer to seek professional leadership in developing a new group, or to join preexisting groups.

The leader in an experiential group, says McCollum, is able to help the members adapt to various means of coping as acceptable, and help develop a sense of trust within the group. Unlike others who write of parent groups which concern themselves with medical problems, McCollum (1975) excluded the hematologist as group leader so that the focus would be almost entirely on emotional problems. It has been this author's experience that it is difficult to prevent parents from centering their discussion on medical rather than psychosocial issues when a physician or a nurse is part of the leadership.

McCollum addressed herself to one further therapeutic delineation. She separated single parents into a group of their own because marital partners have each other, while single parents "lack even this. It can be bleak, lonely, and frightening to raise a healthy child without a marital partner . . . Much more difficult is the plight of a single parent whose child's health is seriously impaired." In Pittsburgh, divorced parents do attend group meetings on a regular basis. Their experiences may be different from couples, but they have no problem identifying with the common medical and psychosocial issues.

THE PITTSBURGH GROUPS

At Children's Hospital of Pittsburgh, an affiliate of the University of Pittsburgh School of Medicine, group work has been a part of the oncology service for the past three years. The need for such treatment was first felt after a series of parent interviews of newly diagnosed cancer patients revealed that emotional support during the early phase following diagnosis was often not available from spouses, family, physicians, or staff, but from other parents on the floor, not necessarily those of children with cancer. It seemed useful, after discharge, to get the parents together on a regular basis so that they could support and sustain each other with the aid of professional leadership. In a major health center, this is not an easy task, but it is possible. Children's Hospital serves sections of three states. A survey revealed that only about one-third of our patients come from Allegheny County, where Pittsburgh is located. Travel and expense were issues, as was resistance on the part of parents; but the need for parents to maintain contact with other parents whose problems were similar made it imperative to try.

The first several inpatient groups were formed of parents of children with several different oncologic diagnoses. They met on an *ad hoc* basis whenever there were enough hospitalized patients whose parents constituted a group of six to ten members. They were led by the social worker with nurse specialists attending, but limited to issues that dealt with treatment, complaints about hospital care, wondering what to tell the grandparents, and fear of death. Postdiagnostic shock was too great, depression too intense to immediately begin to learn the new skills necessary to lead a different, yet still constructive life-style. Parents received tremendous strength from one another. "Knowing you weren't alone," as one parent said, "took away the feeling of isolation. When my child was first diagnosed I was sure I was the only one this had ever happened to."

One of the major issues discussed at the initial in-house meetings was re-entry into the community. All parents were concerned about being accepted by neighbors, and were overwhelmed by the responsibility of caring for the sick child at home. "What should I look for? How will I know if Billy is all right? What do I tell grandparents who want to overindulge him with inappropriate gifts because 'he hasn't got long to live'?" Though the perceived severity of problems was eased somewhat by initial discussion and mutual reinforcement, the work toward finding solutions had really just begun. There were many more adaptations that had to be made. Almost everyone who attended agreed that if it were possible, they wanted to return after discharge for group meetings on a regular, on-going basis. Once their children had achieved remission, parents were far more receptive to learning new coping mechanisms.

STRUCTURING THE GROUPS

Perhaps the most difficult administrative component of all is the pulling together of a cohesive group. It is time-consuming. It is frustrating. It is sometimes disappointing. But when it is done successfully, it is worth it.

The first step is making known to parents that groups exist to meet their needs. This is done at the first office visit after diagnosis. It is important to recognize that at that moment most parents are too deeply enmeshed in other emotions such as shock, depression, anger, to recognize, let alone be ready to prepare for, future needs. The initial hospitalization is a time for building trust between the therapist and the parent. It is important to make yourself known, early, to show that you care and to extend a helping hand so that when the time comes to offer a formal invitation to join a group, rapport has been established. Some will welcome the group experience and some will find it threatening. Others find strength through extended family and social relationships, some through religion. Personal phone calls to all parents who live within reasonably easy access to the hospital are more effective than letters or questionnaires.

MIXED VS. SEPARATE DIAGNOSIS

Many colleagues have argued that there is no point in separating parent groups by diagnosis since "Cancer is cancer and the problems are all the same." Cancer is cancer, to be sure. The outcome is often the same, but different prognoses and different treatments do involve different problems. On two separate occasions the choice to combine was offered to both the AML and the ALL group for consideration. Neither group wanted to mix. The AML parents didn't want to hear about children who could possibly live for five years, while the ALL group said they would be "too guilty knowing" the other had only eighteen months to live. Since additonal guilt and anger were not among the issues we needed to deal with, this decision was respected.

While groups can function with a mixture of diagnoses, they may not function with the same intensity. This proved to be the case in a bereavement group as well, which was, with one exception, composed of parents of children who had died from AML or ALL. The exceptions in this group were parents of a child who died of osteogenic sarcoma, who found it frustrating to be unable to communicate successfully the problem of phantom pain associated with amputation, or the rapidity with which the tumors took over their child's body. My clinical impression was that the mixed group meetings were therapeutic for this couple, but in a much more limited way than for the parents of leukemic children.

PATERNAL INVOLVEMENT

Speculations as to why fathers' needs are often overlooked by group leaders are fascinating, but are best not gone into in a chapter of this nature. In Pittsburgh, group meetings are intentionally scheduled on weekday evenings and Sunday afternoons so that the fathers who want to can attend. Telephone calls to the mothers are made during the day, but invitations to the meetings are explicitly extended to both parents. Very often mothers say: "I'll come. But I know my husband won't." The reply: "That's okay. But invite him anyway." In all but two cases, invited husbands have attended. After two sessions, one of the two absent fathers joined the group. The other husband, himself a leukemia patient, was never able to meet with the group, although it is interesting to note that two weeks before he died he asked his wife if she thought I could get together a group of adult leukemia patients with whom he could talk.

TIMING

It is important in the early stages to develop a relationship of confidence and trust between therapist and parents and patients, and in doing so, it is important to allow time and space to breathe by not rushing quickly into exploration of emotional conflicts. Parents can become overwhelmed. Patients and parents need time to go through a private, personal time of grieving before they are ready to expose themselves to strangers, no matter how well-intentioned. Sometimes a mental health professional is less persuasive than another parent, a doctor, a nurse.

Times for meetings, maximum number of members, and how often to meet are all things the Pittsburgh groups collectively decide. So that everyone has a chance to participate, I prefer a maximum membership of ten or twelve. The parents sometimes feel differently. We had a Sunday afternoon meeting of sixteen at one time which I found unwieldy. The parents did not. It was left at sixteen. On the other hand, there were times when only one or two parents were able to meet. Those groups turned out to be productive, too. There are no hard and fast rules. Leaders, like members, learn as they go, with every group teaching something new.

GROUP PATTERNS

Certain common patterns arose in all the groups. The newness made people uncomfortable, the reason for being there made them angry. Parents asked, "Why should I have to attend meetings where everyone's child has leukemia?" Or adolescents asked, "What am I doing in a roomful of kids with cancer? Are they going to be my future friends?" But the anxiety wore off and the closeness began. Leaders, too, experience anxiety. Will the group mesh? Can I help them help each other? Without the experience and working through of intense anxiety, how can we help allay it in others? In spite of the motivation that drew them there, most members came into the group a little suspiciously, if not negatively. Slowly the doubts began to diminish as commonalities arose and parents began to identify with each other. There followed a long period of worry about the future, talk about the side effects of treatment — such as hair loss, bone pain, nausea — teasing and isolation by other children, sibling problems, fear of relapse, and reassurance that their children are getting the best possible medical treatment.

Cassem (1975) addressed one of the most important phases of group work. He viewed the bereavement process as synonymous with ego development, i.e. personal growth ("All loss is narcissistic bereavement because all loss is personal." p. 10) and focused his attention on narcissistic injury and growth. There is perhaps no blow stronger to a parent's narcissism than that of producing a defective or a terminally ill child. There is nothing more damaging to the budding ego of an adolescent than to know that he is different from his peers. It remains, therefore, for the group to spend as long a time as needed to nurse wounds, redefine individual roles, and then move on to task orientation. When the time had been reached to progress, members often said that they were tired of complaining, tired of talking about problems.

SEPARATE PSYCHOSOCIAL AND MEDICAL MEETINGS

By trying to cover both in the same group, the medical and the psychosocial issues suffered. It became important to separate them entirely.

In the fall of every year there were two Sunday afternoons set aside for meetings conducted by one of the attending physicians. One was open to all parents of children with ALL, whether or not they had indicated an interest in being a part of an on-going small therapy group. The other was open to parents of the children with solid tumors. Physicians described what medical progress had been made, redefined treatment, and generally made themselves available to answer any and all questions which came up. Parents appreciated the time the doctors invested and found it easier to ask questions when their children were not there. The presence of others in the same situation made it easier to ask questions which produced difficult or unwelcome answers. Questions usually started out on a global basis, but ended up being highly personal. This gave an opportunity — for some parents the only chance they would allow themselves — to explore their own child's disease. From the physicians' point of view, there were benefits, too. There was a chance to foster a stronger bond between them and the parents. Feedback to them was positive and attendance was good.

From the author's vantage point, this separation offered a means of limiting the on-going group work to emotional and psychosocial issues. It should also be added here that in Pittsburgh, most patients are treated by an association of four private pediatricians who make themselves available twenty-four hours a day, seven days a week, to answer questions so that parents' anxiety is allayed. This, too, helped maintain the focus of our self-help groups.

THE GROUPS

Parents of Children with ALL

Although it meets now only on an ad hoc basis, this group has had the longest life of all. It met bimonthly for well over a year on Sunday afternoons. Its membership numbered sixteen, seven couples and two single parents, both divorced mothers, representing nine patients who ranged in age from four to sixteen years. It crossed all socioeconomic lines and included a Ph.D. in engineering, a newspaper editor, two nurses, a teacher's aide, a waitress, a business executive, an assembly line worker, and a welfare recipient.

One couple, whose son was in remission and doing very well, was felt to be an abrasive influence on the rest of the group. Almost everyone agreed that while this seemed, at first, cause for disbanding the group, its end result was a useful experience.

> Mrs. G. was a bitter, vindictive woman, who attacked everyone who cared for her son, from floor nurses to the radiation therapist who, she told her son, "is the man who made your hair fall out." Other parents felt no such disdain for their children's physicians, but their protests were unheard by Mrs. G. The group considered disbanding because of her bitterness, which she admitted was there before her son's diagnosis. They finally resolved their conflict by ignoring her vituperations. They listened, unmoved, to her destructive remarks, then continued their discussions as though she were not among them. The development of tolerance was seen as a positive experience.

When the group arrived at a point at which they wanted to do something task-oriented, they set their goal as fund-raising, with the proceeds to be given directly to leukemia research. They incorporated, began their drive toward raising $10,000, and, at the time of this writing, have amassed more than $8,000. As the focus shifted, so did the number of meetings. They were cut from twice to once a month. Since it did not seem like the best use of my time, I asked to be excluded from the business portion of the meetings and requested that they be held elsewhere and at another time. These occurred in the hospital, one hour prior to the therapy sessions. Although there was ample opportunity given to bring up problems in therapy, few arose. The group did rally cohesively around an emotional issue when the first child relapsed. With the exception of one couple who saw the experience as too anxiety-provoking, the members felt it important to support the parents of the patient who had relapsed and felt a need to be informed of his progress between meeting times.

It is important that members have the feeling that the group can be reconvened whenever the need arises. Situations are constantly changing and parents and patients are always adapting to new stresses which need outside support. Without fostering dependency, members need to know there is mutual help available. Thus, all the members of the group continue to meet on a once-every-three-months basis just to keep in touch.

Parents of Children with AML

Socially and economically, this group was more homogeneous than the ALL group. Most members were salaried, working class people with the exception of the wife of a self-employed advertising executive.

The AML group met for over a year on a bimonthly basis. Its core membership was three couples and one mother whose husband, a leukemia patient himself, did not join us. Occasionally, there were two other mothers who came to meetings on an irregular basis. Four children were represented who ranged in age from six to twelve years of age. The feelings of closeness were unusually strong and many of the members still maintain contact even though the group no longer meets. This group sustained itself through the deaths of all the children. When the parents of the child who was the first to die returned to a meeting, apprehension was high, but it diminished fairly quickly. As one of the fathers said, "It's reassuring to see that even though Kathy has died, her parents are still able to function."

In this setting, too, there was one abrasive member, a mother whose presence and barbed remarks taxed everyone's patience. But again, most parents came to see this as positive. One father said that her negative viewpoints reinforced his own positive position. He had previously felt somewhat ambivalent about discipline, but when he saw how destructive a parent's lack of control could be, he found the reinforcement he needed. Parents, in this group particularly, felt they got the support they needed which their spouses were unable to give. They learned that it was often impossible for husbands and wives to give because each was involved so intensively with personal pain, anticipatory grief, that there was little compassion left to give, nor did they want to burden spouses with additional problems.

The issues discussed in both parent groups were quite similar and covered, mainly, the problems involved in getting the family back to as normal a life as possible. The loss of the child's hair was the most traumatic experience for everyone, no matter the age of the patient. Coping with siblings' needs was another area which required an important investment of time. One remarkable difference between the two groups was the intensity with which emotional overlays related to medication came up in the AML group. AML treatment is more intense, is given more frequently, requires more potent drugs than treatment for ALL. Therefore, the time consumed in finding suitable ways to deal with treatment time was quite appropriate and decidedly worthwhile. No two families coped with their child's discomfort in exactly the same way, but that difference in itself was a stimulus for teaching tolerance. One mother's feeling of helplessness produced anger when her son vomited after treatment, but she learned from another parent to carry a bucket, towels, and tissues in the car on treatment days.

Though the issues were parallel to those of the ALL group, the intensity in the AML group was much greater. Long and involved

discussions centered around the parents' inability to allow themselves
social reinforcement or a sex life. While their children were sick, and
indeed after their deaths, pleasure was something they did not feel
entitled to. One father, whose wife felt the world was passing her by,
said that the group meetings offered a semi-acceptable social life. It was
a way of getting out of the house, but the focus was still on the child's
illness. Sharing of such intimate problems was helpful, and in some
cases, remedial.

> Despite her husband's protests, Mrs. A. would not go out to dinner or bowling
> with him and their friends because, she said, she was unable to find a sitter who
> could care for their child. The group saw through this, expressed their empathy,
> encouraged her to go for only an hour or so at first, then for longer periods later
> on. The understanding and support of others who had experienced the same
> reluctance gave Mrs. A. the permission she needed.

Adolescent Group

The composition of this group was eight patients with diagnoses
including Osteogenic Sarcoma (1), Hodgkins Disease (2), ALL (4) and
Lymphoma (1). Ages ranged from twelve to seventeen. The first year
we met on a once-a-week basis, then, as issues were resolved,
bimonthly. The focus here was entirely different from parent groups
since we were dealing directly with patients and patient problems.
Nevertheless, we tried as much as possible to eliminate medical comments from the discussion. This was not hard to control since most of
what came up for discussion was adolescent-oriented anxiety exacerbated by the disease.

Hair loss and reentry into school with wigs was a major concern. The
two female Hodgkins patients found it difficult to deal with the knowledge that they would not wear bikinis because of the scars left by
staging laparotomies. We dealt with overprotective parents, feeling
different from other kids, secondary gains, developing a priority list of
goals that could be met within a limited life span. We talked about
growing up very quickly. As one fifteen-year-old ALL patient put it, "I
went from thirteen to thirty-one overnight." One of the most time-
consuming discussions centered around the adolescents' common
fears of radiation. Children in Pittsburgh are radiated in the adult
hospital of the medical center where they come into contact with older
patients so sick that adolescents often become overwhelmed. Many of
them wondered if radiation were the cause of this debilitation, if it
would happen to them, or if brain cells could be killed just like cancer
cells.

After several weeks of this kind of anxiety-laden discussion, they
were asked what they wanted to do about it. What would help allay
some of their anxiety? They undertook as a joint project, writing
individual letters to the chief of radiation. He was invited to come to
one of their meetings, speak with them, and answer their questions.
Reassurance was given but their request for a separate waiting room, or

at least special appointment times when only children would be present, was denied. They learned that from the hospital's point of view, it was not feasible either physically or financially.

The adolescent group was the only one in which there was a co-leader, a clinical nurse specialist, who had worked with all the members during their inpatient phase and who knew them well. She agreed not to wear her white uniform. She did not encourage medical discussion. We worked well together and in many instances enhanced each other by picking up nuances that the other had missed.

This group, too, lasted for well over a year. One young man has gone away to college, four patients have died, and one has moved out of town. Unlike the adults, the adolescents were unable to cope with a member whose needs were so overpowering that they usurped everyone else's. The problems of a pathological family which one of the patients was bringing to the group were inappropriate and overwhelming to the rest of the membership so it was suggested that she avail herself of one-to-one therapy until the next adolescent group took shape. Movement and progress were stopped. It was unfortunate, but necessary, to refer her to our psychiatry clinic for a different kind of help. She has done well working alone and is now ready to join a newly formed group.

Bereavement Groups

Two bereavement groups ran simultaneously and were experimental in nature. These meetings were to have been a joint effort between the hospital and the local chapter of Candlelighters, a national organization of parents whose main interest is childhood cancer.

Lay leadership of these groups seemed appropriate. I was certain that parents would have more credibility than I, since they knew the devastating experience of a child's death first-hand. My original contract was to work with two couples, one to lead each group, sit through two sessions with each, then turn the meetings over with the knowledge that I would always be available for consultation. It seemed like a perfect solution for everyone. But it failed. McCollum's (1975) remarks, quoted earlier in the chapter about the struggle for power and control of leadership, were borne out in the weeks that followed. Disputes between parents arose and questions like "Who says your way of coping is any better than mine?" came up over and over again. During holidays, when feelings may have been strongest, bereavement group meetings were called off because leaders were unable to handle their own depression, let alone untangle that of other members. One woman wanted desperately to discuss the guilt that arose from sex after her son's death, but that issue was too threatening for a group to handle, so it, too, was dropped.

Without question the membership got help from meeting others who shared a common experience, but that was the extent of the benefit. After several meetings led by the lay couples, both groups asked that professional guidance be restored. It is clear after this experience that what is needed from a leader is not so much a shared experience, but objectivity and the ability to maintain distance, assess covert messages, and bring them out into the open at appropriate times.

Another unique aspect of the bereavement groups was time-limitation. While it is important for patient and parents to feel that other groups can be reconvened at any time or can continue as long as new needs arise, it is just as important to time-limit bereavement groups. The original contract can be set for as many weeks or months as the group deems necessary, and renegotiated, but if, at the end of the second contract, the membership is still not able to restructure the fragments of life, it is the author's feeling that there is something wrong. Either the group has been ineffective because the leader has been remiss or there is pathological mourning present. Both possibilities need to be examined. The goal for this group is different in that the end product is independent functioning, not ongoing support.

While support is intrinsic to any group process, it is important for bereavement groups to focus on rebuilding. Here the process revolves around parts of a life that have been fragmented and putting them back together so the business of living can begin again. Here we see the narcissistic wound at its deepest. New roles have to be defined. Death has brought a rupture. Ego damage has to be repaired. Relationships with spouses and existing children have to be reestablished. Voids need to be filled. New satisfactions can be learned.

Timing is important here, too. I wait a minimum of three months postmortem before an invitation is extended to join a bereavement group. Parents need time for privacy, to recover from the shock, to regain lost strength.

Fischhoff and O'Brien (1976) reported on a parent bereavement group which met bimonthly to share individual experiences. They felt the need for such groups arises from several factors: (1) Our mobile society denies us the emotional support of an extended family. (2) Children die less frequently today so that death is unique and most often unshared with others in the community. (3) There is a misconception among the general population that the mourning process lasts only a few weeks or months. I would also add that our own sociological taboos around death isolate parents even more. In bereavement groups, parents often talked of what they had to go through to educate their friends and neighbors, to appease them, and offer solace and reassurance, when it should be the other way around.

One mother told of insisting that her friends tell stories about her dead son, in spite of the fact that the friends felt that it would upset her. The mother liked hearing things about him she had never known before. Most parents do.

Just as with premortem coping, there is no right way or wrong way to grieve. Who is to say that six weeks or three months is the right time to go through a dead child's cherished possessions and give them away?

Who is to say that the second Christmas after death should be joyful because the family has been through one year of anniversaries? Anniversaries and holidays will be painful spots forever. The goal of the group is not to erase the memories, either good or bad, but to restore the family to productive functioning in spite of them.

SUMMARY

Nothing in our culture prepares parents for coping with the unique problems of fatal pediatric illness, but the resources within a hospital setting can be mobilized to this end. One of the most effective means of restoring family homeostasis is through group therapy. Whether the group process focuses upon parents or the patient, an objective, professionally-trained leader can help tap into natural resources of members who can help each other through mutual support and understanding.

Groups can be used for a range of problems from staff needs in the hospital wards to siblings of the patients. Our next project will be to offer the group experience to latency age patients and to siblings, both of living patients and to those who have died. In other settings, groups would be helpful to parents of children who are contemplating experimental or relatively new procedures such as bone marrow transplantations. While groups will not and cannot serve all the needs of everyone, they are a most satisfying, efficient, and highly adaptable treatment modality which offers the participants and leader a truly creative outlet.

My own experience has been experimental. I grew by helping others. I learned from interviewing that there is much more to know. Because there have been patients whose needs were not as satisfied as they might be, I will be more alert to this in the future. When it is feasible, I will ask for a co-leader, a male if possible, to achieve a better empathic balance.

Additional studies might elucidate the effects of such factors as leader's style, age, and sex upon group process, as well as objectify the nature of therapeutic change. Finally, the question needs to be asked concerning the effects of patient self-selection: does this create a bias either for or against therapeutic efficacy?

REFERENCES

Ablin, A. R.; Binger, C. M.; Stein, R. C.; Kushner, J. H.; Zoger, S., and Mikkelsen, C.: A Conference with the Family of a Leukemic Child. *Am J Dis Child, 122:*312, 1971.

Binger, C. M.; Ablin, A. R.; Feuerstein, R. C.; Kushner, J. H.; Zoger, S., and Mikkelsen, C.: Childhood Leukemia: Emotional Impact on Patient and Family. *N Engl J Med, 280:*414, 1969.

Bozeman, M. P.; Orbach, C. D., and Sutherland, A. M.: Psychological Impact of Cancer and Its Treatment. III. The Adaptation of Mothers to the Threatened Loss of Their Children through Leukemia. *Cancer. 8:*1, 1955.

Cassem, Ned: "Bereavement as Indispensable for Growth." In *Bereavement: Its Psychosocial Aspects.* Edited by B. Schoenberg, I. Gerber, A. Wiener, A. H. Kutscher, D. Peretz and A. C. Carr. New York, Columbia University Press, 1975. 9-17.

David, A. C., and Donovan, E. H.: Initiating Group Process with Parents of Multihandicapped Children. *Social Work in Health Care. 1 (2):*177, 1975-76.

Fischhoff, J., and O'Brien, N.: After the Child Dies. *Pediatrics, 88:*140-146.

Hamovitch, M. B.: *The Parent and the Fatally-Ill Child.* Los Angeles, Delmar, 1964.

Heffron, W. A.: Group Therapy Sessions as Part of Treatment for Children with Cancer. In *Clinical Management of Cancer in Children.* (Carl Pochedly, Ed.) Acton, Mass., Publishing Sciences Group, 1975.

Heffron, W. A.; Bommelaere, K., and Masters, R.: Group Discussions with the Parents of Leukemic Children. *Pediatrics, 52:*831-840.

Kartha, M. and Ertel, I.: Short-Term Group Therapy for Mothers of Leukemic Children. *Clin Pediatr, 15:*803, 1976.

Kelly, O.: "Make Today Count" In *New Meanings of Death.* (Herman Feifel, Ed.) New York, McGraw-Hill, 1977. p. 181.

McCollum, A.: *Coping with Prolonged Health Impairment in Your Child,* Boston, Little, Brown, 1975.

Natterson, J. M. and Knudson, A. G.: Observations Concerning Fear of Death in Fatally Ill Children and Their Mothers. *Psychosom Med, 22:*456, 1960.

Stephen, S.: "Bereavement and Rebuilding of Family Life." In *Care of the Child Facing Death.* (L. Burton, Ed.). London and Boston, Routledge & Kegan Paul, 1974. 207-217.

Chapter Sixteen

NIGHT TERRORS IN A LEUKEMIC CHILD*

P AVOR NOCTURNUS, or night terror syndrome, has been described as a disorder in which the following pattern is observed: A sleeping individual wakes, sits up, screams, exhibits a high degree of motility, cannot be comforted, and returns to sleep with little or no recall of the incident (Broughton, 1968; Christozov and Dascalov, 1970; Fisher et al., 1970; Guilleminault and Anders, 1976; Hersen, 1972; Kales and Kales, 1974). Broughton (1968) has noted that such terrors can be differentiated from REM nightmares in that they occur during arousal from slow-wave sleep, most frequently Stage IV sleep. As such, he posits that pavor nocturnus is a disorder of arousal rather than a sleep disturbance, per se.

Little data exists regarding the incidence of night terrors. Hersen (1972) cites a 1935 study reporting occurrence of monthly nightmares in 32 percent of a sample of normal children, but this figure refers to several types of nightmares and does not consider pavor nocturnus as a separate entity. Other authors (Broughton, 1968; Guilleminault and Anders, 1976) feel that true night terrors are rare. It is clear (Guilleminault and Anders, 1976; Kales and Kales, 1974) that such episodes are most common in children, particularly preschool children, and that the condition is almost always a transitory one of short duration. Concomitance with other disorders of sleep-arousal, most notably somnambulism and enuresis, has been observed (Christozov and Dascalov, 1970).

With regard to etiology, several authors consider prior psychological trauma a major factor (Christozov and Dascalov, 1970; Fisher et al., 1970; Hersen, 1972; Kales and Kales, 1974; Marshall, 1975). One study examining the relationship between EEG findings and night terrors and somnambulism, found evidence of both diffuse and focal EEG abnormalities, and psychological trauma in a sample of 150 children with these problems (Christozov and Dascalov, 1970).

Successful treatment approaches have included the use of medication (Comly, 1975; Golick et al., 1971; Marshall, 1975; Persikoff and Davis, 1971) and behavior therapy (Cautela, 1968; Handle, 1972; Silverman and Geer, 1968; Taboada, 1975). With regard to the former, drugs that have been reported to bring about quick remission of night terrors include imipramine (Comly, 1975; Marshall, 1975; Persikoff

---

* Reprinted with permission from the *Journal of Nervous and Mental Disease*, 167, 182-185, 1979.

283

and Davis, 1971), diazepam (Golick et al., 1971) and methylphenidate (Comly, 1975).

Behavioral approaches have concentrated upon the reduction of sleep and dream-associated anxiety and have included systematic desensitization (Cautela, 1968; Silverman and Geer, 1968), implosion (Handler, 1972), and hypnosis (Taboada, 1975).

The present case reports upon the successful behavioral treatment of a three-year-old girl with acute lymphocytic leukemia (ALL) in remission who presented with a one-month history of persistent, recurring night terrors. This case is of interest due to the long-term, recurrent nature of the disturbance and the diagnosis of malignant disease. An attempt is made to relate psychological aspects of childhood leukemia and its treatment to the development of the night terrors and to specific treatment approaches that were effective in eliminating the disturbance.

Case One

The patient was a girl three years four months who had been diagnosed with ALL a few days before her third birthday. Remission was induced with therapy according to Children's Cancer Study Group Protocol 141. Chemotherapy was interrupted temporarily during the early maintenance phase due to development of a submandibular abscess which required inpatient antibiotic treatment. The patient has remained in complete continuous remission since.

Three weeks prior to psychological referral, the patient's mother reported that she was having recurrent nightmares and that her "bottom hurt." Therapy for probable pinworm infestation was administered, and when this did not bring about abatement of the nightmares, the patient was referred for psychological evaluation and treatment.

At the time of initial evaluation, the patient's mother reported a one-month history of recurrent nightmares occurring from one to six times nightly. The patient had not slept through the night once during this time. The mother's description of the nightmares conformed to the pattern of pavor nocturnus, in that the patient sat up, screamed "T. scared!" or "T. doesn't want to!," appeared extremely anxious, and then went back to sleep.

The parents had been previously advised to take the patient into their bed contingent upon occurrence of the nightmares. This unfortunate bit of advice had been discontinued for two weeks prior to initial psychological evaluation, when it appeared to be ineffective in reducing the night terrors.

The hypothesis was made that the night terrors represented an anxiety reaction. Trauma in this child's life included diagnosis of leukemia and the multiple medical procedures related to its treatment.

Other factors to consider in the assessment included the child's young age, and the submandibular abscess which required minor surgery during which the patient was restricted by having her arms and legs bound with bandages.

It has been noted that anxiety in children this age takes the form of separation fears. This is true for children with malignant disease as well (Spinetta et al., 1973). Thus, I attempted to find out if any outstanding separations had taken place in this child's environment prior to the appearance of the night terrors. The mother informed me that due to her own anxiety at watching her daughter undergo bone marrow aspirations, she left the treatment room during this procedure. This was not the case for venipunctures, lumbar punctures, or the child's surgery for her abscess. The mother also noted that on nights following bone marrow aspirations (BMA's) the patient's sleep appeared to be more disturbed than usual.

Working on the assumption that the night terrors were related both to this separation and to the child's subsequent generalized anxiety reaction to BMA's, medical procedures, and the hospital setting, the following behavioral treatment plan was devised:

1. The parents were to keep written records of the incidence of night terrors including stimulus events proceeding and following the episodes,
2. I explained to the parents the importance of separation anxiety in young children and trained the mother in the use of progressive muscle relaxation to reduce her anxiety to the point where she would be able to remain in the room with her daughter during BMAs.
3. The patient was seen for twice-weekly sessions during which the mother was gradually removed from the treatment room so as to increase the child's tolerance of separation. During these sessions, she was offered the opportunity to engage in play with syringes, swabs, and other medical apparatus and could simulate medical procedures on a variety of dolls.
4. At the point where the patient first began to experience one restful night of sleep without nightmares, a positive reinforcement system was set up in which the patient was able to earn a specified treat each morning following a restful night. This was done to counteract any potentially reinforcing qualities the nightmares may have assumed in terms of eliciting parental attention.
5. When the patient did experience a nightmare, the parents were instructed to offer minimal reassurance using the phrases "Mommy's here" or "Daddy's here" and to refrain from hovering over the child for prolonged periods or removing her from her bed.

RESULTS

Figure 16-1 shows the incidence of night terrors in terms of weekly totals. As can be seen, there was a slight increase of terrors during the second week of treatment. During this period, the patient underwent a BMA. Her mother, having practiced progressive relaxation exercises, was able to remain with the child. It was noted by the nurses who administered the BMA and by the mother that the procedure went much more smoothly than had been observed prior to this time. The patient cooperated, and after completion of the procedure, got up, smiled, and began to talk. This was in sharp contrast from previous post BMA periods during which she was withdrawn and depressed for several hours.

For the next nine weeks there was a steady decline in the weekly incidence of night terrors with the patient experiencing her first completely restful night on the twenty-fourth day following the initiation of treatment. From Day 24 to Day 46 she experienced intermittent nightmares no more than once a night. From Day 47 to Day 69 she was free from symptoms. Then, she experienced five nightmares on the two evenings prior to the second bone marrow aspiration on Day 71.

Following this, her pattern fluctuated between weeks of symptom-free nights and periods of intermittent nightmares (never more than once a night). In addition, her mother noted that the waking incidents were less severe, of shorter duration, and accompanied by less vocalization. Following her third BMA, Day 126, she experienced one nightmare and has been symptom-free since that time, for a period of 120 days. She underwent a fourth bone marrow aspiration with no attendant sleep disturbance. Outpatient psychotherapy sessions were gradually tapered off to weekly, bimonthly and monthly schedules.

There were other changes in the patient's behavior. She progressed from being terrified and fearful at the hint of separation from her parents, to being able to play without them for periods of over one hour. During these sessions, she energetically engaged in repeated and aggressive simulated administration of hypodermic injections to dolls. Parents reported that she engaged in similar play at home. During the latter weeks prior to termination of psychological treatment, she lost interest in medical apparatus and began to engage in nonprocedure-related play.

DISCUSSION

This case illustrates the use of behavioral analysis and treatment in the reduction and eventual elimination of persistent night terrors in a child with serious concomitant medical problems. The nightmares experienced by this child were remarkable in their persistence and recurrence. This is not surprising if one adopts the view that night terrors are an anxiety reaction (Christozov and Dascalov, 1970; Fisher et al., 1970; Freud, 1900; Marshall, 1975; Persikoff and Davis, 1971; Cautela, 1968; Handler, 1972; Silverman and Geer, 1968; Taboada, 1975). The typical transitory night terror pattern observed in most children (Guilleminault and Anders, 1976; Kales, and Kales, 1974) may represent a reaction to transitory psychological trauma. The patient described in the present study, however, experienced continuous

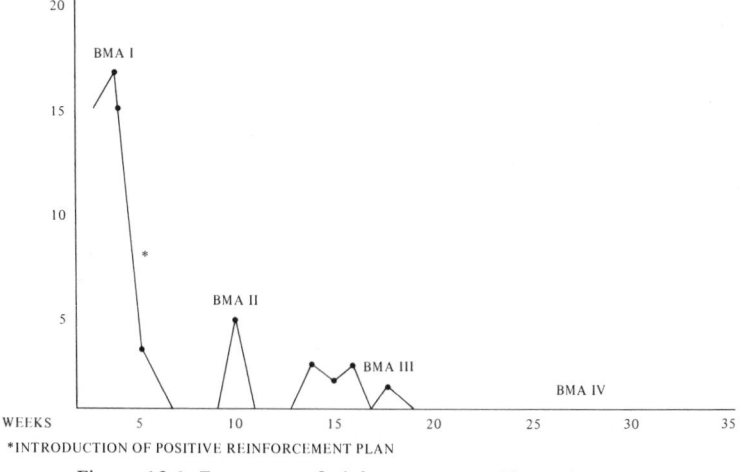

Figure 16-1. Frequency of night terrors: weekly totals.

trauma in the form of illness and treatment related separation, and may have been expected, therefore, to exhibit a continuing reaction. The notion of night terrors as anxiety-mediated receives empirical support from the findings that behavioral methods aimed at anxiety reduction (Cautela, 1968; Handler, 1972; Silverman and Geer, 1968; Taboada, 1975) have proved effective in the management of this disturbance. Marshall (1975) speculates that anxiety stimulates a hormonal reaction that further stimulates the reticular system to bring about heightened arousal. This is in accordance with Broughton's (1968) hypothesis that pavor nocturnus, somnambulism, and related disorders are disturbances of arousal and not of sleep. Glick et al. (1971) posit that the effectiveness of diazepam in eliminating transitory night terrors may be due to its tranquilizing effect. The mechanisms behind the effectiveness of other agents, namely imipramine and methylphenidate, are less clear.

Psychological trauma related to acute leukemia and its treatment has been implicated as an etiological factor in the present study. The question arises as to why this child, in particular, developed night terrors while other children similarly diagnosed and treated, do not. Reactions to psychological trauma are often idiosyncratic, and there is a paucity of data relating individual and environmental characteristics to specific types of reactions. One might hypothesize, however, that this child experienced greater than ordinary stress even for a childhood leukemic, due to a combination of factors: age, a continuous pattern of separation, and medical complications. The submandibular abscess required minor surgery during which the child was completely bound. Such physical restriction may have served to heighten the intensity of emotional trauma.

The basic approach used in the present study was to reduce the child's anxiety. It is important to note that an indirect way of achieving this — reducing the mother's anxiety so that she could minimize or avoid separation from the child during a particular stressful medical procedure — was effective. The relationship between separation anxiety and the night terrors is supported by the finding that this child reacted most strongly to that procedure during which her mother was not present — bone marrow aspirations. The relationship between BMA's and night terror frequency is supported by the data presented in Figure 16-1 where clear peaks around the time of BMA's are observed. No such relationship was found with lumbar punctures, during which the mother was present.

Other treatment components included individual psychotherapeutic sessions during which the child was able to pace herself in densensitizing her anxiety to medical apparatus and in achieving a sense of mastery by enacting medical procedures upon dolls. This is not dissimilar to the alternative response approach utilized in behavioral studies (Handler, 1972; Taboada, 1975). These sessions also aided the child in feeling comfortable for progressively longer periods of separation from her mother.

The use of positive reinforcement for restful sleep was used to counteract potential rewarding aspects of the night terrors including that which may have resulted from an instruction to remove the child from bed and have her sleep with her parents contingent upon interrupted sleep. It has been my clinical observation that such advice is counterproductive and can lead to a persistent pattern of inappropriate sleep in children. What is seen as childhood insomnia is often the result of selective parental reinforcement of disrupted sleep.

Due to the use of a combination of approaches, it is impossible to factor out specific treatment effects. There was a quick reduction of night terrors following the first BMA with mother present though it took several months before the night terrors were eliminated. This may have been due to the child's "need" to experience several mother-present BMA's.

It should be noted that no EEG measurements were taken to substantiate the clinical impression that this child was suffering from slow-wave arousal pavor nocturnus. Behavioral indicators were present, however, that conformed to the description of this disturbance in the literature.

Clinicians presented with children suffering from nightmares would do well to look at the pattern of prior psychological stress in the environment, as well as at potentially reinforcing properties of the disturbance. In addition, the importance of having parents maintain careful behavioral records cannot be over-stressed.

REFERENCES

Broughton, R.: Sleep disorders: disorders of arousal. *Science 159:*1070, 1968.

Cautela, J. R.: Behavior therapy and the need for behavioral assessment. *Psychother Theory Res Pract 5:*175, 1968.

Christozov, C., Dascalov, D.: Correlation between clinical and EEG findings in children with night terrors and somnambulism. *Acta Paedopsychiatrica 37:*61, 1970.

Comly, H. H.: Successful treatment of night terrors. *Am J Psychiatry 132:*76, 1975.

Fisher, C. F., Byrne, J., Edwards, A., Kahn E.: Psychophysiological study of nightmare in adults following trauma. *J Am Psychoanal Assoc 18:*747, 1970.

Freud, S.: The interpretation of dreams. London, Hogarth, 1900.

Golick, B. S., Schulman, D., Turecki, S.: Diazepam treatment in childhood sleep disorders. *Dis Nerv Syst 32:*565, 1971.

Guilleminault, C., Anders, T. F.: Pathophysiology of sleep disorders, part II. *Adv Pediatr 22:*151, 1976.

Handler, L.: The amelioration of nightmares in children. *Psychother Theory Res Prac 9:*54, 1972.

Hersen, M.: Nightmare behavior: a review. *Psychol Bull 78:*37, 1972.

Kales, A., Kales, J. D.: Sleep disorders. *N Engl J Med 290:*487, 1974.

Marshall, J. R.: Treatment of night terrors associated with post-traumatic syndrome. *Am J Psychiatry 132:*293, 1975.

Persikoff, R. B., Davis, P. C.: Treatment of pavor nocturnus and somnambulism in childhood. *Am J Psychiatry 128:*778, 1971.

Silverman, I., Geer, J. M.: The elimination of a recurrent nightmare by desensitization of a related phobia. *Behav Res Ther 6:*109, 1968.

Spinetta, J. J., Rigler, D., Karon, M.: Anxiety in the dying child. *Pediatr 52:*841, 1973.

Taboada, E. L.: Night terrors in a child treated with hypnosis. *Am J Clin Hypn 17:*270, 1975.

Chapter Seventeen

"ALL THE THINGS THAT I DON'T LIKE ABOUT HAVING LEUKEMIA": CHILDREN'S LISTS

BARBARA M. SOURKES

A CHILD WITH LEUKEMIA lives under the constant stress of uncertainty, of trying to lead a "normal" life while coping with the illness and its treatment. While it is critical for the child to articulate different facets of the experience, it may be difficult to express feelings of anger or fear. Within a family or a therapeutic relationship, new doors are opened if the child is given license to talk about the hardships imposed by the illness.

A technique which enables the child to focus on leukemia-related problems without undue stress is the compilation of a list entitled: "All the things that I don't like about having leukemia." Early in the therapeutic relationship, I will say to the child: "Children find all kinds of things difficult about having leukemia. . . . Different things may make them angry. . . . Why don't we make a list of all the things that you don't like or that make you mad about having leukemia?" With the title and the child's name at the top of the page, the child dictates his or her list with whatever elaboration or encouragement is necessary.

Following are the main categories of problems, with examples, cited by six leukemic children in their lists.

Medical Procedures

—I don't like the pain and the idea of needles getting stuck in my back.
—Bone marrows. I don't like all the pushing and pulling.
—The bone marrow and the spinal tap hurt too much — too many needles.
—The numbing medicine is the worst part because it feels like your leg is going to sleep. You feel like you have to move it and you can't because they're holding you down. It's not fun.
—I don't like when my IV infiltrates.
—Shots make my hand sore. And finger pricks bug me because they sting.
—I don't like lying stiff for an x-ray.

School Problems

—I don't know how to read and I'm in second grade.
—Some kids say I don't read as well as they do. They hurt my feelings when they do that. They call me "dummy."

289

—Kids at school ask me questions that I can't answer.
—Because of my relapse, I couldn't go to school at all. And then I couldn't go full-time.

Restrictions on Peer and Play Activities

—When my counts are down, there are restrictions. Like I can't play with kids.
—I used to be afraid of getting hurt. Like slipping on ice, or falling off my bike. I was too careful. Sometimes when you are too careful, you get hurt even more. Now I play more. I even slip on ice and get blacks and blues.
—I miss my friends when I'm sick. I don't like being in the hospital.

Hair Loss

—In first grade, not having hair bothered me. I wore a wig. But in second grade, I was afraid to wear a wig in gym, so I gave up wearing it. I tell kids I like it cut short. The junior high school kids tease me and call me egghead.
—Everyone called me "baldy." I lost my hair because of the IV. I hate that . . . everyone calling me "baldy."

Nausea

—At Christmas I got a "baby-alive" doll. She is really pretty and uses batteries. You can feed her special food. But now she is broken and I can't feed her . . . Sometimes I feel hungry but I just can't eat because I throw up. Afterward it feels sour in my throat.

General Sense of Worry

—I worry about it. It ruins my day because I'm so busy worrying. I get so upset and start to cry and throw up.
—I don't like coming to Clinic and I never know if I have to get a bone marrow.
—I have dreams that I can't be with my mother and I miss her.

The issues enumerated by the child serve as a springboard for discussion, at the time and/or at a later point in therapy. The specific identification of the child's difficulties or upsets can be a first step in their remediation. For example, a child who greatly fears bone marrows can use the list to specify the most aversive aspects (e.g. needle, being held down). These precise factors then become targets for intervention, whether through discussion, desensitization, or hypnosis techniques. In making changes, additions, or deletions in the list over time, the child sees his or her pattern of coping in concrete terms. The child gains a sense of mastery in the evidence of the amelioration of problems or change in attitude.

I have found the list technique most useful with children between the ages of five and ten years; however, these boundaries are obviously flexible. A thematic analysis of lists of pediatric cancer patients who differ with respect to disease, age, and sex could help to delineate the central concerns of each group.

Chapter Eighteen

PROGNOSTIC EXPECTATION AND MAGICAL THINKING

Jonathan Kellerman

S TEVE, THE SIXTEEN-YEAR-OLD brother of fourteen-year-old Marcia, was referred for psychological treatment due to behavioral problems of several months duration. His sister, diagnosed with acute lymphoblastic leukemia five and a half years ago, had remained in initial remission since that time. She gave evidence of having adjusted well to her disease and its treatment.

The behaviors for which Steve was referred were not atypical problems of adolescence — petty vandalism, smoking marijuana, and truancy. What was notable was that they represented a marked departure from his previous conduct pattern. The mother reported that Steve had always been a high academic and athletic achiever, and had won several awards for citizenship and scholarship. In contrast, she had always regarded an older son, from a previous marriage, as overly passive and had been pleased at Steve's successes.

At the time of referral, Steve and Marcia's mother was experiencing a high degree of marital stress in her second marriage and was emotionally depressed. Her initial reaction to Steve's acting out had been panic, and she had subsequently placed him under virtual house arrest. This confinement led to increased frustration on Steve's part, several escapes, and increased problem behavior.

At the time of referral, Steve presented as an intelligent and apparently well-adjusted adolescent. He described relational problems with Marcia that did not appear out of the ordinary. Steve attributed his difficulties with his sister to the fact that she was spoiled and not required to assume responsibilities around the house. This, he felt, resulted in his having to shoulder more than his share of chores. Steve's perception of himself as being overburdened was a consistent theme running through his conversation. He talked of being weary of being a "superkid" and was quite aware of how his acting out had served to shake up his mother's image of him and to frighten her.

Sessions with the mother revealed that there were, indeed, major discrepancies between her expectations of Steve and Marcia and that this was reflected in terms of differential assignment of chores and responsibilities. When it was pointed out to her that both Marcia and Steve were intelligent adolescents and that the one and a half-year age difference between them did not justify such radically divergent treatment, she said that she still regarded Marcia as a dying child.

It was then pointed out to the mother that Marcia had achieved an initial remission over five years ago and that, functionally, she was a healthy young woman and was not dying. At the mention of the words "five years" the mother's eyes misted with tears and she related that when Marcia had been initially diagnosed, in another city, she had asked the attending oncologist what her daughter's prognosis was. She reported that the physician had told her that Marcia had "five years to live."

Since that time, the five-year period had stuck in her mind and she had resigned herself to losing her daughter within that period. Now, despite the fact that Marcia had lived several months past the five-year anniversary, her mother continued to regard her as dying and had downwardly adjusted her expectations accordingly.

What emerged from further conversations with this mother was that the five-year estimation had taken on virtually magical proportions and that Marcia was considered psychologically dead. This, combined with the mother's lack of other sources of emotional gratification, had caused her to place all of her hopes and expectations upon Steve. Such an attribution of excessive responsibility was made easier by the fact that Steve was an innately gifted and competent youngster. Eventually, however, he began to chafe under the pressure and to resent having to do so much more than his sister. Steve was quite explicit about considering his acting out as an overt attempt to climb down from the pedestal upon which he had been placed.

Subsequent sessions with Steve and his mother concentrated upon the unreality of her perception of Marcia as dying or terminally ill and included provision of accurate medical information. Once she began to view Marcia as a living adolescent, the mother was able to begin to adjust her behavioral expectations accordingly. Simultaneously, she was guided toward an understanding of Steve as an adolescent with normal developmental needs rather than as a superhuman, "perfect" child.

This redistribution of expectations and pressures was followed by a cessation of antisocial behaviors on Steve's part.

Professionals who communicate medical information to patients and families need to be aware of how psychological factors can contribute to distortions and misinterpretations. There is often a tendency for patients and parents to attach excessive significance to comments that may be viewed, by the professional, as offhand or unimportant. This is particularly true during times of medical and psychological crises when perceived dependence can be at its highest. Care needs to be taken to monitor the accuracy of information provided to patients and families as well as to gauge subsequent understanding and interpretation.

In the previously discussed case, lack of maternal gratification outside of child-rearing, as well as innate giftedness on the part of a sibling, combined with a distorted understanding of prognosis to create a set of unbalanced expectations. Of interest is the fact that Steve's behavioral rebellion began soon after his sister's five-year anniversary, during the period in which the mother began to regard Marcia as, for all intents and purposes, psychologically dead. One can only speculate as to the significance of anniversaries and this is, clearly, an area for future research.

Chapter Nineteen

DEATH, DYING, AND TERMINAL CARE: DYING AT HOME*

Gordon D. Armstrong
Ida M. Martinson

E NCOURAGING ADVANCES in cancer control treatments have been made; however, the long-term prognosis for many children with cancer is still death. That reality, for parent and child, is in conflict with our cultural tendency to avoid thinking about death, especially the death of a child. It has become somewhat of a cliché to refer to our society as denying of death and dying. Such denial is increasingly less general, however, as we are fast bringing the topic of death into the open. While largely overlooked by psychology and related disciplines until recently, the proliferation of writing, both theoretical and data-based, concerning death, indicates that the social and health sciences are making up for lost time. Kastenbaum and Costa (1977) provide a recent review of the psychology of death. They trace the topic back to ancient times and its emergence as a credible topic of study in the 1950s and the 1960s as well as reviewing recent work. Not surprisingly the focus of existing death literature is on adults.

This chapter will mention selected references dealing with awareness and understanding of death in children and then discuss the clinical management and family response to the dying and death of a child with cancer as part of a home care alternative to hospitalization.

THE CHILD'S CONCEPT OF DEATH

Stages of dying such as those of the pioneering work of Kubler-Ross (1969) postulate a series of responses by adults to their impending death, i.e. denial, anger, bargaining, depression, and finally acceptance. Regardless of the validity or utility of such theorizing for adults, it is of little use when considering the dying child without first considering the child's cognitive grasp of the concept of death. While the development of the child's awareness and understanding of death has not received the attention by researchers it seems to deserve, a not insubstantial literature does exist which speaks to the child's view of death. Many of the studies are fairly old. Most are based on interview

* This chapter was supported in part by DHEW, PHS Grant CA 19490. We wish to thank Lois E. Anderson of our grant staff for her assistance in the preparation of this chapter.

data and lack the methodological rigor one would prefer. However, the consistency of findings does lend support to their credibility.

Children's concepts of death may have changed in the past several generations and may still differ among cultures. In the last century the death of a child was much more common. It was not unusual for a child to lose a sibling or peer group member to death. Any death, child or adult, was likely to occur in the home and thus involve children in the family somewhat. Today fewer children are born and more live, per family. Also, extended families are more spread geographically so that when grandparents die it may be a distant event involving essentially a stranger. Finally, when death does occur it probably takes place in a hospital which most likely forbids the presence of younger children. Thus a child today may grow up with little or no experience with human deaths. Parents compound children's limited opportunity to understand death by attempting to shield them from it. Death, together with sex, are two things which parents may be uncomfortable about themselves. They seek to keep their children innocent despite the fact that both are fundamental aspects of human existence. While rarely succeeding in completely isolating children from death, parents and society certainly can confuse them by providing misleading answers to questions, e.g. "Grandpa is permanently asleep," or answers which are difficult to grasp, e.g. "Grandpa has gone to heaven."

Piaget (1929) inferred that children pass through four phases of animism or understanding of life. He based his findings on observations and interviews of Swiss children. For Piaget the ages of children within the four phases may vary, but the order of the phases through which the child passes is fixed. He theorized that the child's attribution of life to inanimate objects results from a deficient boundary between the child and surrounding objects. That is, children attribute their own notions of being alive to other things in the environment. As the child develops, the notion of what is alive becomes more restricted. In the first stage, which includes children up to about six or seven years of age, life is equated with general activity, i.e. anything active is viewed as being alive. At ages seven or eight the child reaches the second stage and life is restricted to things which move, e.g. bicycles are alive. By ages eight to eleven years, life becomes viewed in the third stage as spontaneous movement, i.e. bicycles are not alive, and finally in the fourth stage, also within this age group, life is restricted to plants and animals.

Safier (1964) studied the relationship between animism and death in thirty children aged four to five, seven to eight, and ten to eleven. She asked them questions about various stimulus words, e.g. "Is a baseball alive?" "Does a baseball grow up?" "Does a baseball die?" If a child thought the stimulus object was alive this was scored as an animism response; if the child thought the object could die this was a death response. Safier found that notions of animism and death were related even in four- to five-year-olds although not in the adult sense. That is, life and death were in flux for those children, with an unlimited number of lives and deaths seen as possible. One is reminded of children's cartoons which depict the bad guy as repeatedly blown up, run over by a truck, falling off a cliff, and then returning in the next scene to be killed again.

Ages seven to eight years appeared to be a transition period since the scores on animism and death were less correlated than at the earlier ages. Finally by ages ten to eleven years, animism and death were again related, by now in the adult sense, i.e. death ends life.

Nagy (1948) in a classic study, interviewed 378 children, ages three to ten, living in and around Budapest, Hungary. She inferred three stages of development of the concept of death. Her stages, while stressing different elements, are not contradictory to Piaget's notions. Nagy found that children under five years of age did not recognize death as an irreversible fact. Death was a departure; a sleep. It is likely that children, in our contemporary culture, are assisted in equating sleep and death by adults. For example, etched on tombstones is the legend "rest in peace" and more recently "just asleep."

For children ages five to nine, Nagy found a tendency to personify death, i.e. death is a man or death is the dead, rather than something which happens to oneself. By age ten death was generally recognized as a process which happened in accordance with certain laws, i.e. the inevitable cessation of corporal life.

Another pioneering study was done in Britain in the 1930s by Sylvia Anthony (1971). She tested and interviewed a large number of children, both normal and disturbed, and demonstrated that young children "discover" death. They attempt to integrate notions of death, including separation and sorrow, into their conception of the world. Anthony noted that even children five years of age were familiar with the word "death." She also stressed differences among children within every age level, i.e. significant individual differences.

Cultural elements contained in religious beliefs and tradition may at times cloud the child's concept of death. A study by Schilder and Weschler (1934) pointed to the problems posed by religious dogma concerning death and afterlife. Their sample consisted of seventy-six children, aged five to fifteen years, with physical or psychological problems. Schilder and Weschler argued that the notion of life after death presents a contradiction which the child accepts but, in doing so, opens the door to the incorporation of other inconsistent notions.

A relevant, more recent study was done by Gartley and Bernasconi (1967). They interviewed sixty Roman Catholic children aged five and one-half to fourteen years and did not find that religious beliefs confused the children nor did they find a tendency to personify death during the ages five to nine as Nagy did. These authors attributed these discrepancies from earlier findings as due to differences in religious training and the influence of television. Personification of death may be a dated (1930s) or cultural (Hungarian) tendency. However, the important finding was that the children viewed death as something external rather than as a process or event which would happen to them.

Childers and Wimmer (1971) studied seventy-five children aged four to ten years. Their method included individual discussions with the subjects including a set of questions about death. Examining the notion of universality of death, e.g. "Will everybody die?" and irrevocability of death, e.g. "Can they come back to life?," they found a significant relationship with age for the former but not the latter. That is, in this sample, universality was a function of age with cognitive understanding established generally after age nine. However, through age ten the irrevocability notion was more independent of age.

The importance of developmental level rather than chronological age in determining conceptualization of death was further stressed by Koocher (1973). Koocher questioned seventy-five children aged six to fifteen years and found a more realistic view of death in children as they moved from the Piagetian levels of preoperational to concrete-operational to formal-operational.

Mauer (1966) goes so far as to postulate the origins of a death concept to the sensorimotor developmental period. He believes that the game of peek-a-boo seen in three-month-old babies shows an awareness of being and nonbeing which is the first in a series of adaptations to the finite nature of life.

Tallmer, Formanek, and Tallmer (1974) studied 199 children between the ages of three and nine years. Half were lower class urban slum dwellers and half were middle class. They administered a questionnaire dealing with animate and inanimate concept acquisition to the children and questioned the parents about their orientations toward death and their explanation of death to their children. Additionally half the children in each social class were given projectives, i.e. three Thematic Apperception Test (TAT) cards and a sentence completion test.

Tallmer and her colleagues found that the concept of death developed more slowly than did the differentiation between animate and inanimate. Parent orientation toward death or parent reported experiences of the child with death were not related to adequacy of the concept of death. There was a significant difference between the lower and middle class children in adequacy of concept of death. The lower class children were more aware of the concept. This finding is in marked contrast to other studies (cf. Figuerelli and Keller, 1972) which have found delayed acquisition of concepts by lower class children. In explaining their unusual findings, Tallmer et al. speculate that lower class children attempt to deal more realistically and sensibly with their environment. The fact that lower class children are exposed to more violence did not seem to be a factor in that they were no more likely than middle class children to associate death and violence in their fantasy content.

In summary, the aforementioned studies have in common the finding that at about age nine to eleven years children (who are not faced with an immediate threat of death) have an adult-like cognitive conceptualization of death. At younger ages, the concept of death follows the child's less rational general developmental conceptualization of the world.

Natterson and Knudson (1960) studied thirty-three children aged zero to thirteen who were dying of cancer or aplastic anemia. They found that the primary source of distress in these dying children differed by age-group. For children aged ten years and older, fear of death and distress over the death of other children in the hospital was the most upsetting factor. Children age five to ten years found traumatic procedures, such as venipunctures, the most distressing, while younger children aged zero to five years found separation from their mother the greatest cause of distress.

Waechter (1971) studied sixty-four children, six to ten years of age, distributed among four groups. One group consisted of children with life-threatening illness including cancer; a second group consisted of children with a chronic disease, but good prognosis; a third group consisted of children with a brief, nonchronic, illness. These three groups of children were hospitalized. The fourth group was made up of healthy, nonhospitalized children. The data were scores on the General Anxiety Scale for Children, four pictures from the Thematic Apperception Test (TAT), and four pictures depicting hospital scenes which were used with the TAT pictures. The parents were also interviewed concerning what their child had been told about the seriousness of the illness. The poor prognosis group showed more anxiety and more thematic content relating to threat to body integrity than did the comparison groups. Children in the poor prognosis group included loneliness, separation, and death content in their stories even when they had not talked about death with hospital staff, or even if their parents believed their child did not know the prognosis. Waechter's finding of increased anxiety and threat to body integrity in her six- to ten-year-old sample is congruent with the finding of Natterson and Knudson (1960) for children of that age. Waechter herself equates these findings with preoccupation with death.

Spinetta, Rigler, and Karon (1973) report a study similar to Waechter's and with similar findings. They studied fifty children six to ten years of age. Half were hospitalized with leukemia and half had chronic but nonfatal illnesses. Spinetta and his colleagues administered four projective pictures depicting hospital scenes, a three-dimensional replica of a hospital room with doll figures which was also used to elicit fantasy, and an anxiety inventory adapted from the State-Trait Anxiety Inventory for Children. The children with leukemia related significantly greater preoccupation with threat to body integrity and functioning on the projectives and significantly more anxiety than the group of children with nonfatal illnesses. Spinetta et al. also supported Waechter's findings that these children were aware of the seriousness of their conditions even if parents had attempted to shield them from such knowledge.

These authors did not go as far as Waechter did in equating the anxiety and threat to body integrity to a preoccupation with death. Spinetta et al. argued that while children do not conceptualize death in an adult manner, they are aware of death on a less cognitive level.

It is reasonable to assume that some of the nine- or ten-year-old children who were included in both the above studies would have realistic cognitions about death and respond to their situation in light of this. For younger children it seems safest to make few inferences beyond the data since anxiety and preoccupation with threat to body integrity are responses to their situation well within the developmental level of these children. It is not necessary to equate these responses with preoccupation with the (unrealistic) notion of death most of the younger children would have as Waechter did. Also it may be questionable methodologically to equate a child with cancer with a dying child. The children in the Waechter and Spinetta et al. studies had an illness which disrupted their activities and threatened their bodies as well as their existences. The children in these two studies were not necessarily in the terminal stages of their illness. In fact, some may have had a prognosis of several or many more years of life.

The three studies cited above whose subjects were children with cancer provide valuable insights into the problems faced by such children. How their notion of death (rational or irrational), or anticipation (conscious or unconscious) of their own death, influences their response to their situation is less clear.

The child with cancer has had unusual opportunity to develop sophistication in conceptualization of death. Children with cancer are hospitalized and hospitals may be equated with the death of a grandparent or neighbor. In the hospital the child with cancer may have been acquainted with another child with cancer or other serious disease who has subsequently died. From the reaction of parents and others and the intrusive treatment procedures, the child with cancer realizes something serious is happening. At the same time we must be wary of the younger child's ability to verbalize a fairly sophisticated notion while not understanding it on a rational level. For example, if a five or six-year-old child with cancer is in the same hospital room as a child who dies, the event may be explained by stating that the child died and now "lives" in heaven. The living children with cancer may then note that they are in a similar situation, i.e. the hospital, and express fear that they, too, will die and go to heaven. That verbalization does not mean that the child understands and fears that a permanent end of corporal life is entailed. Rather, the child realizes something very unknown may happen. The bad part, from the five-year-old's standpoint, is not that one is dead, whatever that is, rather that the child will undergo separation from mother while in heaven.

THE TERMINAL STAGE OF CHILDHOOD CANCER

The care of the child with cancer who is in the terminal stages of the disease has been discussed in the literature. Programs of good psychological care prior to the terminal stage are often extended to the dying process. For example, Green (1967) proposes competence, availability, continuity of care, personalized care and preparation of the family about what is going to happen. Knudson and Natterson (1960) provided for the presence of the mother in the hospital during the child's waking hours, and 'round the clock when the child was dying. Easson (1974) emphasized the need to consider the child's level of understanding. He noted that children about eight years of age may view their condition as punishment and should therefore be reassured that this is not so. Easson believed that adults should be honest and supportive. This allows dying children to ask questions as much or as little as they can emotionally handle. Evasive answers are not likely to shield the child from the reality of the situation since so many other cues that something serious is happening are available, e.g. adults speaking with quivering voices, averting their eyes, forcing smiles; and there is also the child's own physiological deterioration.

HOME CARE

It is common for pediatricians to avoid hospitalization, unless absolutely required, given the adverse fear reaction that children, especially young ones, have to the hospital situation. Allowing a child to go home to die is practiced by some physicians and hospitals and is not a new idea. However, the overwhelming majority of children who die of cancer do so in the hospital. The following describes a research study on the feasibility of home care for children dying of cancer. For other reports of this research, see Martinson et al. (1978a; 1978b).

Method

Children aged up to seventeen are accepted into home care when their cancer control treatments are no longer effective and their physician considers them to be dying. Predicting the final stages of cancer in children is difficult, but dying generally means that the child is likely to die within one month. Further, no treatment protocols which require inpatient hospitalization of the child are anticipated. The option of returning to the hospital is open but not planned. Children still receiving cancer treatment but who are not expected to live will be accepted provided those treatment procedures are given on an outpatient basis. Children in remission or receiving outpatient treatment but not expected to die shortly are not accepted for home care services for purposes of this research.

Parents and other family members are the principal providers of comfort care to the dying child at home. In most cases the child's mother has provided the majority of the care. A nurse is on call for the family twenty-four hours a day, seven days a week. She answers questions over the telephone and serves as a liaison between the family and the physician. The nurse makes home visits whenever and as often as the parents request they be made. Most home visits are made at mutually convenient times. Some, however, have occurred late at night and on holidays. The focus of the nurse is to help the parents care for the child. During home visits the nurse may assess the child's condition, provide technical nursing services, e.g. catheterization, teach the parents methods of care for their child, or provide emotional support to the parents or child. Needed furnishings, e.g. bedpans; disposable supplies, e.g. oral hygiene swabs; equipment, e.g. alternating air mattresses; oxygen and apparatus; and medications are secured or arranged for by the nurse. Physicians are informed of the child's status and prescribe medications, such as analgesics, as needed. Home visits or direct contact with the family by physicians are not required in our home care program, although some physicians do like to talk with the family directly and even make home visits.

Both hospital and public health nurses have provided the home care. If possible, a single nurse is assigned to the case with another backup nurse available as needed. The level of nursing skill required is not greater than that of the typical registered nurse. However, extra familiarity with analgesics is helpful since pain control is a large component of the child's care. The responsibility and gravity of the nurse's role makes it challenging.

Upon death the nurse assists the family members in whatever way they require. This includes preparing the child's body, arranging to have it removed to the mortuary and seeing that a death certificate is secured. Often the nurse calls the physician, relatives, clergy, etc., to inform them of the death. The nurse at this traumatic time does as much or as little as the family wishes.

Data reported on at this time from this research comes principally from the interviews of the parents at one, six, and twelve months after the child's death and interviews of older siblings; significant others (grandparents, neighbors, clergy) and health professionals (nurse and physician).

Results

Thus far over fifty children have died of cancer while participating in home care. Sufficient data are available on thirty-two of those: twenty boys and twelve girls. Median age was 8.5 years and ranged from an infant of one month to an adolescent of seventeen years. Of these thirty-two participants, twenty-seven (84%) actually died at home while five reentered and died in the hospital. About half of the children had leukemia and half had lymphomas and solid tumors.

The children were referred from the University of Minnesota Hospitals and other hospitals in the Minneapolis-St. Paul area. About half of the children lived in the area, while the other half lived in cities and rural areas throughout Minnesota and neighboring states. The parents represent a wide range of income and education levels. All were Caucasian.

The twenty-seven children who died at home were in the home care project for a mean of 32.7 days, a median of twenty days, and a range of two to 104 days before death. A mean of 11.4 home visits were required with a mean length of 2.3 hours per visit for each child. The mean number of telephone contacts between the nurse and the family was 26.2 per child. Medications, especially analgesics, were required by all but three of the twenty-seven children who died at home. Of the five children who died in the hospital, two were admitted for pain control and died within ten hours of admission. The medication they received in the hospital (morphine) was, however, administered at home to other children in the project. Of the other three children who died in the hospital, one girl with leukemia was hemorrhaging and taken to the hospital where she died thirteen hours later. Another girl had a painful wound which distressed the parents, and she was rehospitalized for care of it. She died there one week later. The other child to die in the hospital was admitted for possible further cancer treatment and spent the next and final five weeks of her life in the hospital.

Not surprisingly there has been great diversity in the form of home care. The children had a broad range of ages and diagnoses, parents approached the situation differently and many different nurses have been involved in the various cases. Our approach centers on allowing the child and family to be together and to maximize the quality of life for the child's final days. The child can be made as comfortable at home as in the hospital. However, some anticipation of need for and prior securing of medication, e.g. narcotic analgesics, is necessary. This requires special cooperation between the physician and the home care nurse.

Case Study

Tim was a nine-year-old boy who died at home from non-Hodgkin's lymphoma. He had one sister, age seven. His father worked outside the home while his mother was a homemaker. Tim had been diagnosed two years previously and been hospitalized sixteen times for a total of 101 days as an inpatient. His tumor was growing rapidly and cancer control treatments were no longer effective. He was referred to the home care project thirteen days before he died. At referral he was in mild pain which was controlled by acetaminophen (Tylenol®) but had a severe cough which required a codeine cough syrup. The parents were given a prescription for hydroxyzine pamoate (Vistaril®), a tranquilizer, to assist the child in relaxing and to help him sleep. The parents were also given a prescription for meperidine hydrochloride (Demerol). This narcotic analgesic was for future use should pain increase to expected levels.

On the day of referral the home care project coordinator nurse met with the family in the hospital and explained the program in greater detail. The next day the home care nurse made the first of nine home visits. She assessed the child's condition and observed that he was comfortable. He spent most of his time either in bed or in the living room watching television. He was able to get up and move around and was eating well. His chest was swollen, tender to the touch, and painful. His respirations were labored and he could not finish sentences due to shortness of breath.

The next day the mother telephoned the home care nurse and expressed concern over Tim's shortness of breath. The nurse contacted the physician who ordered oxygen and the nurse arranged for the tanks and apparatus to be delivered. The next day, day 4 in home care, the nurse visited the home to instruct the parents in administration of the oxygen.

The following day the nurse again visited the home to see that the oxygen was working effectively. All was well with the oxygen, and the nurse spent time talking with the mother and father about Tim's condition and what they could expect in the future, i.e. possible central nervous system involvement and eventual death. Both parents were coping well with the situation. The parents had talked with the younger sister about her brother's dying but not with Tim himself. The younger sister was admonished by her mother not to mention dying to Tim or any of his friends. The home care nurse updated the physician on the child's condition and arranged for a refilling of the codeine prescription.

That same day two of Tim's nurses from the hospital came to pay a social call on him and his parents. Their visit was not in conjunction with the home care program.

The next contact with the family by the nurse was by telephone on day 6 when the mother reported that the oxygen mask was not working properly. The nurse secured a new mask and took it to the home with her. After the oxygen was again working properly, the nurse and the parents talked about whether or not an autopsy would be done. The parents decided to permit an autopsy to be done if it would help others by learning from Tim's case. Later questions about who would pay for the autopsy, since the child would not die in the hospital, resulted in no autopsy actually being done.

Over the next five days the nurse was in daily contact with the family by telephone and visited the home three times. During that time Tim's condition rapidly deteriorated. The Tylenol and the codeine for his cough no longer controlled his pain so the physician recommended they use the Demerol. The dosage of Tim's tranquilizer was also increased during that time. Tim was lethargic, but he still received visits from his friends and was apparently more attentive during their visits.

On day 11 the mother telephoned the nurse to report that Tim was in more pain and the dosage of Demerol was increased. The following day the nurse made a home visit. Tim was in much pain and the dosages of Demerol and Vistaril were further increased. It was obvious to all that the end was near. Late that night the mother called the nurse saying that Tim's condition had worsened and the mother requested that the nurse come again. She returned and remained in the home for the rest of the night. In the early morning Tim took a few very shallow breaths and then stopped breathing. Tim's younger sister was asleep at the time and was awakened later and informed of her brother's death. Other relatives were then informed. The home care nurse contacted the mortician and told him when Tim's body could be picked up. The parents had made prior arrangements with that mortician. The nurse also informed the child's physician.

The family, as well as the nurse, were Roman Catholics and the parents, sister, grandparents and the nurse stood in the living room around Tim and prayed.

Later that day the nurse arranged for the oxygen equipment to be picked up.
This case study was slightly unusual in the high frequency of the home visits.
This is partly accounted for by the rapidity with which the child deteriorated and
the use of the oxygen. It was, however, typical in that no serious problems arose
and the child's death was peaceful.

Our home care approach includes a somewhat directive intervention
with the parents as the child's death approaches. The nurse encourages
the parents to prepare for the funeral, e.g. choosing or contacting a
mortuary; arranging for a cemetery plot. Some parents, even though
they may verbally express awareness that their child will soon die, have
not accepted that reality on an emotional or subconscious level. Even if
they do not actually make any prior funeral arrangements, realizing
that they will be faced with that death dependent task moves them
toward a fuller acceptance of the situation. A few parents refuse to
discuss funeral arrangements while their child is alive and the nurse
does not press the issue. In other cases parents openly talk about the
funeral with their clergyman and mortician. Such open communication about the coming death is also, we believe, beneficial to the children.

The project nurses have raised the issue of parents talking with their
children about death, but the parents decide ultimately whether or not
they do so. Of the thirty-two children, twenty-four were age four or
older. Of those twenty-four, it is known that the parents or someone
else talked with the child about death in ten cases. For the remaining
fourteen children, there was no such discussion in thirteen cases and in
one case data are unavailable. In three of these thirteen cases (ages
seven, nine and ten), the parents would have talked with the child but
were waiting for the child to ask questions which the child never did. In
one case (age ten), the child was aware that he was dying but refused to
talk about it. In six cases (ages seven, ten, twelve, fourteen, sixteen and
sixteen), the children indicated an awareness that they were dying, but
the parents never talked to them about it. In two cases (ages four and
fourteen) the parents did not talk to the child about death and the
children themselves did not verbalize an awareness of dying. One final
case was a thirteen-year-old girl who was very religious and accepted
her fate whatever it would be. She seems to have been aware that she
was dying but hoped for a miracle. Her parents talked with her about it
being in God's hands which was also her acceptance of the situation.
The ten children whose parents did talk about death with their child
were aged four, six, seven, ten, and six at thirteen years or older.

It is difficult for us to conclude from this preliminary data what the
best communication approach should be. Children below the ages of
nine to eleven years who are dying clearly can talk about their situation.
If they do not raise the issue perhaps it need not be brought up. Most
but not all professionals advise an open and direct approach to
disease-related communication with children with cancer. Kellerman
et al. (1977) provided some data indicating that children's talking about

their illness was inversely related to depression, i.e. talking about cancer was associated with a positive mood. With older children who can rationally grasp their situation, additional considerations are involved. First, they are more likely to correctly assess their situation. Second, they are more likely to experience the cognitive impact of dying since they can fully understand it. Third, it may be unethical to not inform older children that they are dying. To try and hide the fact that they are dying from such children may be difficult to do, harmful, and wrong.

The parents of the thirty-two children who died had, with one exception, accepted or were aware of the fact that their child was dying prior to the death event itself. A number of parents who were devoutly religious retained some degree of hope despite acceptance of the probability of death. The one exception mentioned above was the mother of a fourteen-year-old girl with leukemia who was readmitted to the hospital while hemorrhaging and who died thirteen hours later. The mother continually denied that her daughter was dying until only a few hours before the girl died. When the mother finally accepted the reality of the situation she spoke openly with her daughter who herself was quite aware of the proximity of death.

Parents take their child home to die for several overlapping reasons. All of the children old enough to so indicate say that they want to go home. Some have had an almost phobic aversion to the hospital, although one sixteen-year-old boy liked the hospital, especially one of his nurses, and found going home only slightly more desirable. With few exceptions the parents also have been desirous to have their child at home. In postdeath interviews, they report the joys of being together as a family and their ability to control the environment. They are active participants in the care. They are not being interrupted by hospital staff. Their child is not subjected to the numerous laboratory tests which even dying children are inclined to receive in the hospital. When the child dies they are not rushed in their final parting.

The expected death of a child with cancer may be a final relief from the long period of stress created by the disease or a precipitant of further stress and abnormal grief reaction. Response to the death may be a function of the wide variability among parents in the reality with which they face the situation. On the one hand many parents seek to make the most of their child's final days of life. They take each day as it comes and enjoy life together as much as possible. Even children with cancer who are close to death often have a "good day" when they are alert and feeling better. Such days are exploited by families at home. Small events take on significance, e.g. a child who lived on a farm went for a ride with his father on their tractor in his last week of life. The parents cherished that memory a year after the death. If that child had been in the hospital he might have been able to leave for a while with his parents, but their farm was many miles from the hospital so his activities would have been limited.

On the other hand, some parents are less reconciled to the fact of their child's impending death. They have come to rely on the hospital for both treatment and hope. They may not want the responsibility for care since it underscores the fact that cancer control treatment is not being done. Such parents may turn down home care when offered it by their physician, or if they take their child home may be more likely to readmit their child as death finally approaches. In only one case have parents elected to take their child home but declined the services of the home care program when offered.

The demands on time and coping ability are great during the home care of many of the children. The parents, especially the mothers, willingly accept the demands. It is the normal role of parents to care for their child and most very much want to do so, whether at home or in the hospital. Many hospitals allow the parents to provide some of the care but not with the autonomy experienced by being in one's own home.

For home care to be effective, the participants must want it to work. Even if the patient strongly desires to be at home, home care requires (1) a parent or parents who recognize their ability to provide care; (2) a physician who is willing to support the concept and to delegate some responsibility to the nurse; and (3) a capable nurse who is able to work cooperatively with the physician. With those three elements, home care proceeds with surprising smoothness. With one or more participants not firmly committed to the idea of home care, the procedure becomes much more laborious and the child is more likely to be rehospitalized.

Data on the child's experience with dying were sometimes acquired first hand but often had to come from the parents after the death. A primary aspect of the home care option was to intrude as little as possible on the family. Thus primary contacts by the home care nurse are centered principally on the parents. The parents may talk about death with their child or the nurse might do so if the parents request. However, it was not a component of this project to directly counsel the children about their situation.

Insofar as data are available, the response of the dying children is congruent with the earlier literature cited. Infants and very young children (under four years) may have had no real awareness that they were dying. Children under about age ten were very concerned about avoiding the needles which they associated with the hospital. For them home care represented relief from uncomfortable procedures as well as the security of parents and familiar surroundings. It is difficult to know if the process of dying changed their understanding of death. Tentatively we would infer that it did. That is, the awareness of the physical deterioration of their bodies was significant. When their bodies are in poor condition and they also sense that they will not improve, that is a graphic indicator that death is permanent. One seven-year-old boy with leukemia was very ill and required pain medication. While resting quietly he suddenly sat up and called out to his father, "Daddy, Daddy, help me. I'm dying." The father held his son and the child died within half an hour in his father's arms.

Older children and certainly adolescents rationally understood what death would mean. They were aware that they were dying, even if not told. Systematic data are not available on enough subjects to determine if these older children experienced reliable stages of dying. Partly that is due to the brief involvements with some families. Adolescents, in their striving to maintain autonomy, often responded with frustration and anger at their physical condition and dependency. Depression was also evident and, for some, so was acceptance of impending death.

THE FAMILY AFTER THE DEATH

There is some inconsistency in reported literature on the psychological adjustment of parents and siblings to the death of a child. Certainly parents and older siblings grieve the loss, but Friedman (1967) noted that the majority of parents are able to adapt, albeit painfully, to the loss of a child to cancer.

Binger et al. (1969) interviewed the parents of children who died of leukemia and reported difficulty in coping in one or more siblings in half of twenty families studied. In eleven of the twenty families, one or more members required psychiatric help, including several cases of severe depression requiring admission to a psychiatric hospital. In another study Kaplan et al. (1977) reported that three months following the child's death from leukemia, fourteen of forty families had a member under psychiatric care.

In our home care project, one person (a mother) out of the thirty-two families received psychiatric care following the death of the child. Differences between Minnesota and California (where the Binger et al. and Kaplan et al. studies were done) in the willingness to seek psychiatric help may account for some of these marked differences. Additionally, it would be wrong to equate psychiatric care for one's grief as evidence of pathology especially considering Engel's (1977) model of grief and disease. However, the thrust of the Binger and the Kaplan studies is that the frequency of abnormal grief reactions is high in families who have a child die of cancer. Examination of psychosomatic and sleep disturbances and work disruption or school problems in the parents and siblings in our sample revealed, with few exceptions, normal grief reactions which were resolved by twelve months after the death or earlier.

In another study done in the Midwest, Lascari and Stehbens (1973) also failed to find a high rate of adverse reaction in interviews of the parents of twenty children who died in the hospital of leukemia.

Of special concern in our interviews of parents and siblings in the home care project were any signs of unusual reaction due to the child dying at home. These might include special notice made of the couch or bed the child died in, guilt feelings over not hospitalizing the child, or any adverse reactions in the several children who witnessed the death of their siblings. Here again there appear to be no abnormal reactions. The witnessing of the death by some siblings was the parents' choice. In other cases the siblings were elsewhere. The wisdom of the parents' decision either way is debatable. Witnessing a death is, of course, an emotionally stirring event but not necessarily a bad thing. Siblings interviewed report that the thought of death beforehand and the death itself was frightening but that they got over their fear shortly afterwards. Younger siblings became upset because everyone else was crying even though they themselves did not apparently realize what had happened at the time. The death of a sibling can leave emotional scars on the children which affect their later emotional adjustment (cf. Cain, Fast, and Erickson 1964). Some of the siblings studied in the home care project may later in life show adverse reactions to the loss of their sibling and its attendant impact on family life. However, there is no reason to believe at this time that home care has produced extra pathological effects on either sibling or parents. In fact, if anything the opposite is believed to be the case. Death is an unfortunate but real event for these families. Home care seems to help them deal more directly and realistically with their grim situation.

ALTERNATIVE PLACES FOR CARE OF DYING CHILDREN

While home care appears to be a valuable option for dying children, it is not intended to compete with or replace hospitalization. Efforts to include families in hospital routine and make the hospitals more homelike should be encouraged as well. Not all parents will want to take their child home nor is home care appropriate for all dying children. A viable system is to have home care nursing services as a part of the hospital, perhaps affiliated with the outpatient clinic. This provides greater ease of administration and transfer of patient information as well as providing more continuity of care. Hospital staff nurses can also be used at times as home care nurses. In some cases in our study, the child's hospital primary nurse, who had known the child since diagnosis, perhaps years before, was then the home care nurse when the child was dying. At the same time relationships with public health nursing agencies are important since those nurses already are familiar with providing care in the home.

Additional alternatives for terminal care include hospices and special units within acute care hospitals. The hospice concept includes both home care or, where not feasible, inpatient care in a special facility (cf. Saunders, 1976). That facility tries to provide dying patients with a homelike environment and is staffed by specially trained personnel to meet the mental, physical, and spiritual needs of the dying patients. The development of hospices with home care and inpatient facilities is to be encouraged. At present most do not provide care for children, but that too may come in the future. Special terminal care units within hospitals (cf. Mount, 1976), provide a compromise between a standard hospital unit and a hospice. Those, also, are primarily designed for adults.

Most cities in the United States would not have sufficient numbers of children requiring special dying care to justify children's hospices or special hospital units. Incorporation of children into such facilities for adults will probably take time since they are a new idea, even for adults. At the same time, home care is more generally feasible for children than for adults. That is, children usually have one or both parents available to provide the required home care. Such an appropriate caregiver may not exist for adults whose spouse may be dead or unable to provide the physical elements, such as lifting the patient, required for care. The dying adult's children may be unwilling or geographically removed. With dying children, the parents are usually available, capable, and willing care-givers.

Thus in the more immediate future, hospital or nursing agency-based home care programs for children dying of cancer seem to be the best alternative. While inpatient hospitals are necessary and appropriate places for the cancer control treatment of children, when such treatment is no longer warranted nor hospitalization requiring comfort treatments needed, hospital death is no longer preferable. Hospitals, no matter how good and progressive their approaches may be, will likely always be less desirable than the home for children spending their last days of life.

REFERENCES

Anthony, S.: *The Discovery of Death in Childhood and After.* London, Penguin, 1971.

Binger, C. M., Albin, A. R., Feurestein, R. C., Kushner, J. H., Zoger, S., and Mikkelsen, C.: Childhood leukemia: Emotional impact on patient and family. *N Engl J Med, 280:*414, 1969.

Cain, A. C., Fast, I., and Erickson, M. E.: Children's disturbed reactions to death of a sibling. *Am J Orthopsychiatry, 34:*741, 1964.

Childers, P., and Wimmer, M.: The concept of death in early childhood. *Child Development, 42:*1299, 1971.

Easson, W. M.: Management of the dying child. *J Clin Child Psychol, 3:*25, 1974.

Engel, G. L.: The need for a new medical model: A challenge for biomedicine. *Science, 196:*129, 1977.

Figuerelli, J. C., and Keller, H. R.: The effects of training and socioeconomic class upon the acquisition of conservation concepts. *Child Development, 43:*293, 1972.

Friedman, S. B.: Care of the family of the child with cancer. *Pediatrics, 40:*498, 1967.

Gartley, W., and Bernasconi, M.: The concept of death in children. *J Gen Psychol, 110:*71, 1967.

Green, M.: Care of the dying child. *Pediatrics, 40:*492, 1967.

Kaplan, D. M., Smith, A., Grobstein, R., and Fischman, S. E.: Family mediation of stress. In R. H. Moos (Ed.) *Coping With Physical Illness.* New York, Plenum Medical Book, 1977.

Kastenbaum, R., and Costa, P. T.: Psychological perspectives on death. *Ann Rev Psychol, 28:*225, 1977.

Kellerman, J., Rigler, D., Siegel, S. E., and Katz, E. R.: Disease related communication and depression in pediatric cancer patients. *J Pediatr Psychol, 2:*52, 1977.

Knudson, A. G. and Natterson, J. M.: Participation of parents in the hospital care of fatally ill children. *Pediatrics, 26:*482, 1960.

Koocher, G. P.: Childhood death and cognitive development. *Dev Psychol, 9:*369, 1973.

Kubler-Ross, E.: *On Death and Dying.* New York, Macmillan, 1969.

Lascari, A. D., and Stehbens, J. A.: The reactions of families to childhood leukemia. *Clin Pediatr, 12:*210, 1973.

Martinson, I. M., Armstrong, G. D., Geis, D. P., Anglim, M. A., Gronseth, E. C., MacInnis, H., Kersey, J. H., and Nesbit, M. E.: Home care for children dying of cancer. *Pediatrics, 62:*106, 1978a.

Martinson, I. M., Armstrong, G. D., Geis, D. P., Anglim, M. A., Gronseth, E. C., MacInnis, H., Nesbit, M. E., and Kersey, J. H.: Facilitating home care for children dying of cancer. *Cancer Nurs, 1:*41, 1978b.

Mauer, A.: Maturation of concepts of death. *Br J Med Psychol, 39:*35, 1966.

Mount, B. M.: *Palliative Care Service Report,* Montreal, Royal Victoria Hospital, McGill University, 1976.

Nagy, M.: The child's theories concerning death. *J Gen Psychol, 73:*3, 1948.

Natterson, J. M., and Knudson, A. G.: Observations concerning fear of death in fatally ill children and their mothers. *Psychosom Med, 22:*456, 1960.

Piaget, J.: *The Child's Conception of the World.* London, Routledge & Kegan Paul, 1929.

Safier, G.: A study in relationship between the life and death concepts in children. *J Gen Psychol, 105:*283, 1964.

Saunders, C.: *Annual Report,* London, St. Christopher's Hospice, 1976.

Schilder, P., and Weschler, D.: The attitudes of children toward death. *J Gen Psychol, 45:*406, 1934.

Spinetta, J. J., Rigler, D., and Karon, M.: Anxiety in the dying child. *Pediatrics, 52:*841, 1973.

Tallmer, M., Formanek, R., and Tallmer, J.: Factors influencing children's concepts of death. *J Clin Child Psychol, 3:*17, 1974.

Waechter, E. H.: Children's awareness of fatal illness. *Am J Nurs, 71:*1168, 1971.

INDEX

A

Actinomycin-D, 8
Acute lymphoblastic leukemia, 5-8
  discomfort in treatment for, 22
  group therapy for, 273, 275-76
  impact of CNS irradiation on, 171-72,
    176-77, 179-82
  night terrors in (case history), 284-88
Acute lymphocytic leukemia, 22
Acute myelogenous leukemia, 6-7
  group therapy for, 273, 277-78
Acute undifferentiated leukemia, 6
Adaptation
  anger as a means for, 77, 108, 112, 246
  and communication about death, 262
  to death at home, 306-309
  through denial, 116-22
  "external and internal" facets of, 122-23
  need for emphasis on, in sibling studies,
    53
Adolescents, 27
  development of, 70-76
  group therapy for, 278-79
  guidelines for research on, 94-96
  as hyponotic subjects, 216
  response of, to death, 308
  sedation of, 253
  self-help for, 86-90, 95
  separation of, from peers, 159
  sexuality of, 74
Adults
  hypnosis of, 216-17
  sensory deprivation of, 129
  See also Parents
Affect
  extinction of bonds of, 102
  in physical isolation, 145-47
  rating scale for, 140
ALL. See Acute lymphoblastic leukemia
Alopecia. See Hair loss
Aminopterin, 5
AML. See Acute myelogenous leukemia
Amputation, 10, 22

and hypnotic regression, 224
prosthetic replacement for, 188
sibling perceptions of, 56-59
Analgesics, 224, 303
Anesthesia, 252
Anger, 77, 108, 112, 246
Animal studies
  of cranial irradiation, 174
  of separation and isolation, 133, 157
Animism, 296-97
Anticancer drugs. See Chemotherapy
Anxiety
  conditioned by medical procedures,
    25-26, 199-200, 210-11, 284-88
  increases in, 79
  parental, 31, 120-21 (see also Parents)
  of patients about psychosocial care, 199
  prior to diagnosis, 76
  reduction of, 87-88, 204-205, 220,
    243-44
  self-reporting of, by children, 289-91
  due to separation, 31-32, 260
  about sexual development, 75
  situational vs. long-term, 342-44
Appetite, 147
Asexuality, 74-75
Attachment behavior, 102, 109-10
Authoritarianism of some physicians,
  93-94

B

Baldness. See Hair loss
Bedwetting, 145
Behavior
  attachment, 102, 109-10
  of children in isolation, 160-63
  changes in, due to CNS irradiation,
    171-72
  collaborative, 113-14
  high risk-taking, 79
Behavioral
  approaches to night terrors, 284

313